Ethical Analysis
of
Clinical Medicine

A Guide to Self-Evaluation

Ethical Analysis
of
Clinical Medicine

A Guide to Self-Evaluation

Glenn C. Graber, Ph.D.
Department of Philosophy

Alfred D. Beasley, M.D.
Department of Medicine

John A. Eaddy, M.D.
Department of Family Practice

The University of Tennessee

Urban & Schwarzenberg
Baltimore-Munich • 1985

Urban & Schwarzenberg, Inc.
7 E. Redwood Street
Baltimore, Maryland 21202
USA

Urban & Schwarzenberg
Pettenkoferstrasse 18
D-8000 München 2
West Germany

NOTICES

Library of Congress Cataloging in Publication Data

Graber, Glenn C.
Ethical analysis of clinical medicine.

Includes bibliographies and index.
1. Medical ethics. 2. Physician and patient. I. Beasley, Alfred D. II. Eaddy, John A. III. Title. [DNLM: 1. Ethics, Medical. W 50 G728e]
R724.G74 1985   174'.2   85-3337
ISBN 0-8067-0701-1 (cloth)   ISBN 0-8067-0711-9 (pbk.)

Sponsoring editor: Charles W. Mitchell
Compositor: Brushwood Graphics
Printer: John D. Lucas Printing
Manuscript editor: Starr Belsky
Indexer: Authors
Production and design: Norman Och and Karen Babcock

PAPER

ISBN 0-8067-0711-9 Baltimore

ISBN 3-541-70711-9 Munich

CLOTH

ISBN 0-8067-0701-1 Baltimore

ISBN 3-541-70701-1 Munich

To our families,

Caroline, Janna, and Rosalie Graber
Sandy, Stan, and Ann Beasley
Virginia, Scott, and Blair Eaddy

who daily teach us the meaning and
value of caring relationships

Contents

Foreword

For most of this century, clinical investigation has focused intently on the biosciences—and with great rewards to human health. Now the growing power of medicine to sustain health and prolong life has broadened the focus of clinical investigation to include not only health care delivery but clinical practice itself—its efficiency, its effectiveness, and its quality. Such research, while fundamentally based in the biosciences, requires attention as well to the social, behavioral, and ethical aspects of patient care, especially as the burgeoning technology and complex logistics of health care force us to set priorities on our resources. But if the *quality* of clinical care is to be adequately researched as well as its effectiveness and efficiency, how can we avoid the systematic study of the human values that underlie medical practice? Journals now abound with articles, editorials, reviews, and letters about the ethical, philosophical, and legal issues of clinical care, and, indeed, about the ethics of clinical investigation itself. Textbooks of medical ethics of all sizes and shapes are sprouting from our presses, and the medical school curriculum is currently being infused with formal and informal courses in medical ethics, law, and philosophy. Regularly scheduled "ethics grand rounds" and other case conferences are becoming a routine feature of hospital staff educational programs.

The publication of this particular text is representative of the "new" coalition of academic medicine and philosophy. It is a work that has grown out of a living program of the practice and teaching of clinical ethics for more than a decade at the University of Tennessee's medical units at both Memphis and Knoxville. As such, it is designed for those engaged in "primary care," that is, those responsible for the comprehensive and continuing care of the individual patient. Drs. Beasley and Eaddy bring their own clinical authenticity to this volume as two highly effective and experienced providers of primary care. It is my own bias that such clinicians bring a special dimension to the formal study of medical ethics that stems from the habitual process of forging doctor-patient relationships. Such relationships are the substance from which some of the most difficult ethical-medical decisions are forged, often as the product of both patient autonomy and physician paternalism. More often, the intensely humanistic role the physician plays as steward of the secrets of his patient's mind and body fosters a habit of accommodating the patient's values that are not always congruent with the physician's own. Thus, physicians tend to be somewhat protective of their prerogative of representing their patients' ethical positions.

If, however, our physicians' examining rooms are to be opened to patients of all creeds and cultures, the caring doctors should be knowledgeable about this ethical and religious pluralism and open to advice and consultation by others who are experts. In this pluralistic society we sorely need the erudition, wisdom, and guidance of our philosophers. Dr. Graber is a philosopher who has obtained first-hand experience by working for some years as a clinical associate in a medical ethics program, as well as directing a graduate program in medical ethics within a philosophy department. He represents a new breed of disciplinary consultants to medical practice that will soon be, in my opinion, a routine resource of our medical center.

The textbook that has been written by this expert team is highly practical to physicians in its approach and content. It is not only a philosophical exercise in critical reasoning and a lexicon of human values, but it is infused with a personal dedication that emanates warmth as well as light from its pages. Such works may help us physicians in our efforts to make caring decisions for our patients and ourselves.

1985
Gene H. Stollerman, M.D.
Professor of Medicine
Boston University School of Medicine

Preface

The pursuit of clinical wisdom is one of humankind's boldest and noblest undertakings. The physician attempts to understand the awesome mysteries of the inner workings of the human body and to gain control over these powers in order to serve the needs of her[1] patients. This book is written in the conviction that philosophy (etymologically, "love of wisdom")—and especially its branch concerned with ethics and values—can be a helpful partner to medicine in this quest. In the chapters that follow, you are invited to reflect upon the ethical and value dimensions of clinical practice; e.g., your own expectations about medicine, the nature of the physician-patient relationship, features of practice settings, and elements of specific decisions, such as those to limit life-sustaining treatment for terminal patients.

As in life, in the pages that follow you will find that answers are less plentiful than questions. The authors do not presume to offer definitive solutions to the ethical issues discussed. Rather, the emphasis is the development of your analytical processes, through which you can work toward answering specific questions on your own. When concrete recommendations *are* offered, they are to be regarded as material for further critical reflection on your part rather than as the last word on the matter.

This is not meant to suggest that any answer is as good as any other. Such a stance would turn morality into a subjective equivalent of whim. Rather, the presupposition is that the ethical dimensions of concrete cases are extremely complex and often subtle, and thus that the variations between cases make general pronouncements ("cookbook ethics") less than helpful. The goal is for you to develop *your own* clinical wisdom.

Wisdom is objective or interpersonal in its requirement that conclusions be supported by reasons that can be communicated and defended to others (including both colleagues and patients); but it is subjective or personal in that the understanding and acceptance of these reasons must be discovered within yourself rather than imposed from without. They must be both *good* reasons and also *your own* reasons.

To achieve this state requires active exercise of critical reasoning; and thus this book is intended to be approached in this fashion. You are frequently asked to stop reading and think through an issue on your own before you resume reading the text. You should keep in mind your own personal values as well as personal experiences as physician, patient, or friend of patients, and reflect upon the implications of these concrete examples for the issues presented. Above all,

---

1. Masculine and feminine pronouns will be used alternately throughout this book. In each case, they are to be taken as generic terms embracing both genders.

formulate *questions,* and look for the answers as you read on. (If you do not find the answers, bring the questions up in class discussion.) In philosophy, a probing question is far more valuable than a glib answer.

The authors approach this study from a background in both medicine and philosophy. The two physicians combine a career-long involvement in medical education with more than ten years of close association with a program of graduate studies in philosophy, concentrating on medical ethics. The philosopher has served for some years as a clinical associate in medical ethics in a teaching hospital as well as directing the graduate program in medical ethics within a philosophy department.

Note to Teachers: This book is designed to prompt active reflection on the issues. The case studies and exercises found in the text can be employed to bring this about in the classroom as well. The authors have developed additional exercises along similar lines, which will be made available upon request.

Acknowledgments: We express gratitude for what we have learned from our parents, our teachers, our students, our colleagues, our patients, and our friends. The analysis of situations we present in these pages reflects our heritage and life experiences. It is not meant to be definitive or exhaustive, but rather illustrative and suggestive.

Glenn C. Graber, Ph.D.
Alfred D. Beasley, M.D.
John A. Eaddy, M.D.
Knoxville, Tennessee

Sources and Permissions

The authors acknowledge the following sources used throughout this book and thank the publishers for permission to use the material.

Henry J. Aaron and William B. Schwartz, *The Painful Prescription: Rationing Hospital Care,* copyright © 1984 by, and excerpted by permission of, The Brookings Institution.

American College of Physicians Ethics Manual, printed in *Annals of Internal Medicine,* vol. 101, 1984. Copyright © 1984 by, and excerpted by permission of, the American College of Physicians.

Tom L. Beauchamp and James F. Childress, *Principles of Biomedical Ethics,* ed. 2, copyright © 1983 by, and excerpted by permission of, Oxford University Press.

Sisela Bok, *Lying: Moral Choice in Public and Private Life,* copyright © 1978 by, and excerpted by permission of, Pantheon Books, Division of Random House, Inc.

Howard Brody, *Ethical Decisions in Medicine,* ed. 2, copyright © 1981 by, and excerpted by permission of, Little, Brown and Company.

Charles M. Culver and Bernard Gert, *Philosophy in Medicine,* copyright © 1982 by, and excerpted by permission of, Oxford University Press.

Current Opinions of the Judicial Council of the American Medical Association, 1984, copyright © 1984 by, and excerpted by permission of, the American Medical Association.

Norman C. Dalkey, *Studies in the Quality of Life—Delphi and Decision-Making,* copyright © 1972 by, and adapted by permission of, The Rand Corporation.

Elmer L. DeGowin and Richard L. DeGowin, *Bedside Diagnostic Examination,* ed. 3, copyright © 1976 by, and excerpted by permission of, Macmillan Publishing Company.

J. Lowell Dixon and M. Gene Smalley, ''Jehovah's Witnesses: The Surgical/Ethical Challenge'' in the *Journal of the American Medical Association* 246:2471, 1981, copyright © 1981 by, and excerpted by permission of, the American Medical Association.

Leon Eisenberg, ''What Makes Persons 'Patients' and Patients 'Well'?'' in the *American Journal of Medicine* 69:277–286, 1980, copyright © 1980 by, and excerpted by permission of, the American Journal of Medicine.

''Ethical Concepts Applied to Nursing'' excerpted by permission of the International Council of Nurses.

John R. Evans, Karen Lashman Hall, and Jeremy Warford, ''Shattuck Lecture—Health Care in the Developing World: Problems of Scarcity and Choice'' excerpted by permission of the *New England Journal of Medicine* 305:1117–1127, 1981.

Charles Fried, *Medical Experimentation: Personal Integrity and Social Policy,* copyright © 1974 by, and excerpted by permission of, Elsevier Science Publishers B.V., Biomedical Division; *Right and Wrong,* 1978, Harvard University Press, excerpt reprinted by permission of Harvard University Press.

Victor R. Fuchs, ''The 'Rationing' of Medical Care'' excerpted by permission of the *New England Journal of Medicine* 311:1572–1573, 1984.

William A. Glaser, *Paying the Doctor: Systems of Remuneration and Their Effects,* copyright © 1970 by, and excerpted by permission of, The Johns Hopkins University Press.

Erving Goffman, *Asylums,* copyright © 1961 by Erving Goffman, excerpts reprinted by permission of Doubleday & Company, Inc.

Lucien Israel, *Conquering Cancer,* translated by Joan Pinkham, copyright © 1978 by, and excerpted by permission of, Random House, Inc.

Albert R. Jonsen, Mark Siegler, and William J. Winslade, *Clinical Ethics: A Practical Approach to Ethical Decisions in Medicine,* copyright © 1982 by, and excerpted by permission of, Macmillan Publishing Company.

Chapter One

Physician-Patient Relationships

1 General Features

The goal of this section is to reflect on the nature of the physician-patient relationship and to assist you in understanding the basic values that you can draw upon in discussions of specific issues and in your thinking about ethical dimensions of medicine. This relationship embodies certain important elements. We agree with Mark Siegler:

> If moral certainty exists in medicine (that is, if it is possible to determine which actions in a medical context are moral and ethical, which are right and wrong), such moral certainty will be discovered not by recourse to formal laws, moral rules, or moral principles, but rather in the context of the particularities of the physician-patient relationship itself. (Siegler 1981a, 56)

What Siegler is speaking of is a moral counterpart to "clinical wisdom." A proper understanding of and appreciation for these traditional medical values provide sound guidance in the face of influences (both societal and personal, some now on the scene and others on the horizon) that threaten to undermine them.

1.1 Fantasies: A Thought Experiment

Think back a few years to when you first envisioned going into medicine. Try to remember the answers to the questions below as a way of reconstructing your image of medicine at that time. [NOTE: Check the appropriate items on the page as you go through the exercise (or, if you have a psychological block instilled by elementary school teachers against writing in books, make notes on paper). You will be asked to reflect on your answers throughout this chapter.]

Instructions: For each question, indicate by some symbol as many items as apply; if one item on the list has been *dominant* in your fantasies, indicate it by a *double* symbol. Symbols to choose from include

√　　　　　†　　　　　—　　　　　*　　　　　X　　　　　+

Several symbols are included to encourage you to return to this exercise periodically to measure changes in your image of medicine. Date the symbol you use now, and choose another the next time you work through this exercise.

1. What was the *setting* in which you imagined yourself practicing medicine?
   ___ an office
   ___ a hospital ward
   ___ an operating room
   ___ an emergency room
   ___ at the scene of an accident
   ___ a social setting (e.g., at someone's home, at church) in which an emergency arises
   ___ a social setting in which someone asks for your advice and counsel
   ___ making a house call
   ___ practicing medicine in a research laboratory
   ___ other (specify): _____

2. What was the nature of the *interaction* that represented your image of "practicing medicine"?
   ___ a procedure (e.g., sewing up a wound, CPR)
   ___ writing a prescription
   ___ giving an injection
   ___ giving advice
   ___ acting to comfort a patient
   ___ listening to a patient
   ___ other: _____

3. What was the *outcome* of these interactions in your fantasies?
   ___ always favorable and dramatically so
   ___ usually favorable, but often not dramatically so
   ___ unfavorable as often as favorable, routine as often as dramatic
   ___ generally or always unfavorable
   ___ other: _____

4. What was the patient's *reaction* to this interaction and outcome?

    ___ dramatic relief and gratitude
    ___ quiet relief and gratitude
    ___ relief but not gratitude
    ___ indifference
    ___ quiet sadness
    ___ dramatic ingratitude and anger
    ___ other: _____

5. Who were *observers* of the scene (besides yourself and the patient)?

    ___ an assorted throng
    ___ your family and/or friends
    ___ the patient's family and/or friends
    ___ others: _____
    ___ no one else

6. What was your *personal reaction* to the interaction and outcome?

    ___ relief
    ___ happiness
    ___ pride
    ___ sadness
    ___ guilt
    ___ anger
    ___ other: _____

7. Which of the following were *never* included in your fantasies?

    ___ being called out in the middle of the night
    ___ resenting being called out in the middle of the night
    ___ informing a patient of a diagnosis of a terminal illness
    ___ sending a bill
    ___ a patient's nonpayment of a bill
    ___ an angry patient
    ___ a patient you found yourself disliking
    ___ a personal feeling of uncertainty over what to do for a particular patient
    ___ uncertainty within medical science over what to do for a particular patient
    ___ a bad outcome
    ___ a personal feeling of failure at a bad outcome
    ___ certifying a psychiatric commitment
    ___ finding a patient's problem uninteresting or boring
    ___ committee meetings
    ___ "pulling the plug" on a patient

___ dictating patient records
___ filling out forms
___ being sued by a patient
___ sexual attraction to a patient
___ subduing a combative patient
___ being chosen for a medical honorary society
___ informing the family about the death of a patient
___ winning the Nobel prize
___ other items: _____

_____

_____

1.2 Expectations

These fantasies have their basis in your process of growth and development. Examination of them is worthwhile, for this process gives clues to your view of medicine. Take some time to probe what lies *behind* these images, i.e., what particular events prompted you to think of medicine in this way, as well as what aspirations and life plans they reflect.

What elements of these fantasies remain with you? (Go back through questions 1–7 in Section 1.1 and use a different symbol to mark your *present* images of medical practice.)

Compare the two sets of answers and consider what images you are disappointed to have lost in your present, more realistic, understanding of medicine. Is your present understanding of medicine wholly realistic, or might your picture of it change as much in the next ten years as it has since you first entertained these fantasies? Most important, which of these thoughts about the medical enterprise represent *fundamentals* of being a physician, and which represent the "trimmings"? These are questions to tackle in depth in the next sections.

1.2.1 What Do You Expect from Yourself as a Physician? Reflection on the elements of your fantasies can reveal your expectations of medicine as a career and of yourself as a physician.

A. *Motivations* Examine these and try to determine whether your motivations are adequate to the tasks ahead.[1]

1. If reflection reveals, for example, that your expectation is for medical practice to be an unbroken series of dramatic successes, then you are bound for frustration.

---

1. Helpful reflection on motivations for and emotional reactions to medical training and practice is found in Knight (1981), especially Chapter 1: "The Decision to Become a Doctor."

2. If, on the other hand, your expectation is for an uninterrupted flow of dramatic failures accompanied by reactions of anger from patients and guilt on your part, then you should check yourself for masochistic tendencies.
3. If a dominant motivating force for you is the expectation of esteem and gratitude from patients as a prerequisite for a sense of accomplishment, you may have difficulty coping with reactions of anger or indifference from patients. The emotional reaction may hamper your capability to carry out adequate care of such patients. What motivating, moderating, or restraining resource is available within yourself that you can draw upon in such a situation?

   a. Resignation to self-sacrifice or martyrdom? If so, do you really undergo this to help patients, or are you acting for the sake of the good feeling *you* get from having practiced self-sacrifice?
   b. Unbounded love for humanity? Has this been tested and shown adequate to the task? If not, perhaps you had better not count on it.
   c. Dogged determination to "do a job right" once you have undertaken it? Has this been tested in prolonged and difficult tasks such as those facing you in a medical career?
   d. Curiosity about human nature, allowing you to create an emotional distance from certain situations by intellectualizing them? Could this not result in "bottling up" your negative reaction to this type of patient, perhaps allowing it to "spill over" into your private relationships?
   e. Self-discipline, by which you adhere to a code of professional behavior? How can you be sure what the code requires in every situation?

Some of these responses may sound cynical, but they are not meant to be. The point is to make you aware that not every motivation is adequate to the tasks you will face as a physician. However, physicians do manage to cope with situations like these, so it must not be impossible to find the motivating force to do so. It is likely that different motivations, and combinations of them, function in different people and in changing situations.

Considerations of motivation are relevant to judgments about a person's *character* but in most systems of ethical theory, they are not directly relevant to judgments about the rightness or wrongness of a person's *actions*. In other words, the fact remains that a person did the right (or wrong) thing, irrespective of the motivation that prompted the action. If Alberta and Alfred perform identical actions in identical circumstances, then their actions are subject to identical moral assessments—even if their motives were radically different. Differences in motive might lead to differences in assessments of the agents' character, but this does not affect judgments regarding the rightness or wrongness of their actions. For example, suppose Alberta and Alfred each jump into a lake to rescue a small child who has fallen into the water. Examination of their motives reveals that Alberta acted solely (or primarily) out of concern for the life of the infant, whereas Alfred's primary motivation for acting was the realization that television news cameras were rolling, recording the event, and that he is likely to receive a public acclaim as a hero. Both did the right thing in saving a life, but we regard Alberta with a moral respect (a character judgment) we would not confer on Alfred.

Even in the domain of character judgments there may be alternative motivations that are equally morally respectable. Immanuel Kant, an influential moral philosopher from eighteenth century Germany, denied this. He maintained that the only morally worthy motive was a "sense of duty," i.e., doing a thing because of acknowledgment that it is one's duty. However, most moral theorists would allow for a wider range of morally worthy motives. Consider Biffy and Buffy, who also rescue drowning infants in circumstances much like the pair in the previous paragraph. Biffy's primary motive for rescuing the infant was a sense of affection and helpfulness toward small children. (This motivation also prompts him to go out of his way to push children sitting alone in swings on public playgrounds, for example, or to rescue balls gone astray from children's games.) Buffy's primary motive was a sense of concern for the parents and a recognition of the blow they would experience if their child drowned. (The influence of this motivating force could also be detected in other actions. Buffy does not bother to push children in swings or to return balls that fly over the fence and land at her feet, but she has exerted a lot of energy to develop a "Parents' Day Out" program at the community center.)

Surely both Biffy and Buffy merit respect for their actions, in pretty much equal degrees. Both of these motivations are worthy and, indeed, laudable. Alfred "spoiled" his action, in character terms, by the unworthiness of his motive; but Alberta, Biffy, and Buffy would all be regarded as morally praiseworthy.

You may detect a variety of motives underlying the interest of your colleagues in medicine as a career (and there may even be a mixture of motives within yourself). However, many of these may be morally acceptable alternative forces prompting right action when the occasion calls for it. On-going self-examination can help determine the adequacy and soundness of your own motivating forces.

B. Specific Expectations   To give some concreteness to these reflections about your expectations, allow us to offer a scenario of our own as a focus for discussion:

> Lynn Languish sits in the waiting room. You sit in your office, dictating notes in the previous patient's record. As you finish your dictation and leaf quickly through the morning's mail, the nurse calls Lynn from the waiting room. They journey past the office scales; finally Lynn is installed in an examining room. You move down the hall to the room, remove the record from its rack on the door, and place your hand on the door handle. The clinical drama is about to begin.

What do you expect from this encounter and the many others like it, in which you will participate in your career in medicine? First, what is your primary focus in this sort of situation?

1. *Do you think of what is about to happen chiefly in terms of an* intellectual puzzle *of diagnosis and management of a disease process?*

If so, your focus is primarily on the disease rather than on the patient. You need to develop the habit of remembering that the patient is a *person* with a disease, and you must pay attention to the person's emotional reactions as well as to the pathophysiology of the disease.

2. *Does it occur to you that this interaction might be the source of a case report for a medical journal, or the start of a research project, or some other means to increase your professional laurels?*

This is an extension of the previous pattern, and the same warning applies.

3. *Do you think of this patient encounter in terms of the contribution it might make to the success of your department or university? Do you think in terms of how you will be evaluated by your resident or the supervising faculty, or perhaps of the impact it might have on your being chosen for advanced training or selected as chief resident, or the like?*

If so, you are reflecting patterns of socialization that have an important influence in medical training, but you must not lose sight of the needs of this particular patient in the process.

4. *Do you think of what is to come chiefly as an occasion for* helpfulness *to the patient?*

If so, what will be your reaction if you are unable to accomplish any helpful result? Will it be enough to have made an earnest attempt? What demands do you make on yourself in terms of intellectual preparation for this helping role?

Furthermore, you should examine the underlying basis of this attitude. *Why* do you seek to be helpful? Is it because of a sense of religious obligation, a felt professional standard, some past social experience, or some other source?

5. *Do you think of the encounter chiefly as an occasion for* socialization *and/or an opportunity to satisfy your* intellectual curiosity *about people?*

Here you must consider whether the questions you ask the patient are intended to give information essential to render care, or whether their *only* function is to satisfy your curiosity.

6. *Do you think of the encounter chiefly as a* chore? *Is your only (or primary) motivation for acting to generate income, to fulfill a corporate contract, to satisfy the demands of a teaching program?*

These sorts of external motivations are inevitable from time to time; but if they become recurrent, it may be difficult to maintain the motivation to provide an adequate level of care.

7. *Do you think of the encounter predominantly as an occasion for exercise of* technical prowess?

If so, be sure not to overreact to the clinical signs in a way that creates opportunities for the exercise of technical skill when intervention is not strictly necessary. Sometimes prospects for monetary gain can enter here as well, as can the role expectations of your specialty field. ("If I am a(n) _____ologist, I am supposed to be doing _____oscopies!")

8. *Do you think of the encounter predominantly as an "ego trip," i.e., an occasion to be lionized by grateful patients?*

This expectation may have been created by the actions of patients in the past. But you need to guard against coming to *expect* this reaction. Doing so might cause you to neglect the needs of the ungrateful patient.

C. Self-Reflection on Other Categories of Expectations In connection with each of the categories listed below, answer the following questions:

— What specific expectations do you have of yourself in this area?
— What barriers or difficulties do you foresee in your attempts to meet these expectations?
— What steps could you begin taking now to overcome these barriers and/or prepare yourself to meet these expectations?

1. Moral behavior

    a. honesty
    b. compassion
    c. desire to help
    d. courage[2]

2. Hard work, self-discipline
3. Skill, current knowledge, relevance; recognition that patients may not follow your advice, even when it is soundly based
4. Resourcefulness
5. Priorities for time use
6. Economic achievement

---

2. For an interesting interpretation of the role of courage in medical practice see Shelp (1983).

7. Having your own psychological needs fulfilled; social recognition
8. Peer group recognition
9. Other: _____

D. Professional Standards Do you expect yourself to abide by professional codes? What guidance do they provide in defining your expectations of yourself as a physician?[3]

1.2.2 What Do You Expect from Patients? It might be ideal if you could look forward to treating only patients with whom you can relate comfortably and easily. This would involve their being like you in the following respects:

— similar moral values
— similar social position
— similar cultural history
— similar religious views
— willing to act on your recommendations
— other: _____

However, this ideal is not likely to be realized. You will probably encounter many patients who are different from you in important ways; you must begin to develop the ability to work with them effectively. What traits can you *reasonably* expect from patients?

Think of specific patients with social, cultural, religious, and sexual values that differ from yours. Answer the following questions about your relationship with these patients in connection with each of the traits listed below:

— What specific expectations in the area mentioned do you have of patients?
— What barriers or difficulties might be created by differences in expectations between you and your patients?
— What steps could you take in your dealings with patients to overcome these barriers?

1. Honesty
2. A desire to be well
3. A need that can be met by your skills
4. Trust

   a. that you bring adequate knowledge and skill to your work with them
   b. that your credentials are acceptable, giving you credibility
   c. that you will preserve confidentiality, and thus they speak openly
   d. that you have their best interests as a primary value

---

3. Chapter 2 will examine professional codes in some detail: the Hippocratic Oath in Section 1.1, the AMA Principles of Medical Ethics in Section 1.2, and the American College of Physicians Ethics Manual in Section 1.3.

5. A recognition that you are fallible and that medical science is limited, and thus that a good result is not guaranteed

6. Gratitude
   a. for your hard work
   b. for your concern and compassion
   c. for your expertise

7. Cooperation in paying your bill
8. Other: _____
   _____

Even these more limited expectations will not always be met. You must prepare yourself for dealing with patients who fail to meet your expectations and who thereby frustrate your attempts to work with them. Significant categories here include patients who are

— belligerent
— noncompliant
— repugnant
— seductive
— ungrateful.

Remember when you encounter these sorts of patients that even the patients who do not meet your expectations may benefit from their encounter with you. The ungrateful patient may not acknowledge the value of your clinical contribution, but it may still have its effect, and thus that patient may get well as quickly as the grateful patient. This is one place to ask yourself what your fundamental goals are. Would you count the outcome of healing without gratitude as a success or a failure? Surely there is an important element of success here, even though there is also frustration.

1.2.3 What Do/Should Patients Expect from You? Just as your image of the "ideal patient" may be far removed from the type of patient you actually encounter, patients may have an image of the "ideal physician" that is unrealistic and cannot be satisfied by you or anybody else. In the following discussion, elements of many patients' expectations will be examined critically to ascertain what patients have a *right* to expect from physicians.

Among the roles patients may expect physicians to fulfill (in addition to the obvious) are the following:

— parent
— magician
— actor
— confessor
— advocate

— gatekeeper
— accomplice
— oracle
— technician
— barrier or hurdle
— friend
— teacher
— other: _____

_____

In connection with each of these, answer the following questions:

— How often have you encountered patients who expect you to fulfill this role? Think of specific examples.
— When is this expectation appropriate?
— What difficulties does this expectation present?
— What steps could you take in your dealings with patients to reduce unrealistic expectations?

1.2.4 The Experience of Illness   In this section the typical progression of steps toward and within patienthood is described in detail. Consider concrete examples throughout this discussion. If you or someone close to you has had experience with illness, think about how the various steps were exemplified in that situation. Otherwise (or also), think of examples of these elements in connection with patients you have treated, or in literary or biographical accounts of illness you have read.[4] Excerpts from one biographical account are interspersed throughout the discussion to provide a concrete example. At each stage continue identifying specific expectations and difficulties, as well as means to resolve them.

A. The Preclinical (or Nonclinical) Phase   It is important to keep in mind that "patienthood is a psychosocial, not a biologic state. A person becomes a patient by consulting a physician, or a surrogate for one, in the officially legitimated health care system" (Eisenberg 1980, 279). The psychosocial history of persons before they become patients can be a significant element in the course of clinical encounters.

A.1 "Dis-ease"   The path toward patienthood begins with some "dis-ease," i.e., some experience of distress or "an experience of unexpected discomfort, decrease in previous functional capacities or a change in physical appearance" (Eisenberg 1980, 279). The following description offers a dramatic example of this stage:

---

4. Several such accounts are listed in the "Further Reading" section at the end of the chapter.

> He woke at 7 A.M. with pain in his chest. The sort of pain that might cause panic if one were not a doctor, as he was, and did not know, as he knew, that it was heartburn. (Lear 1980, 11)

This state of "dis-ease" should not be identified with states of organic pathology (which may or may not underlie it). Eisenberg (1980, 278) makes the distinction in the following terms:

> Modern physicians diagnose and treat diseases, that is, abnormalities in the structure and function of body organs and systems; whereas patients suffer illnesses, that is, experiences of disvalued changes in states of being and in social function. Disease and illness do not stand in a one-to-one relation. Similar degrees of organ pathology may generate quite different reports of pain and distress;[5] illness may occur in the absence of disease, as witness the high proportion of visits to the physician for complaints without an ascertainable biologic basis. The course of disease is distinct from the trajectory of the accompanying illness.[6]

However, the occurrence of "symptoms" does not, by itself, turn the person into a patient. There are several intermediate steps along the way, each involving decision making by the prospective patient, "almost always with the participation of important others" (Eisenberg 1980, 279).

A.2 Interpretation   To quote Eisenberg again: "The first decision must be made: is the change a 'significant' deviation or is it a 'normal' part of living? Can it be dismissed as transient? Is it to be attributed to some recent event: the 'wrong' thing eaten, having 'strained' a muscle, 'that time of the month'?" (Eisenberg 1980, 279).

If the symptoms can be explained away in some such manner, the person may attempt to cope with them on his or her own (at least for the present) without seeking outside help. To illustrate, the story of Dr. Harold Lear continues.

> He went into the kitchen to get some Coke, whose secret syrups often relieve heartburn. The refrigerator door seemed heavy, and he noted that he was having trouble unscrewing the bottle cap. Finally he wrenched it off, cursing the defective cap. He poured some liquid, took a sip. The pain did not go away. Another sip; still no relief.
> Now he grew more attentive. He stood motionless, observing symptoms. His breath was coming hard. He felt faint. He was sweating, though the August morning was still cool. He put fingers to his pulse. It was rapid and weak. A powerful burning sensation was beginning to spread through his chest, radiating upward into his throat. Into his arm? No. But the pain was growing worse. Now it

---

5. See Coulehan (1980) for a fascinating description of three patients with identical diagnoses but markedly different courses of illness.
6. For further explication of this distinction between "disease" and "illness," see Cassell (1976).

was crushing—*"crushing,"* just as it is always described. And worse even than the pain was the sensation of losing all power, a terrifying seepage of strength. He could feel the entire degenerative process accelerating. He was growing fainter, faster. The pulse was growing weaker, faster. He was sweating much more profusely now—a heavy, clammy sweat. He felt that the life juices were draining from his body. He felt that he was about to die.

On some level he stood aside and observed all this with a certain clinical detachment. Here, the preposterous spectacle of this naked man holding a tumbler of Coke and waiting to die in an orange Formica kitchen on a sunny summer morning in the fifty-third year of his life.

I'll be damned, he thought, I can't believe it. (Lear 1980, 11–12)

A.3 Seeking and Choosing Help   If no satisfactory explanation can be found, the person may decide to seek outside help. But the question is still open whether the help sought will be *medical*. "Once it has been decided that something must be done, one has to identify the appropriate type of help: a family remedy, a folk healer, the local druggist, a chiropractor, a doctor. The choice is not unconstrained; it will depend upon the resources, both financial and cognitive, available to the person and upon the culture in which that person is imbedded" (Eisenberg 1980, 279).

Terrence Ackerman (1982) describes some of these constraints, although he focuses primarily on the clinical phase. The four kinds of constraints he enumerates—physical, cognitive, psychological, and social—all come into play in the pre-clinical phase as well. The emotional impact of illness (psychological constraint) is felt from the first recognition of dis-ease and the attempt at its interpretation.[7] The limits to the patient's understanding of the situation (cognitive constraints) have a strong influence on the decision about whether to seek help, and where to go for it. Social and physical constraints limit the possibilities for seeking help even when it is decided that medical institutions are the appropriate recourse.

> Slowly he tugged on a robe, staggered back into the foyer and pressed for the elevator. At this hour it was on self-service. When it arrived, he entered, pushed 1 and CLOSE DOOR, and braced himself against the wall. Suddenly he knew that if he did not lie down he would fall. He lowered himself to the floor. When the elevator door opened, he rolled out into the lobby and said to the startled doorman, "Get a wheelchair. Get me to the emergency room. I am having a heart attack."
>
> "An ambulance, Doctor? Shouldn't we get an ambulance?"
>
> "No. No time. A wheelchair." [The hospital—his hospital, where he was on staff—was nearby, a few blocks from his home.] Then he lost clarity. (Lear 1980, 13)

---

7. On this notion of the "vulnerability" of the ill person, cf. Cassell (1976), especially Chapter 1, and Pellegrino and Thomasma (1981, 207–209).

Lear chose to seek medical help (wisely, given his condition). However, many who experience illness do not seek medical assistance. "Up to this point, a whole series of transactions have occurred outside the official health care network and may never be known to it, unless it extends its purview beyond the door of the doctor's office and the hospital. Community studies indicate that some 75 to 90 percent of episodes self-identified as illness are managed entirely without recourse to the medical system" (Eisenberg 1980, 279).

A.4 Reasons   The remaining 10% to 25% do cross the threshold to patienthood. Ian McWhinney (1972) offers a useful set of categories that he claims are exhaustive and mutually exclusive, for classifying these episodes:

1. Limit of tolerance: "The patient comes because his symptoms are causing pain, discomfort or disability that have become intolerable."
2. Limit of anxiety: "The patient comes, not because his symptoms are causing distress, but because of their implications . . . because he, or a relative, fears the consequences of his symptoms."
3. Problems of living presenting as symptoms (heterothetic): The decision to come is "due to a problem of living that has disturbed the equilibrium that the patient has established with his environment."
4. Administrative: "This category covers doctor-patient contacts whose sole purpose is administrative, even though the patient is ill," e.g., excuses from school, filling out an insurance form, or certifying a period of disability.
5. No illness: "This category includes all attendances for preventive purposes, such as antenatal or well-baby care, or for general medical assessment when no symptoms are offered."

B. The Clinical Phase   Just as the prospective patient must make a judgment, on the basis of a complex of factors, about the appropriateness of seeking medical help, "similarly the physician now embarks on the difficult task of disentangling these multiple factors to determine whether the patient has found his way to the proper institutional setting, i.e., a medical setting, and whether the patient's problem is properly 'medical' rather than being a social, religious, political, or economic problem" (Siegler 1981b, 635).

B.1 Clinical Method

What usually follows after the patient's initial presentation is a process which we have come to call the clinical method . . . [which] has two central components: 1) data-gathering, and 2) data-reduction and diagnosis. Both of these features of the clinical method, but especially the data-gathering phase, require a considerable amount of personal interaction and an exchange of information about both technical and value-laden concerns between the patient and the physician. (Siegler 1981b, 635)

Gathering and organizing data requires special sensitivity when (as frequently happens) the patient is unsure about the details of symptoms and/or interprets them in an unusual way. Furthermore, patients may not have made up their own minds about the value priorities involved in clinical choices. Thus, even here,

> while the physician wears his persona of objective scientist, an enormous amount of human, personal, subjective interaction is occurring between patient and doctor. The eliciting of a medical history is not a job for machines and requires the profound subtlety that only trained, sensitive humans can bring to it. . . . Nor do I believe that the data-reduction phase which generates a diagnosis and a differential diagnosis is a mechanical process. The apparently scientific, mechanical [process] . . . is full of personal drama, and it leads inexorably to the individualization of the patient. . . . (Siegler 1981b, 636)

B.2 Recommendation and Negotiation Ideally, the clinical method will yield a firm diagnosis for which some treatment regimen (or perhaps any one of several alternative approaches) is likely to be effective. Often, however, things are less clear-cut, and sometimes it will tragically become clear that no curative treatment is possible. In any case, the physician will be expected to offer recommendations. Pellegrino and Thomasma (1981, 211) speak especially of this clinical moment:

> The end of medicine . . . is therefore a right and good healing action taken in the interest of a particular patient. All the science and art of the physician converge on the choice . . . a choice of what is *right* in the sense of what conforms scientifically, logically, and technically to the patient's needs, and a choice of what is *good,* what is worthwhile for the patient.

Not only must the therapeutic course settled upon *be* worthwhile for this specific patient, but it must also be *recognized* as worthwhile by the patient. This is accomplished by the process of persuasion and negotiation that Siegler calls "the doctor-patient accommodation" (or DPA).

The careful physician will learn as much as possible about the expectations, values, and beliefs of the specific patient (insofar as these are settled in the patient's own mind) and will take this information into account in formulating recommendations for this case. (This shows the merits of a complete psychosocial, religious, and sexual history.)

However, it is not enough to formulate a recommendation that is both right and good. If the patient cannot be made to *see* its appropriateness, he is unlikely to carry it out, and thus it will have as little effectiveness as a medically non-therapeutic regimen. Our legal and social structures leave the decision about cooperation with the physician's recommendation to the patient.[8]

The physician and patient must come to agreement about the elements of their cooperative endeavor through a DPA.

---

8. See Section 3 of this chapter for further analysis of the legal and ethical requirements of informed consent, the primary social structure referred to here.

The process is one of communication and negotiation—sometimes short and to the point, sometimes extended—on what rights and responsibilities each of the participants wishes to retain and which will be relinquished in the context of their medical relationship. From the moment the patient originally presented to the physician's attention, testing has been undertaken by both parties to decide whether this patient and this doctor wish to work together. (Siegler 1981b, 637–638)

This is the point at which you can communicate your expectations of patients (see Section 1.2.2) as well as your self-expectations (Section 1.2.1). If there are serious discrepancies between what the patient expects of you and what you are willing to provide, then perhaps no DPA can be reached between you and the patient, who should be advised to seek care elsewhere. If there are less serious discrepancies, compromise on both sides may be necessary to reach a DPA satisfactory to both parties. You need to define the points on which you are (and those on which you are not) willing to compromise your expectations in the interest of reaching accommodation with specific patients.

Often the patient remains unclear about *what* he wants, and he may abdicate his responsibility in the DPA. ("Just do whatever you think is best, Doctor.") However, it is unwise for the physician to accept this invitation to paternalism at face value. The patient is the one who must live (or perhaps die) with the choices arrived at in the DPA, and he should be gently guided to work out a basis of values for participation in these choices. Otherwise, as the situation develops, the patient is unlikely to honor the choices through compliance, since he feels no "ownership" of them.

B.3 The Physician-Patient Relationship   Siegler describes the physician-patient relationship as "characterized by mature and enduring exchanges of trust between the patient and the physician, which establish an almost inseparable bond. If such an exchange of trust occurs, it serves as a stabilizer of the medical relationship even during periods of new and difficult stresses" (Siegler 1981b, 639).

The classic "chicken and egg" problem arises: Which comes first, the accommodation between physician and patient with regard to a specific treatment approach, or this deeper, more enduring relationship? Siegler insists that the former is prior:

In contrast to previous descriptions of the doctor-patient relationship [following Siegler, let us abbreviate this as DPR] which tend to regard it as an established, static arrangement between doctor and patient, the DPA provides a more dynamic and realistic model of the medical encounter. Perhaps DPRs as such rarely exist; rather, what we regard as a DPR may really be repeatedly negotiated DPAs. More likely, a DPR represents a specific, and increasingly uncommon variant of the DPA. It may be distinguished from the DPA by its duration, depth, and maturity. (Siegler 1981b, 639)

Certainly it is important to recognize that the relationship between patient and physician is dynamic and changing, but it is no less vital to recognize that many (though not all) such relationships contain from the start elements of a mutual bond of trust, depth of relationship, and expectation of an enduring continuation of the relationship. Without these, the physician cannot gain access to intimate information or cooperation for onerous treatment regimens.

It is true (as Siegler says elsewhere) that developments in technology, medical specialization, and institutional structures of health care create barriers to the early establishment of a "traditional" DPR. A full-scale DPR rarely occurs on the first encounter with a patient. Its development may be influenced by the setting of practice (Compare, for example, the clinic setting, an HMO structure, a group practice setting, and an individual practice: in which of these is a DPR likely to develop most quickly and naturally? Compare, also, a long-term relationship with a primary care provider to encounters with a specialist.) However, in spite of these difficulties, it is important to acknowledge that (1) the traditional relationship is still possible in many settings, and (2) it is still a goal to be vigorously pursued. Without the basis of trust and mutual regard, the DPA Siegler describes could not easily be achieved.

C. Extraclinical Elements   Even during the clinical phase, there are elements of the patient's life that are external to the immediate concerns of the health care system. These may have significant influence on the clinical course. Again, one important aspect of this is well illustrated in Dr. Harold Lear's story:

> Then, dimly, he felt himself being lifted onto a stretcher, sensed noise and light and a sudden commotion about him. They were giving him nasal oxygen, taking his pulse, taking his blood pressure, starting an intravenous, getting a cardiogram—the total force of modern emergency care suddenly mobilized; a team clicking away with the impersonality of an overwhelmingly efficient machine.
>
> He understood that at this moment he was no more than a body with pathology. They were not treating a person; they were treating an acute coronary case in severe shock. They were racing, very quickly, against time. He himself had run this race so often, working in just this detached silent way on nameless, faceless bodies with pathologies. He did not resent the impersonality. He simply noted it. But one of the medical team, a young woman who was taking his blood pressure, seemed concerned about *him*. She patted him on the shoulder. She said, "How do you feel?" It was the only departure from this cool efficiency, and he felt achingly grateful for it. Ah, he thought in some fogged corner of the brain, she must be a medical student. She hasn't yet learned to depersonalize. She will. We all do. What a pity.
>
> (Later—he thought it was that same day, but it may have been the next—she came up to the coronary-care unit, and took his hand and said, "How are you doing, Dr. Lear?" and smiled at him. He never knew her name, and he never forgot her.) (Lear 1980, 14)

The patient will interpret events in terms of his cultural, educational, religious, and social categories of thought; and other people may contribute interpretive elements in communications with the patient. Furthermore, the patient may be preoccupied with events occurring outside the institution. It has been shown above that life stresses in the patient's environment contribute to the step into patient-hood. These events must not be forgotten by health professionals in the course of care, for they are a source of concern for the patient and may frustrate the best therapeutic efforts. The disruption the hospitalization produces in the patient's social system may add new stresses, e.g., concerns about employment respon-sibilities or child care, financial worries, etc.

D. The Postclinical Phase   Except for those who remain in institutions per-manently (whether for long-term custodial care, or in a short-term wait for death), patients have a life *after* the direct clinical interactions of patienthood. This can be divided into two sub-phases: recuperation and return to active life.

D.1 Recuperation   During the recuperation phase, the person is still *partly* a patient, for there are medical restrictions and/or treatment regimens to be carried out. However, the patient is no longer under the sort of total medical supervision that is possible during hospitalization, so the responsibility for carrying out these medical procedures is left to the patient and his or her social group.

This is an important part of the reason why cooperation, negotiation, or accommodation is to be preferred to an authoritarian or paternalistic approach. If you hope to influence patient cooperation after he or she has left direct medical supervision, it is important that the patient understand the issues and agree with the necessity for the procedures. (This may not, of course, be enough to guarantee cooperation, but without it noncooperation is virtually certain.)

D.2 "Back to Work"   The DPA and DPR are important even after the episode of illness, when the patient has returned to active life. Life-style changes that may prevent future illnesses can be a significant part of any DPA that has been reached. The trust characterizing the DPR (and the patient education stemming from this DPA) may be a significant influence in the patient's decision to seek medical help the next time symptoms occur.

1.2.5 Expectations of/by Society   It is impossible to be a physician in isolation from others. This follows from the concept of a physician. If one of your colleagues jets to an uninhabited tropical isle immediately following graduation from medical school, before treating her first patient, to live a Robinson Crusoe existence, she would be "medically trained" but would not "be a physician."

Medical practice depends upon society in more concrete ways as well. The government supports medical education through financial subsidies. The licensure system permits those appropriately trained to practice and enhances the prestige of the profession by providing legal barriers against practice by untrained, self-styled healers (or even those whose training does not conform to the letter of United States standards).

Members of society make practice possible by submitting themselves for treatment, and special social and economic status is granted to members of the profession. Several authors have drawn ethical implications directly from this relationship of reciprocity, contract, or covenant between the profession and society (Ballantine, 1979; Chapman, 1979, 632; Veatch, 1981).

Even if one does not draw central ethical principles directly from the professional's relationship with society, certain expectations of society must be acknowledged.

1. Society expects one who has accepted the training subsidized by its contributions to use these skills to promote the general welfare. A medical school graduate choosing not to employ those skills through practice, research, or teaching medicine tests this trust.
2. How much control over the location and form of one's practice is society entitled to exert because of its contributions to medical training?
   a. Is it legitimate to provide scholarships conditional upon service obligations, while those who can afford to pay full tuition can avoid such obligations?
   b. Is it reasonable to require service obligations from all medical graduates, on grounds of national interest and/or some degree of governmental subsidy of virtually all medical education programs?
3. How important is the value of independence when balanced against society's claims and needs?

These questions are considered at some length in Chapter 5.

Society also has specific expectations from physicians. It expects you to serve social institutions by certifying illness, disability, eligibility for various services, and the like. Society expects physicians to contribute to social decisions in matters relating to health. Consider other expectations by society you have encountered or expect to encounter in practice.

What specific things do *you* expect from society? What things do *your patients* expect? (Some answers to these questions will be discussed in Chapter 5).

1.3 Conclusion

Look back over this section to spot discrepancies between different elements you have examined. Do your expectations of yourself (Section 1.2.1) match likely patient expectations of you (Sections 1.2.3 and 1.2.4)? Do your expectations of patients (Section 1.2.2) match what patients are willing to offer as their part of the DPA (Section 1.2.4)? Are there serious discrepancies between what you and patients could agree on and expectations of society at large (Section 1.2.5)? If you find significant discrepancies on any of these points, you need to begin to develop resources to deal with them.

You will examine specific elements of these expectations in the remainder of this and other chapters. Keep in mind the conclusions you have reached in this section, for you should bring them to the issues to which the discussion now turns.

2 Information Exchange

2.1 Relationships

As background for discussions of information exchange in the DPR, consider the expectations and obligations for providing information in the following relationships.

2.1.1 Casual Encounters   You are flying home to visit your family. The person sitting next to you on the plane is a stranger, and is friendly. You chat casually from time to time, though you are both reading. When asked "what you do," you say only that you are "a student" and do not mention that you are in medical school. (Perhaps you are tired and not in the mood for the health history or the catalogue of gripes about doctors you know could follow your giving this information.) Then your neighbor calls your attention to a magazine advertisement for an acetaminophen tablet and asks, "I wonder if this stuff is really safer than aspirin? What do you think?"

How would you respond to this question? What is expected of you?

This stranger is clearly "making conversation." She may be genuinely interested in your opinion, which may influence her opinion on the matter. As a layperson herself (apparently), she has heard enough about this subject to have some concern about the relative safety of aspirin, and she assumes that you (whom she assumes to be a layperson) have been exposed to similar information. Her interest seems to be in hearing (1) something about what you have learned about this issue ("I have heard . . . ") and/or (2) something about the impact this information has had on your own thinking about what pain reliever to take yourself ("I intend to keep taking my old reliable aspirin."). She would undoubtedly be shocked by either (3) an authoritative pronouncement from you without explanation (e.g., "Look, just ignore these 'scare pieces' in the popular press. Go ahead and take your aspirin and don't worry about a thing!") or (4) an elaborate explanation couched in scientific terminology.

If you give the sort of response she is expecting, your reply might have an influence on her thinking, but it will not be particularly great. She will consider what you say alongside what she has read and heard from others and, on that basis, she will make a decision.

Matters would be significantly different, however, if you responded: "As a matter of fact, I am a medical student, and I have just been going over the studies dealing with the comparative safety of aspirin and acetaminophen. I can tell you with assurance that . . . " Obviously, this would gain you a much greater influence on her decision. But it would not guarantee that she would follow your advice. For one thing, it makes a difference that you are a medical *student,* not a practicing physician (although, in fact, your knowledge base may be more extensive and more up-to-date than many physicians in practice). Second, you are not *her* physician, so the trust and reliance built into established physician-patient relationships does not exist, which affects the weight she will give to your response.

Let us carry this scenario further. Suppose that you do not reveal your background and dig into your medical knowledge for a detailed answer to her question. Further suppose she proceeds to make a choice, which might have been different if you had given detailed and convincing advice—and that this choice leads to a harmful result (e.g., she continues to take aspirin and a life-threatening hemorrhage develops).

Would it be appropriate to say that you were in any way *responsible* for this harm? Did you have any *obligation* to provide a detailed answer to her question? It would certainly be ethically wrong to give her an answer you knew to be *false,* but it is difficult to see how you have any obligation to give her detailed medical advice. It would probably be inappropriate to ask the questions whose answers you would need in order to give a response fitting the particularities of her physical condition. You would do her a service if you gave an answer drawn from your study of the issue, but you have no obligation to launch into a detailed recital of medical science.

A related issue is the respect for and authority of medical pronouncements that are regularly part of commercial advertising. (The epitome of this is the actor who formerly played the role of a kindly physician in a television series who now trades on that role to assure viewers of the health benefits of caffeine-free coffee). Here, even when the claims have some connection to medical information (which is not common), they are not specific enough to count as solid "medical advice." All too often the appeal to a medical basis for a claim is wholly unfounded. This is the fallacy of "appeal to authority," in which a figure who has attained a position of authority due to genuine achievements is used to lend credibility to claims that fall outside the arena of his expertise.

2.1.2 Friends   You are "shooting the breeze" in a group with which you have maintained a close friendship since high school days. None of its members is in a field related to medicine. (Perhaps that is one reason you look them up periodically, for it is good to escape from the preoccupation with medical science shared by your medical school friends.) One of them points out a billboard advertising an acetaminophen product and says to you, "Hey, Doc, is this stuff really safer to take than aspirin? What do you think?"

How would you respond to this question? What is expected of you?

Your friends may be interested in giving you a chance to "show off" your knowledge. They may be less interested in the *content* of your answer than in (1) the authoritative tone and/or (2) the impressive-sounding scientific terminology in which your explanation is couched.

However, you would be remiss if you launched into meaningless "double-talk" (unless you eventually made it clear to everybody around that you were doing so) because your friends undoubtedly do respect your knowledge and they might quote your answer to others or take it into account in making decisions about painkillers. However, if a bad result occurred (either from following advice given in this sort of casual situation or from your not having given a detailed answer), you could not really be held responsible, either legally or morally.

2.1.3 Patients   You are seeing a patient in the hospital outpatient clinic. After you have taken care of the presenting complaints and as the patient is gathering things to leave the examining room, he turns to you and asks, "Doctor, what is this I hear about XYZ (an acetaminophen product). Is that stuff really safer to take than aspirin?"

How would you respond to this question? What is expected of you?

This is a request for professional advice. This patient is likely to take your answer seriously, quote it to neighbors, and base his pain reliever purchases and administration habits on your response. The trust and reliance on your authority that is a component of the physician-patient relationship is present here.

However, it is your general knowledge of medical science being sought, not a diagnosis of any particularities of the patient's condition. (Although you would be wise to think through the patient's history to determine if there might be any special risk factors present.)

It is possible (but not probable) that this is more than a casual question. Sometimes the question asked at the examining room door as the patient is leaving is the *primary* reason that brought the patient in. If there is any indication that this might be the case here—that, for example, the patient is especially worried about this issue, or perhaps that he suspects that some harmful effects have occurred from taking one or the other pain reliever—then it might be good to bring him back into the examining room to explore the matter in detail.

However, it is more likely that the question is a casual one, asked for the purpose of settling doubts in the patient's own mind, or perhaps to settle an argument with a friend. Thus, a generalization is a sufficient response.

Let us carry this scenario further. Suppose this patient acted on the basis of your recommendation and a harmful result ensued. What would be your responsibility?

If there had been a specific contraindication in the patient's medical history you overlooked in formulating your advice, there might be legal liability. However, if no such contraindication had been revealed, you would probably not be expected to conduct further examination and tests to provide a specific basis for answering this question, and you probably would not be held legally responsible for a bad outcome that could have been prevented only by further examination and tests. Moral responsibility is congruent with legal responsibility in this situation.

2.1.4 High-Risk Patients   A patient you are treating for nasal polyps asks whether it would be safer to take acetaminophen rather than aspirin for frequent headaches.

How would you respond? What is expected of you?

Here a full-scale medical judgment is called for—general scientific information as well as the application of that information to the particularities of this patient's condition. There are higher stakes involved than in the other cases we have looked at because there are significant risk factors present in this case. You would be well-advised to review the patient's medical record carefully and draw on the full range of your knowledge of medical science in formulating a reply.

2.2 Obligations

Some fundamental principles about moral obligations regarding information exchange can be derived from the foregoing scenarios:

1. There is a general moral obligation *not* to give *mis*information or tell a direct lie. This applies in dealings with everybody.
2. There is *no* general moral obligation to tell "the whole truth," i.e., to give to others information we happen to possess, even if what we could tell them would be beneficial to them. It might be commendable to assist others in this way, but this seems more like a matter of "Good Samaritanism" or action "above and beyond the call of duty" rather than a moral *obligation*.
3. A moral obligation arises to provide beneficial information in the physician-patient relationship. This is an aspect of the duty of care, recognizing that providing information is a significant element of medical treatment. This includes especially information about things the patient could do to speed recovery and/or to prevent a recurrence of the condition being treated, but it also includes providing information about the rationale underlying recommendations for treatment, since this may be the best way to impress on the patient the importance of following these recommendations.
4. Furthermore, the obligation to provide care includes an obligation to
   a) *acquire* the information needed to provide adequate care, and then
   b) share this information with the patient for his benefit. If the stakes are

high, this may require elaborate steps (e.g., high-technology diagnostic tests and/or an extensive literature search) to acquire the needed information.
5. You will see in the next section that the legal and moral requirement of informed consent imposes an obligation on the physician to impart information to the patient.

These principles do not settle the matter of information exchange, however. A number of questions are still left unanswered.

1. What are the obligations of the *patient* to give information to physicians?
2. What (if any) are the *limits* of the obligation to provide information to patients? Must a physician impart "the truth, the whole truth, and nothing but the truth"?
3. What are the moral guidelines about imparting information to *persons other than the patient?*[9]

2.3 Fulfilling These Obligations

Consider a concrete example of the transactions of information exchange. Many people think of this as occurring exclusively in the phase of clinical interaction that was earlier called "Recommendation and Negotiation" (Section 1.2.4.B.2).[10] However, much of the most important information exchange takes place in the part of the clinical phase that was earlier called "clinical method" (Section 1.2.4.B.1), so let us begin there.

> Lynn Languish[11] sits on the edge of the examining table when you enter the examining room. She is a well-groomed woman in her mid-thirties. She appears not to be in acute distress at the moment, but that she is worried is obvious.
>
> She explains her reason for coming in: "The other day, I noticed this lump in my armpit. When it did not go away after several days, I got concerned about it. I would like you to examine it and tell me whether it is anything to worry about."
>
> Your examination reveals a small, firm node in the axilla. You do a thorough breast exam, but no mass is palpable and no dimpling is observed. You question her about a history of infectious diseases or localized infections, but she reports no signs of anything along these lines.

What should you do next? (Pursuing details of the clinical work-up is beyond the scope of this book. The focus here is on the *ethical* dimensions of practice. However, the ethical dimensions cannot be separated from the clinical, so you should think through the clinical dimensions as you are guided to address the ethical issues here.)

---

9. Discussion of this issue is found in Section 4 of this chapter.
10. This component of information exchange is linked closely with the legal and ethical requirement of informed consent, which is the subject of Section 3 of this chapter.
11. See Section 1.2.1.B for the initial scene in this patient's story.

More central to the ethical issues, what should you *say* to Lynn at this point? Look over the list of items below. For each item,

1. Consider whether you would tell this to Lynn at this time.
2. Consider *why* you would or would not tell her this.
3. Consider whether you would express it to her in *just this way*. If not, indicate in the space provided *how* you would put it.
4. Consider *in what order* you would explain these items. Number them in the order in which you would proceed.

<u>Tell Lynn?</u>   <u>In what order?</u>

Y / N   Say, "The nodes might be a sign of cancer of the breast."   _____.
         Why or why not? _____.
         How to put it: _____.

Y / N   Say, "The nodes might be a sign of AIDS."   _____.
         Why or why not? _____.
         How to put it: _____.

Y / N   Say, "I don't think this is anything serious."   _____.
         Why or why not? _____.
         How to put it: _____.

Y / N   Say, "This could be something serious."   _____.
         Why or why not? _____.
         How to put it: _____.

Y / N   Say, "This *could not possibly* be anything serious."   _____.
         Why or why not? _____.
         How to put it: _____.

Y / N   Say, "I am sure this is *not* cancer."   _____.
         Why or why not? _____.
         How to put it: _____.

Y / N   Say, "This is nothing to worry about."   _____.
         Why or why not? _____.
         How to put it: _____.

Y / N   Say, "I'm not sure what caused the swelling in this node."   _____.
         Why or why not? _____.
         How to put it: _____.

Y / N   Say, "We need to do some tests to find out the cause."   _____.
         Why or why not? _____.
         How to put it: _____.

Y / N   Describe the risks and discomforts of the test(s).   _____.
         Why or why not? _____.
         How to put it: _____.

Y / N   Say, "Here's how much the test(s) will *cost*."   _____.
         Why or why not? _____.
         How to put it: _____.

Y / N   Ask, "What do *you* think the problem is?"   _____.
         Why or why not? _____.
         How to put it: _____.

ADD: Say, _____   _____.
         Why add this? _____.

ADD: Say, _____   _____.
         Why add this? _____.

ADD: Say, _____   _____.
         Why add this? _____.

ADD: Say, _____   _____.
         Why add this? _____.

2.3.1 "The Truth" This discussion takes a "Golden Rule" approach to the issue of information exchange. It begins by considering examples of miscommunication by the patient and asks you to examine your reaction to these; on that basis, you should consider the parallels between these incidents and certain practices by physicians.

A. Patient Suppose you discovered that Lynn had lied to you in her account of the node. Suppose she told you that it was extremely tender and painful (perhaps even feigning a wince or a groan when you palpated it), whereas, in fact, it was not painful at all. Perhaps she said this hoping you would prescribe pain medication (which she enjoys using when it is available, although she does not seek it on a regular basis). If you discovered this subterfuge, you would no doubt be angry and disappointed to learn that a patient had told you a direct lie. You expect patients to tell you the truth when you ask them questions. You feel that you have a *right* to the information and a right to be trusted with the information. You are employing your diagnostic skills for her benefit, but a lie subverts this goal.

Would your reaction change if you discovered that the reason for her lie was that she had heard that nontender lumps are a sign of cancer and she could not bring herself to face the possibility that this might be cancer? *Think about this question for a minute before you continue.* A sensitive reaction would include empathy for her fear, but some frustration and disappointment is likely to result in even the most sympathetic clinician, for her misinformation could steer you down the wrong diagnostic trail entirely. In addition, her failure to communicate fully with you shows that (at some level, perhaps subconscious) she is not willing to be open with you and trust you to handle her fears sensitively and assist her in dealing with them. Even with the most favorable interpretation, her lying shows something is lacking in the relationship between you and her. As indicated in Section 1.2.2, honesty and openness are expected of patients.

Of course, some kinds of patients' lies are so common as to be expected; thus they are treated as part of the clinical data. Patients' reports about how much they smoke or drink are routinely "corrected" upwards. Or patients present with a complaint so transparent in its falsity that it must be regarded as a disguised call for help, and the clinician must explore the *real* reason for their visits. For example, a patient may come to a hospital emergency room repeatedly in a highly intoxicated state complaining of "chest pains" and deny that he has been drinking heavily, although his behavior and the alcohol on his breath clearly show he is intoxicated. Sensitive and patient exploration with the patient might lead him to agree that he is really there seeking help with his drinking problem.

However, the typical reaction of physicians to these situations demonstrates that they are not free of ethical issues. Patients may be excused (at least to some extent) from moral condemnation for this behavior on grounds of their impairment. The physician may be willing to "play the little game" in the interest of helping patients overcome the problems that prompted this behavior. However, the negative attitudes these patients arouse may be due, in part, to a recognition of the questionable ethical character of these actions.

B. Physician   Of course, patients have a similar expectation of you. A serious breakdown of Lynn's trust in you would occur if she discovered you had told her an outright lie—for example, if she discovered that you were aware that there *were* life-threatening possibilities among the differential diagnoses at the time you told her that "It *could not possibly* be anything serious."

And even if she did not discover your lie outright, it is likely that your calculations to maintain the deception would affect the nature of your interactions with her. (For example, you would be forced to try to act casual about the importance of carrying out additional tests, although you would feel a certain urgency about this.) This is likely to produce significant impairment of your relationship at a subconscious level, even if she were not aware of the cause. This result could be avoided only if either you were so adept at lying that no clues at all of your artifice were communicated, or you were so emotionally "cold" toward the patient that she could not detect any difference between an open and honest communication and one clouded by artifice. The former of these requires morally questionable skills, and the latter is hardly to be recommended as a way of interacting with patients. Thus, it can almost never be justified to tell a patient an outright lie.

B.1 Half-Truths   Is there a significant moral difference between an outright, "bald-faced" lie and other forms of expression that might mislead? Consider this question for yourself in connection with the following examples. Do you see a significant moral difference between these responses to Lynn Languish?

1. Telling her "This *could not possibly* be anything serious," when you are well aware that life-threatening conditions are included among the differential diagnoses.
2. Telling her "I am quite sure that this node is not a sign of cancer of the breast" when you are *pretty sure* it is not, but you are not really "quite sure."
3. Telling her "I don't think this is anything to worry about" and reassuring her that you would let her know if you had reason to believe that this was cancer
   a. when *you mean* that there is no point in her worrying about this *now* since there will be plenty of time for worry later if it turns out to be cancer,
   b. but you know that *she is likely to take you to mean* that you are sure that it is *not* cancer.
4. Telling her that you are 95% sure this is *not* cancer
   a. because you feel you cannot honestly give any greater assurance than this on the basis of the evidence available so far,
   b. although you know she is so worried about cancer that she will not be calmed unless you tell her that you are *100%* certain that it is not cancer.

All of these have the same outcome: the patient comes to believe something the physician considers to be false or, at least, unsupported by the available evidence. Only the first, however, is an outright lie. (Following many ethical theorists, we would define a "lie" as a matter of saying something that one believes to be *false*.) None of the other examples involve this, strictly speaking. However, responses 2 and 3 are forms of *deception,* for they involve deliberately causing the patient to believe something the physician regards as false or unsupported. Furthermore, all three responses are contrary to the usual expectation of patients. Indeed, the deceptions succeed (particularly in example 3) only because the patient presupposes that she will be told the truth. So, even if there are moral gradations among these three responses, all raise serious ethical questions.[12]

Response 4 is significantly different from the others. Here the physician cannot be said to be deliberately deceiving the patient, even though the result may still be that the patient comes to believe something the physician regards as almost certainly false. The ethical issue raised by this example is the value and importance of *truth* in itself. Which is more important for the physician: to be honest or to offer

---

12. For further discussion of these questions, see Bok (1978), especially Chapter XV: "Lies to the Sick and Dying".

reassurance? The AMA Principles of Medical Ethics favors the former. Section 2 says: "A physician shall deal honestly with patients. . . . "[13]

2.3.2 "The Whole Truth" *How much* should physicians tell patients? Should patients be informed of all your suspicions? Should you share all your uncertainties? If not, where is the line drawn between what should and what should not be communicated? Look over your responses to the exercise in Section 2.3 and consider what answer to these questions your choices presupposed. Again, let us approach discussion of these questions by first considering your expectations about patients providing information to you.

A. Patient

A.1 Deliberate Omission Suppose you found that Lynn had not lied directly but had *withheld* certain information. (NOTE: We are changing the hypothesis here. Forget about the earlier scenario in which she told a direct lie.) Suppose that she had deliberately refrained from telling you about a bit of bloody nipple discharge she had noticed a few days ago, even though she was (vaguely) aware that this information might be directly relevant to the diagnosis. (Why did she withhold this information? She thought the discharge might be the result of some aggressive sexual play her husband had engaged in, and she felt too embarrassed to tell you about it.) What would be your reaction if you learned she had withheld this information?

A.2 Relevance Unrecognized The situation might be different if the omission were not deliberate. Suppose it became clear that she had failed to recognize this information was relevant to the diagnostic puzzle. It is not that she was trying to mislead you by withholding this information, she merely *failed to recognize the importance* of bringing it up (and was acutely embarrassed to mention it). What would be your reaction?

A.3 Information Overlooked A still different situation results if the information is not provided because the patient *failed to obtain it:* "Have you had any dark stools or frank rectal bleeding?" "I don't know. I haven't looked." What would be your reaction here? Do you expect "the whole truth" from patients?

B. Physician Similarly, do patients expect "the whole truth" from their physician? There are indications that physicians do not always give full information. In a poll conducted by Louis Harris and Associates for the President's Commission for the Study of Ethical Problems in Medicine and Biomedical and Behavioral

---

13. For the full text of the AMA Principles, see Chapter 2, Section 1.2.

Research (1982b, 17–316),[14] physicians reported the following information-withholding practices (Table 1-1):

Table 1-1   Frequency With Which Physicians Report They Withhold Information

	Information Is Withheld About	
Frequency	Diagnosis or Prognosis	Treatment Risks and Alternatives
Once a day	2%	4%
Once a week	7%	6%
Once a month	12%	9%
Few times a year	32%	24%
Almost never	46%	57%

[President's Commission (1982a, 97).]

Approximately one-fifth of physicians admit to withholding key information from patients at least once a month.

One situation corresponding to A.2 in the description of patient miscommunications occurs when the physician omits an item of information because he or she does not recognize that it might be important to the patient. This marks a failure to ascertain the value system of the patient. More serious are situations corresponding to A.1: deliberately withholding information you *know* would be relevant to the patient's thinking. What sorts of reasons might lead one to take such a step? In the following list mark the items you have found yourself exemplifying in your own reasoning in the past, or can envision yourself exemplifying in the future:

1. To avoid the discomfort the patient's reaction is likely to cause *you*.
2. "It would take too long to explain it all."
3. Not wanting to have to get an investigational work-up underway this close to your vacation.
4. Not disclosing how remote the probabilities are for certain frightening but extremely remote possibilities (e.g., AIDS), in hopes of luring the patient into an expensive diagnostic work-up to rule these out.
5. Wanting to wait until you are *sure* before giving her information of this magnitude.
6. Because the family urged you not to tell.
7. Not wanting to cause her needless anxiety.
8. Not wanting to take the time to deal with the patient's ensuing depression.
9. Not wanting to deprive her of hope.
10. Because you judge that giving her this information might prompt her to forego needed therapy.
11. Because you judge that she will not be able to *understand* the information.

---

14. This poll involved standard opinion survey methods. Interviews were completed with a national sample of 805 physicians and a national cross section of 1251 adults.

12. Because you think she is not mentally competent to make any sound *use* of the information.
13. Because you think that although she may be competent *now*, she *will not* be able to make competent use of the information once it is presented to her, because her mental state is such that hearing this information would destroy her ability to make competent decisions on the matter.
14. Because you think her reaction would be *irrational*.
15. Because you are convinced that she really doesn't want to know.
16. Because you think she probably *already* knows.

The professional community has not been silent on this issue. Consider the following statement by the Judicial Council of the American Medical Association (1984, 29–30):

> *8.07 Informed Consent.* The patient's right of self-decision can be effectively exercised only if the patient possesses enough information to enable an intelligent choice. The patient should make his own determination on treatment. Informed consent is a basic social policy for which exceptions are permitted (1) where the patient is unconscious or otherwise incapable of consenting and harm from failure to treat is imminent; or (2) when risk-disclosure poses such a serious psychological threat of detriment to the patient as to be medically contraindicated. Social policy does not accept the paternalistic view that the physician may remain silent because divulgence might prompt the patient to forego needed therapy. Rational, informed patients should not be expected to act uniformly, even under similar circumstances, in agreeing to or refusing treatment. (I, II, III, IV, V)

Let us analyze the reasons cited for withholding information in the light of this statement and other moral considerations.

1. *To avoid the discomfort the patient's reaction is likely to cause* you.

The first rationale for withholding information is likely to operate at the level of unacknowledged motivation rather than as an explicit reason. Surely no one would seriously deny that if the patient's best interests were served by receiving this information, a physician's obligations would include accepting any personal discomfort involved in presenting it to her.

However, even though it is theoretically indefensible, this consideration may continue to influence unconscious motivation. In particular cases, you should examine your own motives to be sure this element is not a determining factor in your decision to withhold information.

2. *"It would take too long to explain it all."*

This rationale functions much like the first, and it too can be readily seen as unjustified when stated explicitly. Allocation of one's time is a necessity, but it is not appropriate to neglect important needs of patients in the process. If it is beneficial to the patient to receive this explanation (and it is argued below that it generally *is*), you have an obligation to find the time to provide it.

3. *Not wanting to have to get an investigational work-up underway this close to your vacation.*

The lack of justification for this consideration is equally obvious when it is articulated openly. Physicians certainly have a moral right to meet their own needs for relaxation and relief from vocational stresses, but they have the obligation to see that this does not interfere with meeting the needs of their patients. If the work-up cannot be completed before vacation, then some appropriate referral should be arranged to ensure that the dangerous possibilities are expeditiously pursued, and either ruled out or confirmed and treatment initiated.

4. *Not disclosing how remote the probabilities are for certain frightening but extremely remote possibilities (e.g., AIDS), in hopes of luring the patient into an expensive diagnostic work-up to rule these out.*

This clearly would be a blatantly unethical practice. The Judicial Council of the AMA (1984, 11) condemns it in these terms:

2.16 *Unnecessary Services.* It is unethical for a physician to provide or prescribe unnecessary services or unnecessary ancillary facilities (II, VII)

Only your own self-scrutiny, however, can reveal the extent to which improper economic considerations are motivating factors in particular decisions.

5. *Wanting to wait until you are* sure *before giving her information of this magnitude.*

The question to ask yourself, if you are persuaded by this rationale, is whether this policy is consistent with your practice regarding other sorts of information. Do you, for example, wait until you are certain before giving a patient indications about the prospect of *good* news, e.g., telling a couple working at pregnancy for some time that it appears that they have finally succeeded?

Psychologists describe the value of "preparatory worry" as a mechanism for coming to grips with bad news. Thus it seems that some preliminary indications, at least, of negative possibilities should be communicated.

6. *Because the family urged you not to tell.*

A recent poll of public opinion showed that nearly half of those surveyed (49%) thought it would be justified for a physician to withhold information at the request of the family; and 8% reported having made such a request of a physician regarding a member of their own family (President's Commission 1982a, 98). Furthermore, 21% of physicians polled reported that the wishes of patients' families were the most common reason for them to withhold information (President's Commission 1982a, 96–97). However, the Commission hastens to point out: "There is no recognition in law for withholding information from patients at the request of a family member" (President's Commission 1982a, 98–99, note 41).

7. *Not wanting to cause her needless anxiety.*

A French oncologist forcefully states a form of this view concerning revealing a diagnosis of cancer:

> For many complex reasons, Western man has a deep-seated conviction that cancer is the sickness that can never be cured. . . . To say to a patient "You have a cancer" is to say much more than "You have a serious disease"—even, sometimes, more than "You have a disease that may be fatal." . . . Doctors have always felt this, and up until now the vast majority of them have refused to tell the naked truth. As everyone knows, they are subject to all sorts of pressures. They are even accused of robbing their patients of their deaths. (Israel 1978, 155–156)

In contrast, the President's Commission (1982a, 99) reports:

> There is very little empirical evidence to indicate whether and in what ways information can be harmful. Clearly there is a need to define "harmful" or "negative" consequences better and to distinguish between situational anxiety (caused by illness or hospitalization) and anxiety resulting from information. In addition, the mere fact that some information may be "upsetting" in and of itself does not justify withholding information.

Similarly, Bok (1978, 247) reports:

> The damages associated with the disclosure of sad news or risks are rarer than physicians believe; and the *benefits* which result from being informed are more substantial, even measurably so. Pain is tolerated more easily, recovery from surgery is quicker and cooperation with therapy is greatly improved. The attitude that "what you don't know won't hurt you" is proving unrealistic; it is what patients do not know but vaguely suspect that causes them corrosive worry.

Furthermore, this reaction may result from a short-sighted view of the consequences of receiving unsettling information. Although there is little doubt that the immediate result will be a degree of unhappiness and anxiety, it may be possible (with counseling and support) for patients to move through this and other negative reactions to a more positive accommodation with their life prospects. It may even be possible for them to come to an active "acceptance" of their situation.

8. *Not wanting to take the time to deal with the patient's ensuing depression.*

Of course, to support the patient through these negative aspects or stages of accommodation requires time, skill, and compassion. And, as discussed in Chapter 3, these aspects of care are often devalued because they fall away from "the moral center" of medicine. However, we have already seen in Section 1.2.4.C that these "extraclinical elements" have an importance to patients equal to (or, in some situations, greater than) the clinical aspects of treatment; thus they must be provided as a part of adequate care. A team approach, in which nurses, medical social workers, and other appropriate professionals cooperate to help the patient work through these reactions, can lighten the burden of time and energy for the physician.

9. *Not wanting to deprive her of hope.*

This is undeniably an appropriate goal, but its realization depends more on *how* information is imparted than on *whether* it is shared. A harsh truth, blurted out in a clumsy way after the diagnosis has been fully confirmed and without any prior hint of serious possibilities is more likely to engender hopelessness than gradually making the patient aware of the degree of seriousness of the condition as it is ascertained through the diagnostic process.

Hope means different things to the patient at different stages of terminal illness. The physician probably should never close the door entirely on the remote possibility of recovery. But for many patients in advanced stages of illness, hope becomes focused on alleviation of pain and isolation rather than on prospects for recovery. Hence assurances that you and other caregivers will continue to be with the patient and that you will continue measures to maintain comfort for him or her may be more reassuring than groundless promises of recovery.

10. *Because you judge that giving her this information might prompt her to forego needed therapy.*

In the poll of the public, only a minority (38%) thought it justified for a physician to withhold information from a patient on the grounds that it might make the patient unwilling to undergo treatment the physician thinks is necessary (President's Commission 1982a, 98). The policy statement by the AMA Judicial Council, quoted a few pages back, explicitly condemns this justification and identifies what is objectionable about it—it is paternalistic.

11. *Because you judge that she will not be able to* understand *the information.*

Twenty-eight percent of physicians polled listed the patient's inability to understand the information as the most common reason for withholding it (President's Commission 1982a, 96–97). However, rather than a justification for not providing information, this should be viewed as imposing an additional task on the physician, i.e., instructing the patient about the *meaning* of the information. In some cases, it may not be easy to educate patients to the level of comprehension necessary for informed consent, but if it is accomplished, it may have salutary effects on their cooperation with treatment and their psychological outlook.

12. *Because you think she is not mentally competent to make any sound use of the information.*

Just as there is no obligation to initiate futile treatments,[15] so also there can be no obligation to provide information that cannot be used by the recipient. In the discussion of informed consent in the next section of this chapter, determinations of incompetency and procedures for decision making in this situation will be addressed.

13. *Because you think that, even though she may be competent* now *she* will not *be able to make competent use of the information once it is presented to her, because her mental state is such that hearing this information would destroy her ability to make competent decisions on the matter.*

The chief difficulty here, as in item 12, is in evaluating the evidence on which this prediction is based. Can you have *sufficient* assurance that you know how the patient is likely to react in this situation? Perhaps she has strengths of which you are unaware. Furthermore, even if her initial reaction is to "fall apart," perhaps (with supportive counseling) she will be able to "pull herself together" in time to take an active part in decision making.

You must guard against tendencies to *overrate* the dangers here. Be sure that you are not reading into the situation either (1) elements of *your own* reaction to such a prospect, (2) anecdotal evidence from one or a few uncharacteristic cases,[16] or (3) your own unwillingness to engage in the needed counseling (see item 8).

14. *Because you think her reaction would be* irrational.

The danger here is in imposing on the patient *your own* judgments of what is rational and irrational. As the policy statement of the AMA Judicial Council reminds us, "rational, informed patients should not be expected to act uniformly, even under similar circumstances." If the patient does react in a way you regard as irrational, this may be negotiated in the process of doctor-patient accommodation (described in Section 1.2.4.B.2 and Section 3).

15. *Because you are convinced that she really doesn't want to know.*

It is tempting to draw this conclusion hastily from indications of denial or resistance on the part of the patient. However, this may be only *one side* of an ambivalent attitude, and the dominant wish of the patient may be to face the truth. Paradoxically, the claim that the patient does not *want* to know is usually stated in association with the claim that the patient *already knows,* which is addressed in the following item.

---

15. See Chapter 4 below for a discussion of this issue.

16. For an example of how a strong case against truth telling is built upon one dramatic anecdote, see Collins (1927).

16. *Because you think she probably* already *knows.*

Again, Israel (1978, 156–157) puts this issue forcefully:

> We must also add to this debate another aspect that's often forgotten: There are an infinite number of patients who, without ever admitting it to others or to themselves, "know." Something in them knows. Yet for a variety of reasons they don't seek to clarify the situation. They don't speak of it to their family. They don't ask their doctor about it. There is, after all, in reply to the advocates of truth at any price, one fact that must be emphasized: the patient very seldom asks for the truth. He undergoes all sorts of treatments, sees his condition fluctuate, is surrounded by menacing problems, and asks nothing. Often he even adopts a complex strategy, proposing explanations and diagnoses first, so that the doctor won't be tempted to supply his own. Is the doctor supposed to break down this resistance and, in the name of the intellectual constructs of persons who are not suffering, to destroy the defenses of those who are? What is the meaning of these defenses? That the patient has a doubt, a doubt he can encapsulate and repress if given the chance, and that he desperately wants to repress. In such a situation, with such a defense mechanism at work, I have never felt I had the right to tell the truth, and I am prepared to defend that position against the criticisms of my contemporaries.

There are several comments to be made about this. First, a "chicken-and-egg" problem arises in interpreting these situations: Israel assumes that patients develop these defense mechanisms for reasons of their own, and thus his attitude toward withholding information stems from a desire to respect these preexisting psychological needs. However, interviews with cancer patients (including children) reveal that their perception is often that things work the other way around. They sense that the physician (and often the family as well) "don't want to talk about it"; thus they develop veiled forms of communication as a way to prevent disruption of relationships vital to them.

Furthermore, even when patients independently develop this sort of defense mechanism, it is questionable whether they ought to be supported in such a reaction of denial. What Israel derides as "intellectual constructs of persons who are not suffering" includes some careful psychological analysis drawn from observation of persons who are suffering, as well as some moral analysis of these situations. Many psychologists hold that the psychic energy expended in maintaining a defense of denial is so great as to make it counterproductive and thus that the suffering of the patient is minimized in the long run if he is guided to face the truth and helped to deal with its emotional impact in a more open way. Similarly, moral analysis stresses the value of honesty in relationships, as well as in one's self-understanding.

Finally, even if we grant that this defense mechanism should be supported on some occasions, there is a danger of *overrating* its prevalence due to our desire to avoid facing the unpleasant emotional reactions likely to result from working past denial. But this brings us full circle, back to the first rationale on this list.

2.3.3 "Nothing But The Truth" Of course, both patients and physicians communicate more than "the truth" or "the bare facts" to each other. *Patients* not only impart the facts about their experience of dis-ease, they convey their interpretations of what it means to them and their worries about it. The sensitive physician listens to this part of the patient's story no less carefully than the details that have direct clinical relevance, because it is upon these that one builds both the "recommendation and negotiation" phase of the physician-patient accommodation and the comforting aspect of patient care.

Similarly, *physicians* convey more than "the truth," especially in their role as comforters. Patients draw clues from the physician's air of confidence and concern. Such clues make an important difference in their mental attitude toward their bout with illness. These aspects of communication are as fraught with moral implications as the technical tasks of arriving at the diagnosis and formulating plans for treatment, and thus they deserve as much care in planning.

2.4 Placebos and the Placebo Effect

Truth is also an issue in the use of placebos. The use of chemically inert or ineffective substances as medications with the expectation that they will have effect through the power of suggestion (Leslie 1954) also involves deception. Even if an outright lie is avoided, e.g., by saying something carefully worded, such as, "I am going to give you a substance that has been proven effective in helping people in your situation" (which is not, strictly speaking, *false*), it *is* still a matter of deception. The statement and the substance have effect only because the patient believes that the substance is chemically therapeutic.

In addition to the fundamental objection to deception in a therapeutic relationship, there is further difficulty with the use of placebos in that the power of suggestion may be *too* effective: (1) Placebos may mask organic conditions in some cases. Studies suggest that some patients genuinely cease to feel the pain of organic conditions such as a myocardial infarction when given assurance that a placebo will relieve the pain. (2) They may cause serious side effects. The full range of side effects of potent medications have been reported from placebos, including such "objective" manifestations as skin rash, diarrhea, urticaria, and angioneurotic edema (Leslie 1954).

The situation is not much different, in moral terms, if a subtherapeutic dose of an active drug is substituted for an inert substance. If the physician believes that the medication will not be chemically effective but makes use of the patient's belief in its effectiveness through the power of suggestion, a form of deception is still the result. Of course, it is *possible* that the chemical properties of the medication contribute to the effect; but if the physician does not believe this will occur and leads the patient to believe it, a form of deception has occurred.

2.4.1 The Placebo Effect Matters are different morally, however, in uses of the power of suggestion in combination with chemically effective regimens. If a physician attempts to ensure or enhance the effectiveness of a chemically potent medication she has prescribed by stating an endorsement of it in a confident tone ("I believe you will get relief with this."), no deception is involved. The physician is merely conveying to the patient something she *believes* (or has solid reason to *hope*) to be the case. This may amount to "manipulation" of the patient, but not in a deceptive way. Indeed, it is not clear that such artifice in a relationship is morally objectionable. A suitor dresses in his best clothes and employs his best manners when calling on his sweetheart to evoke a favorable response from her; we do not object and insist that he has an obligation to wear his shabbiest clothes and use his worst manners (or even to wear ordinary clothes and use ordinary manners). A professional seeking to enhance the patient's confidence in a treatment regimen is doing no more than this—"putting the best face on" the situation. There is an obligation to warn the patient of possible side effects of the regimen, but this does not preclude presenting the recommendation in the most favorable light that is honestly possible.

2.5 Conclusions

There is much more that could be said about information exchange. Additional questions about it will be encountered later in this book, in connection with other specific issues. In particular, the "informed" part of informed consent involves this issue and will be the topic of the next section of this chapter. However, it is time now to summarize the discussion of this section, both as a basis for future sections of this book and for your independent thinking. Let us return to the exercise at the beginning of Section 2.3 and draw answers about what and how Lynn should be told about the possibilities.

2.5.1 What To Tell Lynn Initially First, say *"I am not sure what caused the swelling in this node."* By sharing your uncertainty at this point with the patient, you help her to understand why additional tests ought to be run (to be proposed in the third step) and thus prepare her to accept this recommendation. This admission of uncertainty also introduces the possibility that the cause *might be* something serious, which she ought to recognize even though you are about to calm her concern about it markedly by reassuring her in the next step.

Second, say *"I don't think this is anything serious."* This statement is reassuring to the patient, but not in a way that fails to fit the facts. At this point, there are myriad diagnostic possibilities; most of them are relatively benign. There are, of course, several serious possibilities as well, and by phrasing the reassurance in a somewhat guarded way—"I don't think . . . "—this is communicated without undermining the reassuring general tone of the statement.

Third, say *"We need to do some tests to find what caused the swelling."* Explain the purpose and nature of the tests you propose to do. This is the next step in the process of clinical method, and it is important to enlist the patient's cooperation.

Fourth, ask *"What do* you *think it is?"* This question can draw out additional clinical information. More important, it can elicit the patient's chief worries, which you can address in your counseling and comforting role. An alternative way to phrase this is: *"What is your biggest concern about what this really means?"*

This approach is preferable to hastily reassuring patients on the basis of what you *presume* to be their chief concern, e.g., by saying: *"I'm sure this is* not *cancer."* Not only may this suggest a basis for worry that had not yet occurred to the patient, but the emotional impact of word "cancer" is so strong that (1) she may not hear anything else you tell her, including your reassurances, and (2) the possibility of cancer may become the exclusive focus of the patient's recollection of the interchange.

2.5.2 "As Time Goes By" As the diagnostic process proceeds, Lynn should be given additional information as it becomes available. As the clinical trail leads decisively toward a diagnosis of breast cancer, for example, she can be prepared for this outcome by being introduced to the possibility in a gradually more explicit way. By the time the diagnosis is finally made, it will not be such a dramatic shock. She will have been prepared for the possibility, at least to some extent, by earlier discussions. This is not to deny that there still may be significant emotional impact to hearing a confirmed diagnosis, and steps should be planned to help her deal with this.

The difficult situation, for the approach proposed here, comes in cases in which the diagnosis was made *abruptly* and *unexpectedly*. This would not readily allow time for recommended gradual disclosure of information. However, (1) the same supportive counseling is required (indeed, even more so) in this situation; it can go a long way toward helping the patient cope with unwelcomed news. (2) Similarly, tact in phrasing the information is no less required in this situation. (3) Finally, the approach recommended permits withholding the harsher elements of "the whole truth" *for a short time* in the interest of maximizing the patient's coping systems. Thus, for example, were it obvious from the first examination that Lynn has breast cancer, disclosing this news might be postponed for a day or two, until members of her family or close friends could be present to offer her support. You might schedule a further confirmatory test and ask her to bring appropriate other persons with her to hear the results. This request would indicate that something serious was involved, prompting some preparatory worry that would begin to get her ready for the news.

3 Informed Consent

The following account by an anonymous correspondent describes an incident that takes place away from the setting of clinical medicine and that might seem remote from the issue of informed consent to medical treatment:

> The scene was a church committee meeting. The business at hand was not especially exciting, so my mind was wandering. As I glanced around the circle of people, I noticed that a physician member of the committee (who had obviously also lost interest in the discussion) was staring intently at the young woman sitting next to him. What was unusual was that the object of his attention was the woman's left foot—and he was neither a podiatrist nor an orthopedic surgeon.
>
> I looked at her foot to see what he found so interesting, and I spotted it immediately—a sizeable round bump on the top of her foot. (It looked like the sort of super-large callus which develops as a result of months of crouching on a surf board for long hours every day. However, this woman was certainly *not* an habitual surfer.) As I watched my physician friend study the bump, it occurred to me that he was completely absorbed in this medical puzzle. (The thought occurred to me that this would be a good example to cite sometime to show that physicians can never stop being physicians, even in their off-hours.) However, my idle fascination soon turned to shock and a growing feeling of impending horror, for I saw my friend slowly (and somewhat absent-mindedly) bend and reach towards the woman until, finally, he touched the bump on her foot and began to palpate it.
>
> The result was explosive! The woman screamed and jumped out of her chair to escape this man groping at her foot. This produced startled cries and movements from others in the group, and thus the whole committee meeting was disrupted.

It is clear from the story that the physician intended this woman no harm. He had become absorbed in a medical puzzle and had forgotten where he was and whom he was encountering. After all, he had come to this meeting straight from his office, where he had spent much of the day palpating various body parts of his patients.

However, the woman was surprised and shocked by his act, and she was genuinely offended, in spite of the fact that she had worked with this man on this and other church projects for a number of years and considered him a friend. But palpating her foot was not something she was ready to have a friend do. It might be okay for her doctor to do such a thing, but this man was not *her* doctor—especially not at this place and time.

3.1 The Legal and Moral Requirement of Informed Consent

The impropriety of this physician's action involves more than a breach of etiquette or social convention. Our society acknowledges the seriousness of invasions of physical privacy by making violations criminal acts. The crime of "battery" is defined in the law to include any willful act of touching a person without her or his consent.[17] This is one of the two primary roots of the legal and moral requirement of informed consent; the anecdote illustrates *why* it is important. People do, indeed, feel strongly about the barriers to physical access included in our civil right to privacy.

3.1.1 The Scope of the Requirement This source of the informed consent requirement has important implications for its *scope*. Some form of consent is required for any procedure involving touching the patient's body in any way (including, it might be argued, the prescription of medications to be ingested). However, this contrasts markedly with actual practice, as shown in Table 1-2.

Table 1-2 Nature of Consent Obtained for Various Procedures

Procedure	Written Consent	Oral Consent	Both	Neither
Inpatient surgery	81%	3%	15%	0
Minor office surgery	26%	58%	9%	7%
Setting bones	39%	42%	9%	8%
General anesthesia	83%	3%	12%	1%
Local anesthesia	21%	57%	7%	15%
Diagnostic x-rays involving injections	45%	35%	8%	10%
Blood tests	2%	52%	0	45%
Prescriptions	1%	43%	2%	54%
Radiation therapy	63%	18%	11%	4%

[President's Commission (1982a, 108).]

Current professional practice may not fall as far short of the ideal as these figures suggest. In the first place, there is no legal requirement that consent be obtained in *written form* for any procedure except research protocols. Nor does the moral requirement of informed consent require a written form. What is important is that the patients (1) receive the information necessary to make an autonomous decision, (2) be free from influences that would render their decision involuntary, and (3) willingly agree to the procedure. The chief advantage of written documentation of these elements is that it carries greater evidentiary weight than reports of a verbal exchange. If verbal consent is obtained, a detailed account should be entered in the medical record; however, if the issue goes to court, the patient may dispute accounts of what was said or agreed to, whereas challenging a signed document is more difficult.

Furthermore, it is not clear that even a *formal* process of obtaining oral consent is required in all situations. Opportunities for a patient to register consent to or

---

17. For a thorough account of this legal basis of informed consent, see Fried (1974, Chapter 2).

refusal of treatment recommendations are part of the social structure of health care in a variety of ways. For example, if a patient decides not to follow the medication regimen the physician has prescribed, he may do so by not having the prescription filled, or having it filled but not using it.

Thus, in spite of the fact that 54% of physicians reported that they obtain neither written nor oral consent for prescriptions, there is still opportunity for consent or refusal by the patient. What may be lacking, however, is information on the basis of which the patient can make an *intelligent* decision. Relevant information should be imparted even if no formal process of seeking consent for the prescription is carried out.

Similarly, patients take the initiative to visit a physician; showing up at the physician's office establishes the presumption that patients consent to routine measures of diagnosis and treatment. However, it is a mistake to read too much into this presumption. On the first visit, it is wise to inform the patient in advance of virtually every procedure you propose to perform—e.g., by saying "I am going to check your pulse rate now" just before you reach for an arm. This gives the patient the opportunity to register any objection or refusal if, for some reason, his or her general consent does not extend to this procedure. On subsequent visits, after the patient has had a chance to learn your routines, explaining each and every procedure may not be necessary. This allows you to move more efficiently—for example, by conducting the physical examination at the same time you are talking through the review of systems with the patient, or by conducting multiple elements of the examination at once.

3.1.2. Who Should Obtain Consent? This source of the doctrine has implications for the question of *who* should obtain consent. Written consent forms for surgery or invasive diagnostic procedures are sometimes handled like hot potatoes in hospitals and clinics. Everybody tries to delegate to someone else the task of getting them signed. The root of the requirement in the legal concept of battery makes clear that consent is to be obtained by *anybody* and *everybody* involved in the acts of touching. Carried to the extreme, then, the entire surgical or diagnostic team would come by the patient's room to discuss the procedure and obtain informed consent for their role in it. This may be excessive, but it is at least required that the surgeon (as "captain of the team") confirm the consent, even if some of the formal details are delegated to others.

For other procedures, the specialists or technicians who carry them out must confirm the consent for themselves. It is not enough to rely totally on the assurance of other parties that the patient has been informed about the procedure and has agreed to it.

3.1.3 The Sources of the Requirement In addition to the foundation in the law of battery, Anglo-American law has acknowledged another root of the legal requirement of informed consent. In an important court opinion in 1960, Kansas Supreme Court Justice Alfred Schroeder declared:

> Anglo-American law starts with the premise of thorough-going self-determination. It follows that each man is considered to be master of his own body, and he may, if he be of sound mind, expressly prohibit the performance of life-saving surgery, or other medical treatment. A doctor might well believe that an operation or form of treatment is desirable or necessary but the law does not permit him to substitute his own judgement for that of the patient by any form of artifice or deception. [Natanson v. Kline, 186 Kan. 393, 350 P.2nd 1093 (1960)][18]

Participation by the patient in decision making is also indicated on the basis of several other factors:

1. The potential for personal gain by the professional may offer a temptation to exploit the patient; a requirement for an explanation to and ratification by the patient serves as a countervailing check on professional choice.
2. The requirement for negotiation with the patient serves also as a check against sexist or paternalistic attitudes by the professional. It is psychologically difficult to sustain such attitudes while recognizing the legitimacy of having the patient share in decision making.
3. More fundamental, enlisting the patient's participation in decision making embodies a *respect for persons* important as a general moral principle[19] and as a demand of professional ethics: Section I of the AMA Principles of Medical Ethics reads: "A physician shall be dedicated to providing competent medical service with compassion and respect for human dignity." The last phrase states the principle referred to here as a basis of the consent requirement.
4. The requirement also protects the authority and esteem of the profession by discouraging unfounded claims of knowledge. If explanations and answers to questions must be provided, one is likely to think twice before spouting off an unsupported claim.
5. Taking total responsibility for the patient's life creates a feeling of isolation and an awesome moral burden. This may be necessary on occasions when patient and family are genuinely unable to share in decision making. However, it is unnecessary to impose this burden on oneself when others are capable of sharing it, and it is self-aggrandizing to assume that others are unable to share in this task or to exaggerate one's own importance.

---

18. For a description of this concept of self-determination, see the discussion of autonomy (another name for the same concept) in Chapter 2, Section 2.3.1.
19. For further discussion of this principle, see Appendix I, Section 2.2.

6. The requirement can be seen as an application of democratic principles to the physician-patient relationship. Just as citizens expect to have a voice in political decisions, they expect to participate in medical decisions. And just as we are convinced that political decisions are improved by being shared, the same may be true of medical decisions.[20]

3.1.4. The Spirit of the Requirement The President's Commission captures the spirit of informed consent in a sound and helpful way: "Ethically valid consent is a process of shared decision-making based upon mutual respect and participation, not a ritual to be equated with reciting the contents of a form that details the risks of particular treatments." (1982a, 2; cf. 36–39, 50–51). The Commission's report points out that a focus on the *legal* aspect of the requirement, as it has developed in court cases, shapes our understanding in some unfortunate ways:

1. "Cases that find their way to court invariably involve interventions that did not go well" (p. 25).
2. "Courts see only those cases in which particular allegedly undisclosed risks associated with medical procedures have led to actual injuries" (p. 25). Thus, "the inquiry concerns whether that particular risk was disclosed, rather than whether the overall course of care, and the extended process of disclosure, were properly respectful of the patient's right of self-determination" (p. 26).
3. "Courts must grapple with . . . the impact of hindsight on the litigation process" (p. 26).
4. "Courts must determine whether required disclosures were in fact made" (p. 28), which leads to reliance on written documentation (although this is not otherwise required and may, indeed, become a barrier to useful exchange of information and shared decision making).
5. "The structure of lawsuits requires the naming of particular defendants who will bear financial responsibility" (p. 29).

In contrast, the spirit of the requirement of informed consent focuses not on specific items of medical information or rituals of obtaining signatures, but on "discussions between professional and patient that bring the knowledge, concerns, and perspective of each to the process of seeking agreement on a course of treatment. Simply put, this means that the physician or other health professional invites the patient to participate in a dialogue in which the professional seeks to help the patient understand the medical situation and available courses of action, and the patient conveys his or her concerns and wishes" (President's Commission 1982a, 38). Clearly, this is closely related to the phase of recommendation and negotiation discussed in Section 1.2.4.B.2.

---

20. Cf. "So fundamental is this right of self-determination in a democratic society that to limit it, even in ordinary medical transactions, is to propagate an injustice" (Pellegrino 1979, 98–99).

To see the contribution patients can make here, we need to recognize that management of a patient's illness rests on value judgments as well as technical decisions of medical science. In prescribing medication for pain in the postsurgical patient, for example, not only must you determine which dosage will be effective in relieving the discomfort without risking toxic side effects (essentially a technical problem, although it rests on an assumption that death is a disvalue), but a choice must also be made between fundamental values. Many pain-killing drugs dull the mind, and many such drugs can lead to addiction. Hence the decision about how long to continue such medication rests on a choice between the value of relief from discomfort and the competing values of maximum mental acuity and freedom from the danger of dependency. Furthermore, the mind may be affected by the medication in a way that alters the experiencing of events. (This is one of the arguments offered, for example, by proponents of natural childbirth.) All of these are acknowledged values, but in the situation at hand it is not possible to preserve all of these values at once. Hence a judgment must be made as to which of the sets of values in conflict is the most important.

One obvious reason for *not* taking this decision on your shoulders is that your ranking of these values might not match that of the patient. You might be motivated to favor relief of pain, for example, on the basis of either (1) your own preference between these competing values, or (2) a feeling of kindness, or even (3) your careful judgment of the patient's best interests. In contrast, the patient might have a stoic attitude toward pain and prefer to endure it and maintain a clear head.

However, even if your value rankings coincide perfectly with your patient's in a given case, there is still a moral reason not to make the final decision yourself. There is intrinsic value in controlling one's own life, a value that reveals itself in concrete situations. Suppose, for example, that in the situation described above you recognized the patient's stoicism and made a decision to withhold medication in acknowledgment of the patient's values. This approach leaves out an important moral element. There is a morally significant difference between choosing *for oneself* to face the pain and having the decision made *on one's behalf* by another; the moral quality of the first of these alternatives (which amounts to a sort of courage) is denied to the patient if you, the physician, make the decision entirely on *your* own initiative.

3.2 Practical Applications

How does this translate into practice? Let us follow further the drama of Lynn Languish. The extended, gradual process of information exchange earlier described in her case is a process of multiple informed consents.

3.2.1 Initial Diagnostic Steps   At the outset, when the axillary lump is discovered, the situation is one of numerous diagnostic possibilities, some of which are serious (e.g., breast cancer, AIDS) but most of which are relatively benign. Since various of the benign possibilities are both (1) much more probable and (2) treatable if discovered expeditiously, clinical wisdom would dictate pursuing them first in the diagnostic work-up. Indeed, it was recommended earlier that specific serious possibilities such as breast cancer, tuberculosis, and AIDS not be mentioned explicitly to the patient at this time (although indication should be given that serious possibilities do exist but that their probability is low).

3.2.2 Patient Anxiety   However, if the patient's response to an explanation of this approach indicates that she is extremely anxious about the threat of breast cancer and will not rest easy until it has been ruled out, this may be reason enough not to postpone diagnostic tests to explore this possibility. Undoubtedly this would be the case if the test in question were both low-risk and low-cost.

But what if the test were expensive? This becomes a question of putting a price on achieving reassurance for the patient. There are limits to the level of expenditure justified for this purpose, but those limits are not easy to define. The situation can be explained to the patient (along with a reminder of the low probability of this diagnosis), and she can participate in the determination.

What if the tests were invasive and/or involved considerable risk to the patient? Again, there is no ready basis for determining what degree of discomfort, risk, etc., is worthwhile to achieve reassurance except to consult with the patient about the matter.

If you disagree strongly with the choice favored by Lynn, you face these options:

1. If you are convinced that Lynn is still not fully aware of the relevant medical information or is not taking it into account in formulating her preference, you should continue the discussion until satisfied that she is fully informed.
2. If disagreement persists, you should carefully examine the basis of your conclusions. Be sure that the values at stake are ones sufficiently important to you that compromise would violate your integrity.
3. If the values are *not* this central to you, try to negotiate a compromise position that both you and Lynn could accept.
4. Even if they are central, give some serious thought to the possibility of a "middle ground." Perhaps there is an alternative not considered that could preserve the key values of both parties.
5. If the values at stake are core values for you both *and* there is no way to resolve the conflict between these values, then perhaps no physician-patient accommodation is possible between the two of you on this occasion. Help her find another physician who is more likely to achieve an accommodation with her.

3.2.3 Diagnostic Decisions   Similarly, the patient's wishes can play a central role in determining whether to pursue diagnostic trails involving risky or painful tests that might detect treatable conditions.

3.2.4 Preparation for Knowledge and Action   As the diagnostic work-up proceeds, explanation of the purpose of the various tests can lead naturally to discussion of the nature of the condition that might be discovered, its degree of seriousness, and the range of treatments available for it.

3.2.5 Useless Knowledge   If the stage is reached, for example, in which (1) the possibility of a serious diagnosis is strong, (2) treatment is inadvisable or impossible (perhaps due to other serious health problems the patient has), and (3) the definitive test is risky, then the patient might agree to forego the knowledge of the precise cause of her condition.

3.2.6 Treatment Choices   If the process has proceeded as suggested, then the choice usually identified with an informed consent (i.e., the selection of a major treatment modality) need not stand out as such a momentous event and difficult task. The information to make a decision about treatment will not come to the patient as a bolt out of the blue. She will have been prepared for this decision gradually and thus will have had opportunities (with proper support and assistance) to work through the emotional reaction to the information, and the intellectual task of understanding and weighing the factors relevant to negotiating a decision with her physician.

If informed consent were restricted to a single session in which information were presented and the patient were required to reach a decision on the basis of it (as happens all too often in actual practice), then a standard such as the following would be overwhelming and impossible:

> The Commission believes the core elements [of substantive issues to be discussed by professional and patient] fall under three headings: (1) the patient's current medical status, including its likely course if no treatment is pursued; (2) the intervention(s) that might improve the prognosis, including a description of the procedure(s) involved, a characterization of the likelihood and effect of associated risks and benefits, and the likely course(s) with and without therapy; and (3) a professional opinion, usually, as to the best alternative. Furthermore, each of these elements must be discussed in light of associated uncertainties. (President's Commission 1982a, 74)

However, if the process is gradual, as recommended here, the task of conveying all this information is not nearly so formidable.

3.2.7 Standards of Disclosure   Many discussions of informed consent offer detailed lists of information to be disclosed in the informed consent process. This is especially true of discussions focusing on informed consent to experimental procedures,[21] but the same is often applied to consent to therapeutic procedures.[22] At least two states have incorporated into legislation specific disclosure requirements concerning treatment of breast cancer.[23] Others have tried to develop a specific criterion for disclosure; every risk with frequency greater than 1:1000, for example. Court cases have dwelt on more abstract criteria, such as whether the standard should be the prevailing practice in the professional community, or what the "rational patient" would want to know, or whatever would influence the decision of the individual patient.

3.2.8 Varying the Discussion In contrast to these general criteria, the President's Commission (1982a, 38) "encourages, to perhaps a greater degree than is explicitly recognized by current law, the ability of patients and health care professionals to vary the style and extent of discussion." The spirit of the requirement, as opposed to an exclusive focus on the legal dimensions, allows for variability to fit the interests of particular patients and professionals. The Commission report continues:

> Such variations might take any of several directions: in one relationship, the patient might prefer not to be burdened by detailed discussion of risks unlikely to arise or to affect the decision; in another relationship, a patient might request unusually detailed information on unconventional alternative therapies; in a third, a patient with a long-standing and close relationship of trust with a particular physician might ask that physician to proceed as he or she thinks best, choosing the course of therapy and revealing any information that the physician thinks would best serve the interests of the patient. Inherent in allowing such variations is the difficulty of ensuring they are genuinely agreeable to both parties and do not themselves arise out of an imbalance in status or bargaining power. (President's Commission 1982a, 39)

3.3 The Paradox of Autonomy

The third variation described in the Commission report gives rise to a paradox: automony is compromised whichever way you respond to patients' requests to make decisions on their behalf without their active participation. The request may be assumed to be an expression of the patients' autonomy; to deny it would be a failure to respect their *present* autonomy. However, to grant the request would be to compromise the patients' *future* autonomy, since future decisions would be made on the patients' behalf (as they request), and thus these would be instances of paternalism. Furthermore, even if patients decided that they wanted to share in

---

21. Cf. The Declaration of Helsinki; Health and Human Services Research Guidelines (Code of Federal Regulations, Title 45, Part 46).

22. Cf. The Patient's Bill of Right (American Hospital Association); The Model Patient's Bill of Rights (The American Civil Liberties Union).

23. Massachusetts (Acts of 1979, Chapter 214); California (SB 1893, "The Breast Cancer Informed Consent Law," effective January 1, 1981).

certain decisions in the future, their contribution would not be fully autonomous if some information had been withheld. Thus the question is "Autonomy today or autonomy tomorrow?" Autonomy on both occasions cannot be achieved.

This text argues strongly for bringing patients into an active role in decision making whenever possible, even if this means going against their wishes (and thus violating present autonomy). Informed consent is not a discretionary right to be exercised or waived as one wishes. It is, instead, one legal and ethical expression of a *responsibility* for one's life; this responsibility cannot simply be handed to another. Patients should be guided (gently and with supportive counseling) to accept responsibility for decisions affecting their own lives.

3.4 Mental Competence

Of course, this goal is not always possible to achieve. Some patients lack the *capacity* for autonomous participation in decision making; in these cases, there may be no alternative to having others exercise paternalism by making decisions on their behalf to promote their best interests.

Infants and small children undeniably lack capacity for exercising autonomy. The only serious question arising here is *who* should give "proxy consent" on their behalf. (It should be noted that "proxy consent" is not, strictly speaking, an alternative *variety* of consent by the patient. Rather it is a form of paternalism that serves as a *substitute* for consent by the patient himself.)[24] To see how the AMA Judicial Council deals with this issue in one especially difficult circumstance, see the second paragraph of "Quality of Life" (Section 2.14) from *Current Opinions,* quoted in Chapter 4, Section 2.1.

For older children, determining whether they possess the mental capacity to give consent is much more problematic. For example, in Tennessee no child under age 18 is legally qualified to consent to medical treatment on his or her own behalf (except for abortion procedures and perhaps birth control). Yet many 17-year-olds possess the mental capacity to give consent for almost any medical procedure. However, it is much less clear what to say about a child of 15 or 10 or 7.

More controversial cases arise with patients afflicted with mental dysfunctions; patients whose judgment is clouded by chronic, severe pain; or patients in the grip of overwhelming compulsions such as alcoholism. Consider the following case sketches. Which of these patients are competent to consent to or refuse treatment?

1. A 70-year-old widow living alone in a condemned dilapidated house with no heat was brought against her will to the hospital. Her thinking was tangential and fragmented. Although she did not appear to be hallucinating, she seemed delusional. She refused blood tests, saying "You just want my blood to spread it all over the city. No, I'm not giving it."

---

24. The issue of proxy consent will be discussed in detail in Chapter 4 in connection with life-and-death decisions, where it has its most momentous application.

2. A 60-year-old woman was found wandering on a city street. When questioned, she could not give her home address. She was unable to remember when her sister, her son, and her husband had died. She also showed what were diagnosed as paranoid tendencies, believing that government agencies had taken her pension away from her. When commitment to the state psychiatric hospital was proposed to her, she said: "I don't want to go to that place. Leave me alone and let me go home!" She was diagnosed as suffering from organic brain syndrome with arteriosclerosis.

However, she was able to find her way to her home (smoothly managing a fairly complicated series of transfers on public transportation), even though she could not recite the address. Furthermore, her government pension had indeed been cut off several years earlier, and an active review of this action was underway (and had been for more than a year). The downtown street on which she had been "wandering" was on the route from the bus stop to the governmental office where she had just gone (as she had many times before) to inquire about the review of her pension status. She does have periods of confusion and mild loss of memory, interspersed with times of mental alertness and rationality.

3. A 54-year-old businessman refuses a treatment that had been recommended, saying "I understand that I am running quite a risk by foregoing this treatment, but I have decided that I don't want it. And I don't think I owe you an account of my reasons. I consider the matter closed."

4. When asked why he has not been taking his medicine for hypertension, the 41-year-old man says, "I mean to take it, but I keep forgetting about it."

5. When asked why she has not been taking her medicine for hypertension, the 40-year-old professional woman says, "I have been following a mega-vitamin program someone at work told me about. He said it was a *natural remedy,* and that it would control my blood pressure without any of the dangers of medicines."

What is mental competence and how can it be determined? Charles Culver and Bernard Gert (1982) relate mental competence to more general statements of competence or incompetence (as in "John is a competent architect" or "Henry is incompetent to design a house"). They point out that "to say of someone that he is incompetent demands a context. A person is not simply incompetent; he is incompetent to do *x*, or *x* and *y*, or *x, y,* and *z.* . . . How is one to decide if such a person is competent to do some particular type of activity? The more precisely described the activity, the more likely it is that one can decide whether or not someone is competent to perform it" (Culver and Gert 1982, 54). On this basis, they offer the following elements of a general standard of competence: "Two necessary features for being competent to perform an activity are that one understands what that activity is and knows when he is performing it" (Culver and Gert 1982, 54).

Some view this much as nearly enough to form a sufficient criterion of competence to consent to or refuse treatment:

> The individual in question must have sufficient intellectual capacity to 1) understand the simple nature and purpose of the act itself in lay terms—"My consenting to medical care means that you can't do it unless I say okay."; 2) comprehend the basic facts of the case—"You say I have this disease even though the doctor I saw before said I had another disease."; 3) recognize alternative ways of acting—"The choices are an operation or radiotherapy or both or neither." (Lipp 1977, 66)

However, this seems too broad. Using this criterion, all patients in the case sketches above would be considered competent. Even the woman in case 1 appears to understand that the choice is hers to make, and she also understands the explanation given by the physicians for the blood test—she does not *believe* them, but she does *understand!* Similarly, the patient in case 4 could recite what he has been told about the importance of controlling his blood pressure. (And the patient in case 5 might be able to do the same thing with what she has been told about the nature of the recommended drug treatment.) Thus, at some level, they understand this reasoning. Their problem is in carrying this understanding into action by complying with the recommended treatment.

Furthermore, if this set of criteria is too broad, the same is true of the generalized mental status exam as a test of competence to consent. That the patient is oriented to time, place, person, etc., does not imply that he has the mental capabilities needed to give acceptable informed consent or refusal. More (and other) capacities than this are necessary.

The roots of the requirement of informed consent in autonomy and self-determination suggest that the conditions of autonomy could serve as the standard here. This fits the way of developing a criterion suggested by Culver and Gert.

However, if we consider the conditions of autonomy,[25] it is obvious that *none* of the patients in our case sketches would qualify as autonomous—indeed, none of *us* would qualify as *fully* autonomous, since this requires a complete and coherent set of life goals and deliberation in terms of them for every action we undertake. This is then too strong a criterion. What must be found is a way of measuring the degree of partial autonomy marking the borderline between mental competence and incompetence to give consent to medical treatment.

The President's Commission (1982a, 57) offers such a criterion in the following:

> Any determination of the capacity to decide on a course of treatment must relate to the individual abilities of a patient, the requirements of the task at hand, and the consequences likely to flow from the decision. Decisionmaking capacity requires, to greater or lesser degree: (1) possession of a set of values and goals; (2) the ability to communicate and to understand information; and (3) the ability to reason and to deliberate about one's choices.

---

25. NOTE: These are discussed at some length in Chapter 2, Section 2.3.1.

How would the patients in the preceding case sketches rate in terms of this criterion? The patient in case 1 appears clearly *not* to fit. Her "tangential and fragmented" patterns of thinking show she lacks the capability to reason and deliberate about her choices.

The patients in cases 4 and 5 seem competent by this criterion. For the patient in 4, the problem comes not at the level of ability to reason, deliberate, or understand, but rather in translating the conclusions of this deliberation into action. The patient in 5 is carrying through deliberations, but, tragically, on the basis of misinformation supplied to her by a no doubt well-meaning, but misguided associate.

The problematic cases here would be 2 and 3, since neither of these *demonstrates* the ability to communicate relevant information, especially the results of their deliberation. However, the President's Commission (1982a, 62) adds another element to the criterion: "An assessment of the patient's decisionmaking capacity begins with a presumption of such capacity." On this basis, the patient in case 3 must be regarded as competent to refuse consent. He has not done anything to demonstrate his *inability* to make a deliberative decision, and thus we must assume he is capable of doing so. Similarly, the patient in case 2 was ruled as incompetent prematurely, on the basis of an inability to communicate, which is not crucial for her to manage her daily life, i.e., she can manage to find her way home, even if she cannot recite the address. So she, too, would have to be ruled as competent once her actual capabilities are discerned.

Cases 2–5 must be classified as examples of mistaken decisions, rather than incompetency *per se*. The President's Commission (1982a, 60) offers the following directive: "The obligation of the professional is not to declare, on the basis of a 'wrong' decision, that the patient lacks decisionmaking capacity, but rather to work with the patient toward a fuller and more accurate understanding of the facts and a sound reasoning process."

3.5 Manipulation

"Work with" must be distinguished from "manipulate" (as must "guide," "negotiate," and other related terms). If the result is to be genuine shared decision making, then you as a physician must be on guard against overt or covert forces that influence the patient in nonrational ways. The authority of your position, the vulnerability of the patient due to the emotional impact of illness and the institutional complexities of care, and the strength of your personality and outlook may influence the patient too much.

Some physicians say, "I can get patients to consent to anything I want." This is undoubtedly often true, but it is achieved through manipulation. The challenge is to avoid this nonrational influence—or, at least, to minimize it if it cannot be avoided entirely.

The goal is to move patients toward autonomous decision making, in which they take responsibility for their own lives. This may require steps on your part to neutralize coercive forces and guard against unduly influencing the patient yourself.

4 Confidentiality

Confidentiality is extremely important to patients and has historically been regarded with great respect by health care professionals. In this section, you will explore the values and ethical principles behind the principle of confidentiality. Why does it matter so much to patients? What values does it promote, and what is the source of its importance? The answer may help one decide when the principle has reached its limit so that information about a patient should be revealed.

4.1 The Importance of Confidentiality

"Why should people be so concerned about confidentiality? If they have done nothing wrong, they should have nothing to hide. And, if they have done something wrong, perhaps we should not assist them in hiding it."

This expresses a common sentiment about confidentiality. Some of the cases in this section involve people who do have something shameful or some sort of wrongdoing to hide, and these may confirm this attitude toward confidentiality.

However, there are reasons for privacy that do not necessarily involve shame or wrongdoing, and it is these that provide the background for the principle of confidentiality. Every society has a sphere of life kept shrouded in secrecy, a private realm. The content of this realm may differ from culture to culture (and from person to person within a culture). Some cultures may not be particularly "up-tight" about nudity but will have other areas of life about which they are as reticent and discreet as our society is about nudity. For example, another domain of secrecy in our culture is money. Ask someone his annual income or net worth, and you are likely to be met with elaborate evasion instead of a straight answer. Of course, some do not share this reticence but may be secretive about some other issues, e.g., political leanings or religious attitudes, about which others, in turn, may be more open.

We would guess that *you* have some secrets yourself. Stop and think about it briefly. Use the following questions to guide you.

1. Would you be troubled if your mind suddenly became an "open book," i.e., such that everyone could tell exactly what you were thinking at any moment?

2. Identify three things about yourself you have never told anyone. (CAUTION: Do NOT write these down! Somebody might discover your list, which could be embarrassing.)

3. Think of three things you have told someone about yourself that you would be disappointed to find he had made public. (If you can think of nothing in this category initially, put it this way: suppose everyone you had talked with in the last month were to rent advertising billboards and post on them everything you had told them about yourself.)

4. Think of three things you have told a physician about yourself, or that she has discovered about you, that you would not want made public, e.g., on an advertising billboard.

Theories abound about why privacy is so important to us. One value theorist claims that the right to privacy is a *property right*. As people are possessive about things they own, so they are possessive about their person and information about themselves [Thomson (1975); see replies by Scanlon (1975) and James Rachels (1975) in the same issue].

Harvard Law School Professor Charles Fried (1970, Chapter 9) claims that the importance of privacy stems from its role as "currency" or "capital" by which people establish and maintain relationships of intimacy with others. One does not customarily share intimate information with casual acquaintances. It would be an affront, for example, to turn to the stranger sitting next to you on a bus and ask questions about the person's sex life or financial status. It would also be an affront to you for the stranger to begin telling you details about these things without being asked. By doing this, the person 1) makes the presumptuous assumption that you care about these intimate aspects of his life, and 2) he implicitly imposes upon you obligations of reacting sensitively to this information and exercising discretion with regard to it.

In contrast to the reserve expected toward strangers, one is expected to reveal intimate information to friends; the level of sharing varies directly with the closeness of the relationship. One who refused to reveal her salary to her spouse would be justly criticized, as would one who refused to reveal information about his political affiliation to a friend of long standing whom he proclaims to be his best friend.

According to Fried, the harm done when confidences are violated is that it becomes impossible to regulate these degrees of intimacy. If *everyone* knows *everything* about you, there is no information left with which to establish close relationships.

Some authors go further than Fried and maintain that a sense of privacy is essential to being a person: "If anyone else could know all that I am thinking or perceive all that I am feeling except in the form I choose to filter and reveal what I am and how I see myself . . . I might cease to have as complete a sense of myself as a distinct and separate person as I have now" (Wasserstrom 1981, 113; cf. Reiman 1976). This is, of course, highly speculative, but it underscores the extreme importance of confidentiality.

4.2 The Need for Confidentiality in Medicine

The reason confidentiality becomes an issue in the health care setting is because of the degree of intimacy necessary to provide health care. Physical examination and treatment of patients requires an intimacy of access to their bodies that may be greater than they allow to anyone else in their life. (Today's media attention to sexual openness may be deceptive. Keep in mind that many still conduct their sexual activities under the covers and with the lights off, and even their sexual partners may never have observed them in the bright lights or the state of undress characteristic of the medical examining room.) Medical examination and procedures involve touching of the body in ways that may be more intimate than people allow any other person to do to them.

Furthermore, a medical history involves intimate information. Aside from the obvious elements of sexual history or symptoms of the genitourinary system, even information regarding aches and pains in other body systems is not usually shared in detail with others. The diagnostic label established as a result of the examination, as well as the details of the treatment regimen, are further items many patients handle with discretion and share with few, if any, acquaintances.

Attention to the psychosocial dimensions of illness brings up other intimate issues. The physician who explores the family dynamics and personal adjustments of patients will tread in areas that may not have been shared by the patient with anyone else. Hence there is plenty of material to be confidential about in the health care setting.

4.3 Confidentiality in Medicine

The principle of confidentiality is one of the oldest and most firmly held doctrines of professional ethics. Consider this list of statements of this principle from various professional codes and related documents:

1. *Oath of Hippocrates (Greece, fourth century B.C.):* "Whatever, in connection with my professional practice, or not in connection with it, I see or hear, in the life of men, which ought not to be spoken of abroad, I will not divulge, as reckoning that all such should be kept secret."
2. *Advice to a Physician—Haly Abbas (Persian Code, tenth century A.D.):* "A physician should respect confidences and protect the patient's secrets. In protecting a patient's secrets, he must be more insistent than the patient himself."
3. *Five Commandments and Ten Requirements (China, 1617):* "The secret diseases of female patients should be examined with a right attitude, and should not be revealed to anybody, not even to the physician's own wife."

4. *Code of Ethics—American Medical Association (1847):* "Secrecy and delicacy, when required by peculiar circumstances, should be strictly observed; and the familiar and confidential intercourse to which physicians are admitted in their professional visits, should be used with discretion, and with the most scrupulous regard to fidelity and honor. The obligation of secrecy extends beyond the period of professional services—none of the privacies of personal and domestic life, no infirmity of disposition or flaw of character observed during professional attendance, should ever be divulged by him except when he is imperatively required to do so. The force and necessity of this obligation are indeed so great, that professional men have, under certain circumstances, been protected in their observance of secrecy by courts of justice." (Chapter I, Article I, Section 2)
5. *Principles of Medical Ethics—American Medical Association (1957):* "A physician may not reveal the confidences entrusted to him in the course of medical attendance, or the deficiencies he may observe in the character of patients, unless he is required to do so by law or unless it becomes necessary in order to protect the welfare of the individual or the community." (Section 9)
6. *Principles of Medical Ethics—American Medical Association (1980):* "A physician . . . shall safeguard patient confidences within the constraints of the law." (Section 4)
7. *American College of Physicians Ethics Manual (1984):* "The physician must keep secret all that he knows about the patient and release no information without the patient's consent, unless required by law or unless resulting harm to others outweighs his duty to the patient."
8. *International Code of Medical Ethics—World Medical Association (1949):* "A doctor owes to his patients absolute secrecy on all which has been confided to him or which he knows because of the confidence entrusted to him."
9. *Code for Nurses—American Nurses Association (1950):* "The nurse safeguards the client's right to privacy by judiciously protecting information of a confidential nature." (Section 2)
10. *Patient's Bill of Rights—American Hospital Association (1972):* "The patient has the right to every consideration of his privacy concerning his own medical care program. Case discussion, consultation, examination, and treatment are confidential and should be conducted discreetly. Those not directly involved in his care must have the permission of the patient to be present." (Section 5) "The patient has the right to expect that all communications and records pertaining to his care should be treated as confidential." (Section 6)

There are significant variations in content between the statements on confidentiality cited above. The principle from China (3) especially stresses the observance of confidentiality within the physician's family, but it severely limits the scope of information protected. The Persian code (2) appears the strongest of them all, demanding paternalistic refusals to reveal information even when the patient authorizes its release. Both the World Medical Association Principles (8) and the Hippocratic Oath (1) allow *no* exceptions to a rule of protecting information.

A comparison of changes over the years in statements by the American Medical Association reveals a progressive *strengthening* of the principle of confidentiality. In the 1847 Code of Ethics (4), breaches of confidence were permitted whenever "imperatively required," leaving pretty wide latitude. By 1957 (5) grounds for revealing information had been narrowed (or at least more firmly specified) to include only three circumstances: (a) when the physician is required by law to reveal information; (b) when revelation "becomes necessary in order to protect the welfare of the individual," and (c) when "it becomes necessary in order to protect the welfare of . . . the community." In the 1980 AMA statement (6), the latter two indications for revealing confidential information are omitted. Thus the only ground for breaching confidentiality is when required to do so by law—as, for example, in mandatory reporting laws regarding suspected child abuse, communicable diseases, etc. The American College of Physicians Ethics manual (7) is closer to the 1957 AMA position.

4.4 Confidentiality and the Law

Society (through law) exhibits an ambivalent attitude toward medical confidentiality.[26] On one hand, the patient's right to confidentiality is supported legally in several states by having breaches of confidentiality grounds for suspension or revocation of a medical license. Stronger legal support for this right is supplied in many (but not all) states by provisions classifying physician-patient communications as "privileged," meaning that they cannot be introduced as testimony in judicial or administrative proceedings without permission of the patient.

Conversely, all states also have statutes requiring physicians to breach confidentiality by reporting specific medical conditions to the authorities. Failure to supply such information is also a ground for suspension or revocation of medical license. The list of conditions covered by mandatory reporting laws is extensive. Among those for which such reporting is required in one or more states are the following:

— indications of child abuse
— gunshot wounds
— indications of "foul play"
— criminal actions

---

26. For a review of the legal issues, see Annas et al. (1981, 170–192) and Fiscina (1982, Chapters 4 and 8).

— contagious, infectious, or communicable diseases (usually those contained on a specified list)
— abortions
— births out of wedlock
— diseases or congenital deformities in newborns
— any psychiatric diagnosis, especially those posing a danger to others
— death
— Medicare, Medicaid, OSHA reports.

4.5 Cases

Many physicians allow the principle of confidentiality and loyalty to their patients to override legal reporting requirements in some circumstances. Thus many physicians treat patients and any acknowledged "contacts" for venereal disease without reporting the incident to the public health authorities as required by the letter of the law. Do you think this practice is justified? Consider the following case as an example.

4.5.1 "Please Don't Ruin My Marriage!"

Joan Wentaway is a 40-year-old businesswoman. She and her husband Stone (who is 43) have been your patients for quite a few years; you know them well.

You were surprised three days ago when Joan came to see you for a routine pelvic exam. She had a small amount of purulent cervical discharge, so you took a GC culture that came back positive this morning.

At today's follow-up appointment, you explain to Joan that laboratory tests confirm that she has gonorrhea, and you administer 4.8 million units of penicillin G, IM. You then explain that state law requires that you report all cases of gonorrhea to the Health Department. You point out that her husband needs to come in for the same treatment you have just given her.

With considerable emotion, Joan begs you not to report her disease either to the Health Department or her husband. "I know exactly where I got this," she explains, "I picked up a prostitute a couple of weeks ago when I was in Atlanta for a business convention. I haven't had sex with Stone, or with anyone else, since, so I haven't spread the disease. If you tell Stone about this, he will walk out on me, I know. And if you report me to the Health Department, Stone will find out. A neighbor of ours works at the Health Department handling these reports, and he'll go straight home and tell Stone all about it. I swear, I have never done anything like this before. What rotten luck! One 'fling' and I get VD! Please don't ruin my marriage by telling Stone."

What should you do? Should you tell Stone? Should you report the case to the Health Department? Consider the following options:

1. Insist that Joan tell her husband and bring him in for treatment.
2. Same as 1 plus threaten that unless her husband has called for an appointment

within 48 hours, you will contact him and tell him yourself.
3. Insist that she bring her husband in for treatment but agree to go along with a fictional explanation for the need for him to receive this treatment, if Joan can come up with some plausible fiction.
4. Call Stone on the spot and tell him yourself, while Joan is still in the room.
5. Call the Health Department on the spot, while Joan is still in the room.
6. Call Stone and/or the Health Department as soon as Joan has left your office.
7. Promise Joan that you will not report her either to Stone or to the Health Department. Keep your promise.
8. Other (specify): _____

Choice 6 may be tempting because it minimizes the immediate hassle, but in our view it is among the least satisfactory of the options (although it is certainly legally defensible). Joan is likely to be extremely upset later when she discovers that the information was revealed. Thus the net hassle is likely to be greater here than for the other options. More importantly, on ethical grounds, she surely has a moral *right* to be informed in advance if this is going to be done so she can prepare for Stone's reaction. This is essential if you hope to preserve trust in your relationship with her.

A. Telling the Health Department The law mandates reporting cases of venereal disease to the Health Department or other health officer. The AMA Principles of Medical Ethics demand reporting information when "required to do so by law."

However, this does not settle the issue on moral grounds. One may always decide, on ethical grounds, to disobey the law and professional codes if there are compelling moral reasons to do so. And it is not irrelevant to this case to recognize that (1) many health departments are too concerned with more serious venereal diseases, such as syphilis, to be upset by failures to report gonorrhea, or to do much follow-up with this disease when it is reported, and (2) the practitioner may be more effective in eliciting information about and treating contacts than the public health authorities.

The primary losses if the case is not reported are (1) the distortion of public health data about the incidence of the disease and (2) the loss of any chance the public health authorities have to locate the prostitute and treat the source case for this infection. Both of these goals might be achieved while still preserving confidentiality by reporting the case to the health department anonymously or assigning an alias for the patient, while handling treatment and follow-up yourself.

Of course, taking matters into one's own hands in this way is risky. Society has vested authority for these matters in the health agency, and there may be penalties for the practitioner who does not acknowledge this authority.

B. Telling Stone   The question of whether to tell Stone is more immediately related to issues of personal welfare. If Stone *has* been exposed to the disease and goes without treatment, the consequences for his health could be serious.

How much weight do these consequences carry compared to Joan's right to confidentiality? Clearly they would have to have considerable weight to provide a justification for overriding Joan's right.

In general, rights require strong countervailing considerations in order to be overridden. Otherwise, rights would not be worth much. If, for example, my right to free speech held only until others felt it is better that I *not* be heard, then my right would be limited and my reason for prizing it is reduced. I don't need the support of a right to say things *no one objects* to hearing. I need to appeal to the right to speak when I want to say things *some may prefer not to hear.* The courts have acknowledged this by ruling that the right to free speech is overridden only in those rare and extreme situations in which the speaking poses a "clear and present danger" to others or the social order. (The classic example is yelling "Fire!" in a crowded theater.)

Is the danger of untreated gonorrhea sufficiently serious to justify breaching Joan's right to confidentiality? Let us isolate the point by constructing a hypothetical proposition that varies in some respects from the case at hand. Suppose (for purposes of this argument) we knew that Stone *had* been exposed by Joan and had contracted the disease. Suppose the only way to get him in for treatment is to breach Joan's right to confidentiality. Is the need for treatment sufficiently serious to justify this breach? Most people would agree that it is. In addition, that Stone is also your patient may add weight to your duty to prevent his suffering the effects of untreated disease when you are in a position to prevent it from happening.

On the other hand, you may find yourself inclined to tell Stone because of a desire (or a sense of obligation) toward this patient/friend/fellow-male (if you are male) to inform him of his wife's infidelity. This inclination should not enter into your deliberations. This consideration does not fall within the physician-patient relationship, and thus (even if it might be relevant in other decision contexts) it ought not intrude into clinical decisions.

The next question may be whether you *believe* Joan's insistence that Stone has not been exposed to the disease. We have said that if Stone were exposed, he ought to be treated, even if arranging treatment requires violating confidentiality. Is your degree of confidence in her report sufficient to warrant a decision not to offer treatment to Stone? (NOTE: In making this judgment, try to avoid extraneous factors, such as the inclination to make sure he knows what a "bad girl" his wife has been, or assumptions based upon your own sexual practices or standards.)

If you are sufficiently skeptical of Joan's report to conclude that Stone must be treated, then you must determine the best means to get him in for treatment. Four alternatives are suggested in options 1–4. List the advantages and disadvantages of each. List the moral principles involved in each choice. Which do you think the best approach and why? Choose one of the options and formulate your reasons for favoring it *before* you go to the next section.

C. Reconsiderations Now that you have made a decision in this case, think it through further. A decision, once carried out, rarely ends a matter. Future events may lead you to reflect on the choice you made.[27] Find the choice you made from the following list and consider the information presented. Would you stick with your original decision?

1. If you have chosen *not* to tell Stone, what if he came in a day or two later with dysuria and a profuse, purulent urethral discharge?

2. If you have chosen *not* to report this case to the Health Department, what if a Public Health officer telephoned you a week later and asked whether you had ever treated Joan for gonorrhea, explaining that someone had reported her as their contact.

3. If you have chosen to tell Stone, how would you feel if (1) his GC culture came back negative and (2) he instituted divorce proceedings against Joan immediately?

4. If you have insisted that Joan tell her husband, how would you feel if you read in the paper the next day that Joan committed suicide immediately after leaving your office?

5. If you chose to go along with option 3, how would you respond to Stone if he asked you point-blank what this treatment was for? What would you say if he asked, "This is for VD, isn't it?"

Now that you have begun to formulate a policy for dealing with cases of this sort, test it further by applying it to the following situation.

4.5.2 "Please Don't Tell my Parents!"

On the appointment book, the patient is listed as "Alice Avender—camp physical." Her record reveals that she is 15 years old.

At the end of the routine camp physical, Alice requests a prescription for birth control pills and asks that her parents not be informed of this request. She says she plans to pay for the prescription and any related office visits herself, so her parents will not have to know. (She has a part-time job at a fast-food restaurant; her earnings, with the allowance she receives from her parents, will be more than enough to pay these expenses.)

Alice explains she has read "all about" alternative methods of birth control and has decided she prefers the pill. She volunteers to return for periodic examinations as often as is advisable while she is on contraceptives. Alice's desire for secrecy is surprising in view of her parents' attitudes. More than once, during general

---

27. Some of the general principles involved in these later events are discussed in Appendix I, Section 2.1.3: "Responsibility for Consequences."

discussions of teenage sexuality, Alice's parents have been mentioned as prime examples of parents who champion openness with teenage children about sex. Although they are not sure that teenagers are mature enough to handle intimate relationships, they think that after adequate parental counseling, young people should make these decisions for themselves.

In contrast, Alice reports that her mother told her a few months previously, "If you want to mess around with sex, I guess I can't stop you. Just do two things for me: Be sure that you are protected, and don't let me, or *especially* your father, hear anything about it."

The application of the confidentiality principle to minors has not been firmly established. Parents are generally considered to have a right to medical information concerning their children. Few physicians would think of asking patients under legal age for permission to discuss their illnesses and problems with their parents. They would feel free to disclose information to the parents as a matter of course. However, this policy may be based on factors extraneous to the case at hand. First, in most instances parents are paying the bills for the minor's care; it can be argued that they have a right to know precisely for what they are paying (a line of argument to be challenged in connection with a later case). Secondly, most of these cases involve medical matters less intimate in nature than the illustrative case. Issues of birth control and abortion have been singled out in recent decisions of the United States Supreme Court for special protection under the constitutional right of privacy, and this protection might apply to the medical sphere. It should be noted, however, that the Supreme Court appears to be weakening this protection, especially with regard to abortion, in some recent opinions.

Two issues are central to this situation; both indicate that it would best serve the interests of *the family as a unit* for the parents to be informed. The first issue concerns truth, honesty, and trust. Secrets are ultimately destructive in these situations, as they are in any intimate relationship. If Alice continues to be sexually active and hides it from her parents, a chronic erosion of their relationship could develop. In contrast, the truth may generate an acute crisis in the family. However, as long as caring and trust remain, there is potential for overcoming the crisis, resulting in the growth of all parties individually and a strengthening of the family unit.

The second issue central to this situation is autonomy. A prime goal of any medical interaction is to support, restore, and enhance autonomy. The physician (particularly the family physician) must consider the autonomy of both Alice and her parents—and even the autonomy of the family as a unit.

To enter into collusion with Alice as she requests can be interpreted as supporting her autonomy, but parental and corporate family autonomy would be eroded in the process. In contrast, were the parents informed of Alice's sexual activity, the family disagreement could eventually resolve itself in a way that enhances the autonomy of all parties. The vigorous family discussions that undoubtedly would follow this disclosure would require each party to express views on the issue more carefully than would be necessary for individual thought about the matter. This process could lead to a creative but disciplined autonomy for the teen-ager and her parents, which differs significantly from (and in our judgment is far superior to) the passive and random autonomy they each appear to express at present. Alice and her parents may recognize (and value) a role for the parents as competent advisers. Because these values exist in the family unit, the family physician is obligated to make a concerted effort to see that Alice's parents are informed.

However, the physician's obligation to ensure that the parents are informed varies with the degree of his relationship with them. If he does not know the parents at all, or if they are merely social acquaintances, then Alice's right to confidentiality outweighs any duty the physician might have to the parents. (One might still *urge* Alice to talk the matter over with her parents, but it would not be justifiable to inform them without her consent.)

One mechanism for bringing this information to the attention of the parents is to prescribe the pill under a mild ruse, e.g., saying it is to achieve menstrual regularity. Knowing their daughter is on the pill is bound to start the parents thinking about the possibility of sexual activity on her part.

If the parents are also the physician's patients (and particularly in the specialty of family practice, where the family as a whole is the fundamental unit of care), the obligation to see that the parents are informed is considerably stronger. However, even here unilaterally informing her parents would undermine the physician's trust relationship with Alice. Thus we propose a strategy of strongly urging Alice to inform her parents, offering to be present and assist the family in dealing with the short-term impact of this announcement, and offering supportive counseling to all parties over the long term.[28]

Note On Law This case raises two issues about the relationship between legal requirements and moral decisions. The Department of Health and Human Services proposed in 1982 an administrative regulation that required informing the parents of any minor provided with birth control by a clinic receiving federal funds. Many health professionals wrote protesting this proposal, arguing that it would increase teen-age pregnancies and that this was far more dangerous in medical terms than the use of contraceptives by teen-agers. Some who protested agreed with our suggestion that it is morally right to inform the parents in some cases. However, it is one thing to hold that this is a moral requirement and quite another to enact a legal reporting requirement. The former allows for professional discretion in deciding when the obligation applies and the best approach to meeting it, whereas the latter would significantly diminish these domains of individual professional discretion. The AMA Principles would require physicians to abide by this regulation were it adopted, whereas a moral decision might require civil dis-

---

28. For details of the strategy we propose, see Eaddy and Graber, (1982).

obedience by refusing to notify the parents in cases where the physician is convinced that this would not be constructive.

The *American College of Physicians Ethics Manual* (American College of Physicians 1984, 132), explicitly allows for civil disobedience in the face of a court order: "If the physician thinks that his commitment to the patient's welfare overrides his duty to obey a court order, he may ethically refuse to give to the courts information not released by the patient but must be prepared to accept the legal consequences."

4.5.3 "Please Don't Tell My Family!" In this case, taken from Melvin P. Levine and colleagues (1977, 205), the physician is a nephrologist or transplant surgeon.

A five-year-old girl has been a patient in a medical center for three years because of progressive renal failure secondary to glomerulonephritis. She had been on chronic renal dialysis, and the possibility of a renal transplantation was considered. The effectiveness of this procedure in her case was questionable. On the other hand, it was the feeling of the professional staff that there was a clear possibility that a transplanted kidney would not undergo the same disease process.

After discussion with the parents, it was decided to proceed with plans for transplantation. Tissue typing was performed on the patient; it was noted that she would be difficult to match. Two siblings, age two and four, were thought to be too young to serve as donors. The girl's mother turned out not to be histocompatible.

The father, however, was found to be quite compatible with his daughter. He underwent an arteriogram, and it was discovered that he had anatomically favorable circulation for transplantation. The nephrologist met alone with the father and gave him these results. He informed the father that the prognosis for his daughter was quite uncertain.

After some thought, the girl's father decided that he did not wish to donate a kidney to his daughter. He admitted he did not have the courage and that in view of the uncertain prognosis, the very slight possibility of a cadaver kidney, and the degree of suffering his daughter had already sustained, he would prefer not to donate.

The father asked the physician to tell everyone else in the family that he was not histocompatible. He was afraid that if they knew the truth, they would accuse him of allowing his daughter to die. He felt that this would "wreck the family."

The physician felt very uncomfortable about this request. However, he agreed to tell the man's wife that "for medical reasons" the father should not donate a kidney.

In what ways is this case different from Case 4.5.2? How would your solution here differ? Give this some thought before you read the explanation in the following section.

Here again a key issue is exchange of information within the family. However, one difference is that the physician is being asked not merely to *refrain* from reporting information to the man's family, but to participate actively in *misleading* them about the outcome of the tests. Clearly mere confidentiality would not accomplish the man's purposes. Suppose the physician were to say to the family, "I cannot tell you the results of the tests. He will have to tell you himself." One can imagine the pressure that would be put on the man to reveal the results. Thus he requests the physician's assistance to avoid this kind of pressure, assistance that goes well beyond protection of confidentiality.

The patient requests that the physician lie about the results of the tissue tests. This course of action is inadvisable. A direct lie, if discovered, will undermine the trust relationship between the physician and the family much more than would evasion of the truth. The phrase "for medical reasons" can be construed to cover the truth, that the father's fear of donation might be regarded as pathological.

Does this seem a semantic quibble to you? Do you feel there is no moral difference between a direct lie and an evasion that, while not strictly false, may be no less misleading? Before you dismiss this distinction, think about how it would apply in a *whole range* of situations. In particular, think of the case in which you would regard the distinction as most likely to be justified. Only if it is *never* justified in *any* situation can it be said that the distinction lacks moral significance. On the other hand, if it is justified in some situations, reasons have to be offered for *not* considering it significant in other circumstances.[29]

If the choice is seen as a one-moment, all-or-nothing matter, i.e., between preserving the man's confidentiality *at this moment* and breaching it, then it would be difficult to defend the physician's action. Important as the man's right to confidentiality may be, it does not outweigh the child's right to life, and although there are some doubts about the prospects for success of the transplant, they do not seem serious enough to justify foregoing this life-saving possibility.

However, the best approach may be to protect the man's confidentiality *right now*, and then continue to help him deal with his reluctance to donate a kidney to his daughter. This approach takes confidentiality to be justifed as a means to an ultimate goal.

There are at least two goals to which confidentiality might be subordinated in this way: either (1) persuading the father to agree to donate, or (2) allowing the father to work through his immediate emotional reaction and reach a considered decision. The difference between these goals would show up at a later stage if, after further counseling, the father still refused to donate. One pursuing the former goal would seriously consider breaching confidentiality at that point, whereas one who held the latter goal would be inclined to accept the father's decision, as long as he was convinced it was a considered decision.

---

29. For further discussion of distinctions of this sort, see discussion of "Half-Truths" (Section 2.3.1.B) and Appendix I, Section 2.1.1: "Side-Constraints."

4.5.4 "Please Don't Tell Anybody!" This case is adapted from Barbara Tate (1977, 21–22).

> A young unmarried woman was admitted to the hospital with excessive uterine bleeding, which she explained was connected with her monthly period. She stated that this had occurred several times over the course of the past year and was of great concern to her.
>
> A medical student (who is currently on an externship rotation with the private practice gynecologist treating this patient) established a good rapport with her, perhaps partly because the student was close to the patient's own age, whereas the physician was significantly older.
>
> On the day after admission, the student was chatting with her when she said: "You would keep anything I told you secret, wouldn't you?" After the student's assurance that confidentiality would be preserved, she confided that she had been certain she was pregnant and took some medication that she had been told would bring about an abortion. She insisted she does not want anyone, not even the physician-mentor, to know about this.

What should the medical student do? What would you do? Consider the following options:

1. "Promise anything." Promise her that you will keep the information confidential, then tell the doctor the whole story (but ask him not to let the patient know that you told him).
2. Promise that you will keep the information confidential and do *not* tell anybody, not even the doctor.
3. Promise you will keep the information confidential, then tell the doctor only "There's more to this case than she has told you, but I cannot tell you the details," leaving it to him to get the whole story from her in his own way.
4. Promise only that you will not take the initiative to tell the doctor, but explain that you will have to answer truthfully if he asks you whether you learned anything relevant in your conversations with her. Then honor this promise.
5. Refuse to promise to protect her secret. Explain that proper treatment cannot be carried out unless the doctor knows all the relevant facts about the patient, and thus you must tell the doctor the whole story.
6. Refuse to promise to protect her secret. Encourage *her* to tell the doctor the whole story, explaining that proper treatment cannot be carried out unless the doctor knows all the relevant facts about the patient.
7. Change the subject. Comment on the pretty flowers someone sent to her and try to forget the whole episode ever happened.
8. Other (specify):_____

The first mistake was to agree to an unqualified promise of confidentiality as the patient prepared to reveal the information. It may have seemed innocuous enough at the time, but soon it became clear that her conception of the scope of confidentiality was significantly wider than the medical student had in mind when he offered the assurance. What she wanted is what we call "secrecy," i.e., that information be kept entirely to oneself and not shared with anyone else. We argue below, however, that this is different from the way confidentiality works in the medical setting.

It would probably have been wise for the student to have qualified any assurance of confidentiality: "Of course, I will have to share information with the physician who is caring for you, but the care team will not tell anyone else." (Of course, one result of responding in this way might be that she would not reveal the information in question to the medical student. That may be the price that has to be paid for the difference between confidentiality and secrecy.)

But the promise *was* made, and now the question is what to do about it. This situation might not have arisen had more attention been paid to its consequences and ethical implications before it was made, but it must be dealt with in ethical terms now that it has reached that stage.

A general issue raised by this case is the exchange of information among the various health care professionals treating the patient. Present practice sets few, if any, limits on exchange of information among professionals. The patient's chart is open to a wide variety of hospital personnel. One physician counted the persons in his metropolitan teaching hospital who had access to the hospital record of a particular patient. He reports:

> I was amazed to learn that at least 25 and possibly as many as 100 health professionals and administrative personnel at our university hospital had access to the patient's record and that all of them had a legitimate need, indeed a professional responsibility, to open and use that chart. These persons included 6 attending physicians (the primary physician, the surgeon, the pulmonary consultant, and others); 12 house officers (medical, surgical, intensive-care unit, and "covering" house staff); 20 nursing personnel (on three shifts); 6 respiratory therapists; 3 nutritionists; 2 clinical pharmacists; 15 students (from medicine, nursing, respiratory therapy, and clinical pharmacy); 4 unit secretaries; 4 hospital financial officers; and 4 chart reviewers (utilization review, quality assurance review, tissue review, and insurance auditor). (Siegler 1982, 1519)

The author concludes that "medical confidentiality, as it has traditionally been understood by patients and doctors, no longer exists. This ancient medical principle, . . . has become old, worn-out, and useless; it is a decrepit concept" (Siegler 1982, 1518).

We do not share completely this negative assessment. Confidentiality is meaningful in today's complex health care structure when its nature and scope are properly understood.

The heart of the agreement to preserve confidentiality is found in the physician-patient relationship as a component of the therapeutic bond comprising the doctor-patient relationship or DPR (as discussed in Section 1.2.4.B.3). The patient controls the scope and content of this principle, having the option to select any information for protection under the principle of confidentiality. The physician has no grounds for judgment about what is to be confidential except his or her reading of what is sensitive to a given patient. From this principle it follows that students, who are in the process of acquiring clinical skills, are well advised to treat *all* information as confidential until they become proficient in determining what each patient regards as sensitive.

There are four cases in which information about patients is shared with other professionals.

A. Communication with Other Caregivers   The primary physician enlists other professionals to assist in the care of the patient, and their role in care makes it necessary for them to become familiar with the facts of the case. Those in Siegler's list above fall into this category. Information about the patient is deposited in the hospital record to make it available to these individuals. This is the key difference between confidentiality and secrecy. Keeping information ''secret'' means that it is not shared with anyone. ''Confidentiality,'' in contrast, means sharing information with others directly involved in the patient's care.

This may include a large number of individuals, as Siegler's list indicates. Protection of the patient's privacy results from the circumspect behavior of these individuals. They should be aware that (1) they have the right to access only those charts and that information within a chart that is directly relevant to their care-giving function, and (2) the pledge of confidentiality made to the patient by physicians makes it wrong for them to reveal any information learned from the chart (or from their own interactions with the patient) outside the bounds of the health care team.

Formal procedural safeguards might be devised to enforce some aspects of these rules of decorum, i.e., to prevent hospital employees other than those directly involved in the patient's care from having access to the chart. However, these could never be ''fail safe,'' and they involve a greater loss (by impeding communication between those with a need to exchange information) than the gain to be achieved. There is no substitute for morally sensitive behavior by the individuals involved.

B. Teaching   The second occasion for sharing information in the clinical setting is for purposes of teaching. This is bounded by safeguards in several ways, including (1) obtaining informed consent of the patient before introducing students into his or her care, (2) impressing upon the students the importance of discretion with regard to information gained about patients, and (3) admitting into this role only those students who, even at this stage of their skills, can be of benefit to the patient. The last is why introduction to clinical practice is delayed in health professions training programs until students have mastered requisite preliminary skills.

C. Peer Review   A third occasion for sharing information is peer review, to be distinguished from (A) above. Although these reviews protect and improve the care of the individual patient, they also protect the hospital and thus cannot be brought entirely under the rubric of providing care. Explicit patient consent should be sought for access to the chart for this purpose. This might be included with other forms filled out by the patient upon admission, but it ought to be specifically described.

D. "Shop Talk"   Professionals often share information about patients among themselves in an informal, often anecdotal form. This "shop talk" is similar to that between other intellectuals as a means of enhancing scientific creativity. To communicate the reasoning behind diagnosis and treatment of a specific case to another professional clarifies one's thinking, prompts the listener to useful intellectual exercise, and promulgates information about disease entities, therapies, etc. Compared to a formal consultation, this sort of exchange is much less structured, and the listener is not committed to share responsibility for the decision reached. The patient's privacy is safeguarded in these discussions by keeping the identity of the patient anonymous. Outsiders sometimes criticize health professionals for referrring to patients, for example, as "the gall bladder in [room] '46'"; but this sort of reference confers anonymity and thereby preserves confidentiality.

Returning to the particulars of Case 4.5.4., the key value conflict is between the principle of promise keeping on the one hand and the patient's health needs on the other. The student made a serious mistake in getting embroiled in what the patient regarded as a promise of absolute secrecy. This promise cannot be sustained, given the student's standing in the clinical setting and the health needs of the patient. The student's position in the setting is ancillary to that of the physician-mentor, and thus the physician-mentor *must* be given the information. To attempt to persuade the patient to reveal the information herself might be best; if this fails, though, the student has no recourse but to inform the physician. Hence, option 6 is recommended as the initial approach, followed (if necessary) by option 5.

4.5.5 "Please Don't Tell My Ex-Husband!"

Ms. Meda Mystake is a 31-year-old woman who has been a patient of yours for about ten years. Her marriage to Roland Doughe ended in divorce six months ago. At that time Meda brought a copy of the court decree to you and pointed out the provision in which Roland had agreed to pay "all medical expenses" for Meda for one year following the date of the divorce. You told your business manager to bill all charges to Roland for the one-year period.

A month ago Meda came to your office again. Laboratory tests confirmed your clinical impression that she is pregnant. When you informed her of these findings, she volunteered that the baby's father is a man she has been living with since shortly following the divorce.

You indicated on the chart that Meda should be scheduled for the standard pattern of prenatal visits. As most physicians nowadays, you charge a flat fee for prenatal visits, delivery, and postnatal care. In your case, the fee is $650.

Today, Roland Doughe is on the phone, irate. The business manager tried to handle the situation, but Roland insisted on talking with you. "I demand to know what sort of treatment is being given to my ex-wife that amounts to $650," he says angrily. "Your office staff refused to tell me anything about it. They said that I must ask Meda about it, but I have asked her, and she won't discuss it. I have a right to know what I am paying for. How do I know you aren't overcharging me?"

What should you tell Roland?

This is another situation that could have been avoided. For the physician to get embroiled in this situation was a mistake. When Ms. Mystake came in with the court order, the physician would have been advised to refuse to take part in this arrangement. It should have been possible for her and her ex-husband to work out an arrangement independently for handling his payment of these expenses—for example, by having her pay the physician and then sending copies of the receipts to her ex-husband for collection.

There is little basis for violating her confidentiality by revealing to Roland the details about this bill. Other third-party payers may demand to know what they are paying for, but the physician must obtain a release from the patient before complying with this request; surely the same applies here.

Roland might have a special claim to information here because a substantial portion of the blanket charge covers the delivery of the baby, but this will occur *after* the one-year period for which he had promised to pay medical expenses. If this were brought to the attention of a court (as Roland would be likely to do if he knew these facts), the court might release him from responsibility for a pro-rated portion of the bill corresponding to the delivery charge. Hence, it might be *unjust* to expect him to pay the entire bill. The questions remaining are

1. Is the injustice involved here sufficiently *serious* to justify a breach of confidentiality?
2. Is relieving Roland of this injustice the responsibility of the physician and his or her staff?
3. Meda is clearly not being "fair" or "just" to her ex-husband, but must the physician intervene to rectify this wrong?

Clearly some harm to others is sufficiently serious to justify breaching confidentiality. If you determine that a certain patient is at risk for a myocardial infarction or seizures and his occupation is such that he will jeopardize lives if such an event occurs (e.g., a bus driver, a commercial pilot), you have an obligation to urge him to inform his employer of this condition and to request relief from duties with direct impact on public safety. If the patient does not notify his employer, you have a moral duty to inform the employer despite his protests.

The difficult issue here is to balance the degree of risk with the impact the patient is likely to have on public safety, and thereby to determine *when* to override confidentiality. A person at risk for an MI might injure others if one occurs while he is driving a private automobile. Should physicians, then, notify the state bureau of licenses of every patient with this diagnosis? If this risk is insufficient for abridging confidentiality, should the authorities be notified of all those who drive a good deal more than the average (e.g., traveling salesmen), on the grounds that the chances of an MI occurring under conditions that could be harmful to others is increased? If this is seen as excessively cautious, then where is the line to be drawn between this situation and the airline pilot responsible for several hundred passengers? These are issues of balancing competing obligations: the principle of confidentiality on one hand, and the duty to protect society from harm on the other. There are no easy formulas for resolving these questions. They depend on weighing normative factors in each individual case.

4.6 President's Commission Recommendations

The President's Commission for the Study of Ethical Problems in Medicine and Biomedical and Behavioral Research (1983, 37–38) has issued guidelines dealing with aspects of confidentiality:

(1) Respect for patients' legitimate expectations of privacy is an important part of ethical health care practices, as well as the foundation on which a relationship of mutual trust and benefit can be built between patient and professional.

(2) Health care institutions and providers are urged to educate the public about their expectations and practices on private medical matters.

—In particular, patients need to be better informed about the scope of confidentiality and to be given the opportunity to give waivers for specific information rather than blanket waivers.

—Specific warnings should be made if disclosures of patient information are anticipated without prior consent.

(3) Instances of unconsented disclosures are to be regarded as exceptions to the general norm of confidentiality and require special justification, such as an important public purpose.

(4) When information is provided based upon a general consent by a patient (for example, permission for a hospital to send records to a third-party payer), no more information should be disclosed than is necessary for the function to be performed by the third party.

—Efforts should be made to permit patients to review for accuracy any records to be disclosed.

—Third-party recipients of confidential information are encouraged to find economical methods of notifying patients whose records they are requesting or when they plan to pass along individually identifiable information to other persons or organizations.

4.7 Review Exercises

1. Is privacy a *right* or a *value?* What difference does this distinction make to a) the scope, b) the stringency, and c) the justification of a principle of confidentiality?

2. Design a statement on confidentiality for one of the purposes indicated below. Develop the rationale, in the way you would present it to an administrative committee as part of a proposal that the statement be adopted as official policy, for (1) having such a statement and (2) the specifics of your statement.

   a. A statement for patients, to be included in the admissions forms for a hospital.

   b. A statement for hospital employees, to be included in an employees handbook.

   c. A statement for medical students, to be included in a student handbook.

3. Describe a range of cases involving the decision to breach confidentiality; on the basis of your response to these, develop a principle to determine when confidentiality should be violated.

5 Conclusion

In this chapter, you have explored central issues in the physician-patient relationship. In the next chapter, you will examine some theoretical resources, from both professional ethics and general ethics, that will assist you in examining these issues more thoroughly.

References

Ackerman TF: Why doctors should intervene: Autonomy and the constraints of illness. *Hastings Cent. Rep.* 12:14–17, August 1982.

American College of Physicians: American College of Physicians Ethics Manual. *Ann. Intern. Med.* 101:129–137, 263–274, 1984.

Annas GJ, Glantz LH, Katz BF: *The Rights of Doctors, Nurses and Allied Health Professionals: A Health Law Primer*, Ballinger Publishing, Cambridge MA, 1981.

Ballantine HT Jr: The crisis in ethics, anno domini 1979. *N. Engl. J. Med.* 301:634–638, 1979.

Beauchamp TL, Childress JF: *Principles of Biomedical Ethics*, 2nd ed. Oxford University Press, New York, 1983.

Bok S: *Lying: Moral Choice in Public and Private Life*. Pantheon Books, New York, 1978.

Cassell E: *The Healer's Art*. Lippincott, New York, 1976.

Chapman CB: On the definition and teaching of the medical ethic. *N. Engl. J. Med.* 301:630–634, 1979.

Collins J: Should doctors tell the truth? *Harper's Magazine*, 1927. Reprinted in Mappes TA, Zembaty JS: Biomedical Ethics. McGraw-Hill, New York, 64–67, 1981.

Coulehan JL: Human illness. Cases, models, and paradigms. *The Pharos,* 2–8, Spring 1980.

Culver CM, Gert B: *Philosophy in Medicine.* Oxford University Press, New York, 1982.

Eaddy JA, Graber GC: Confidentiality and the family physician. *Am. Fam. Physician* 25: 141–145, 1982.

Eisenberg L: What makes persons 'patients' and patients 'well'? *Am. J. Med.* 69:277–286, 1980.

Fiscina SF: *Medical Law for the Attending Physician.* Southern Illinois University Press, Carbondale IL, 1982.

Fried C: *An Anatomy of Values: Problems of Personal and Social Choice.* Harvard University Press, Cambridge MA, Chapter 9, 1970.

Fried C: *Medical Experimentation: Personal Integrity and Social Policy.* American Elsevier, New York, Chapter 2, 1974.

Israel L: *Conquering Cancer* (Pinkham J. trans). Random House, New York, 1978.

Judicial Council of the American Medical Association: *Current Opinions of the Judicial Council of the American Medical Association–1984.* American Medical Association, Chicago, 1984.

Knight JA: *Doctor-to-Be: Coping with the Trials and Triumphs of Medical School.* Appleton-Century-Crofts, New York, 1981.

Lear MW: *Heartsounds: The Story of a Love and a Loss.* Simon and Schuster, New York, 1980.

Leslie A: Ethics and practice of placebo therapy. *Am. J. Med.* 16:854–862, 1954. Reprinted in Reiser SJ, Dyck AJ, Curran WJ: *Ethics in Medicine: Historical Perspectives and Contemporary Concerns.* The MIT Press, Cambridge MA, 240–247, 1977.

Levine MD, Scott L, Curran WJ: Ethics rounds in a children's medical center: Evaluation of a hospital-based program for continuing education in medical ethics. *Pediatrics* 60:205, 1977.

Lipp MR: *Respectful Treatment: The Human Side of Medical Care.* Harper & Row, New York, 1977.

McWhinney IR: Beyond diagnosis: An approach to the integration of behavioral science and clinical medicine. *N. Engl. J. Med.* 287:384–387, 1972.

Pellegrino ED: *Humanism and the Physician.* University of Tennessee Press, Knoxville, 1979.

Pellegrino ED, Thomasma DC: *A Philosophi-* *cal Basis of Medical Practice.* Oxford University Press, New York, 1981.

President's Commission for the Study of Ethical Problems in Medicine and Biomedical and Behavioral Research: *Making Health Care Decisions: The Ethical and Legal Implications of Informed Consent in the Patient-Practitioner Relationship. Vol. 1: Report.* US Government Printing Office, Washington DC, 1982a.

———: *Making Health Care Decisions: The Ethical and Legal Implications of Informed Consent in the Patient-Practitioner Relationship. Vol. 2: Appendices: Empirical Studies of Informed Consent.* US Government Printing Office, Washington DC, 1982b.

———: *Summing Up.* US Government Printing Office, Washington DC, 1983.

Rachels J: Why privacy is important. *Philosophy and Public Affairs* 4:323–333, 1975.

Reiman JH: Privacy, morality, and the law. *Philosophy and Public Affairs* 6:26–44, 1976.

Scanlon T: Thomson on privacy. *Philosophy and Public Affairs* 4:315–322, 1975.

Shelp EE: Courage and tragedy in clinical medicine. *J. Med. Philos.* 8:417–429, 1983.

Siegler M: Searching for moral certainty in medicine: A proposal for a new model of the doctor-patient encounter. *Bull NY Acad. Med.* 57:56, 1981a.

———: The doctor-patient encounter and its relationship to theories of health and disease. *In* Caplan AL, Engelhardt HT Jr, McCartney JJ (eds): *Concepts of Health and Disease: Interdisciplinary Perspectives.* Addison-Wesley, Reading MA, 635–639, 1981b.

———: Confidentiality in medicine—A decrepit concept. *N. Engl. J. Med.* 307: 1518–1519, 1982.

Tate BL (project director): *The Nurse's Dilemma: Ethical Considerations in Nursing Practice.* International Council of Nurses, The Florence Nightingale International Foundation, Geneva, 1977.

Thomson JJ: The right to privacy. *Philosophy and Public Affairs* 4:295–314, 1975.

Veatch RM: *A Theory of Medical Ethics.* Basic Books, New York, 1981.

Wasserstrom R: The legal and philosophical foundations of the right to privacy. *In* Mappes TA, Zembaty JS (eds): *Biomedical Ethics.* McGraw-Hill, New York, 109–116, 1981.

Further Reading

General Features

Abrams N, Buckner M: *Medical Ethics: A Clinical Textbook and Reference for the Health Care Professions*. The MIT Press, Cambridge MA, Section II, 1983.

Bayles MD: *Professional Ethics*. Wadsworth Publishing, Belmont CA, 1981.

Cousins N: *Anatomy of an Illness as Perceived by the Patient*. WW Norton, New York, 1979.
Patient's own account of his unconventional self-treatment for ankylosing spondylitis.

Goldman AH: *The Moral Foundations of Professional Ethics*. Rowman and Littlefield, Towata, NJ, 1980.

Halberstam M, Lesher S: *A Coronary Event*. Popular Library, New York, 1976.
Account of the course of an illness, told by both the patient (Lesher) and the physician (Halberstam).

Massie R, Massie S: *Journey*. Warner Books, New York, 1975.
Parents' account of the course of illness of their hemophiliac son.

May WF: *The Physician's Covenant: Images of the Healer in Medical Ethics*. Westminster Press, Philadelphia, 1983.

Parsons T: *The Social System*. Free Press, Glencoe, IL, 428–479, 1951.

Reich WT (ed-in-chief): *Encyclopedia of Bioethics*. Macmillan and the Free Press, New York, 1978.
Therapeutic Relationship
I. History of the Relationship (Entralgo PL)
II. Sociohistorical Perspective (Bloom SW)
III. Contemporary Sociological Analysis (Mechanic D)
IV. Contemporary Medical Perspective (Cassell EJ)

Siegler M, Osmond H: Aesculapian authority. *Hastings Cent. Studies* 1(2):41–52, 1973.

Sontag S: *Illness as Metaphor*. Farrar, Straus, and Giroux, New York, 1978.
Reflections by a former cancer patient on the emotional impact of a diagnosis of cancer, as compared with the rather glamorized image of tuberculosis in the nineteenth century.

Information Exchange

Abrams, Buckner: *Medical Ethics*, Section II.C, 1983.

Novak DH, Plumer R, Smith RL, et al: Changes in physicians' attitudes toward telling the cancer patient. *JAMA* 241:897–900, 1979.

President's Commission for the Study of Ethical Problems in Medicine and Biomedical and Behavioral Research: *Making Health Care Decisions: The Ethical and Legal Implications of Informed Consent in the Patient-Practitioner Relationship. Vol. 3: Appendices: Studies on the Foundations of Informed Consent*. US Government Printing Office, Washington DC, 1982.

Reich: *Encyclopedia of Bioethics*, 1978.
Truth-Telling
I. Attitudes (Veatch RM)
II. Ethical Aspects (Bok S)

Sheldon M: Truth telling in medicine. *JAMA* 247:651–654, 1982.

Placebos

Bok S: The ethics of giving placebos. *Sci. Am.* 231:17–23, 1974.

Brody H: *Placebos and the Philosophy of Medicine*. University of Chicago Press, Chicago, 1980.

———: The lie that heals: The ethics of giving placebos. *Ann. Intern. Med.* 97:112–118, 1982.

Informed Consent

Abrams, Buckner: *Medical Ethics,* III.A, 1983.

Annas G: *The Rights of Hospital Patients: The Basic ACLU Guide to a Hospital Patient's Rights.* Avon Books, New York, Chapters 6 and 7, 1975.

Meisel A, Roth L: What we do and do not know about informed consent: An overview of the empirical studies. *JAMA* 246:2473–2477, 1981.

Miller LJ: Informed consent. *JAMA* 244: 2100–2103 (Part I); 2347–2350 (Part II); 2556–2558 (Part III); 2661–2662 (Part IV), 1980.

President's Commission: *Making Health Care Decisions, Vol. 3,* 1982.

Reich: *Encyclopedia of Bioethics,* 1978.
Informed Consent in Human Research
  I. Social Aspects (Gray BH)
  II. Ethical and Legal Aspects (Lebacqz K, Levine RJ)
Informed Consent in Mental Health (Burt RA)
Informed Consent in the Therapeutic Relationship
  I. Clinical Aspects (Cassell EJ)
  II. Legal and Ethical Aspects (Katz J)
Right to Refuse Medical Care (Capron AM)

Confidentiality

Greenawalt K: Privacy and its legal protections. *Hastings Cent. Studies* 2(3):45–68, 1974.

Grossman M: Confidentiality in medical practice. *Annu. Rev. Med.* 28:43–55, 1977.

Jonsen AR, Perkins HS: Conflicting duties to patients: The case of a sexually active hepatitis B carrier. *Ann. Intern. Med.* 94:523–530, 1981.

Judicial Council of the American Medical Association: *Current Opinions of the Judicial Council of the American Medical Association–1984.* American Medical Association, Chicago, 1984.
  5.03 Communications Media: Press Relations
  5.04 Communications Media: Standards of Professional Responsibility
  5.05 Confidentiality
  5.06 Confidentiality: Attorney-Physician Relation

  5.07 Confidentiality: Computers
  5.08 Confidentiality: Insurance Company Representative
  5.09 Confidentiality: Physicians in Industry
  7.01 Records of Physicians: Availability of Information to other Physicians
  7.02 Records of Physicians: Information and Patients

Parent WA: Privacy, morality and the law. *Philosophy and Public Affairs* 12:269–288, 1983.

Pennock JR, Chapman JW (eds): *Privacy, NOMOS.* Atherton Press, New York, 1971.

Reich WT: *Encyclopedia of Bioethics,* 1978.
Privacy (Greenawalt K)
Confidentiality (Winslade WJ)

Streiff CJ (ed): *Nursing and the Law,* ed 2. Aspen Systems Corp., Rockville MD, 31–33, 95–100, 1975.

Chapter Two

Professional Codes and Ethical Theories

1 Professional Codes

Health professionals have long been concerned with ethical issues arising in practice, and they have developed statements of key ethical principles as guides in making decisions in professional practice. This chapter begins by looking at one of the oldest and most influential of the medical codes.

1.1 The Hippocratic Oath

The following version of the Hippocratic Oath is taken from Owsei Temkin and C. Lillian Temkin (1967, 6).

1. I swear by Apollo Physician and Asclepius and Hygieia and Panaceia and all the gods and goddesses, making them my witnesses, that I will fulfill according to my ability and judgment this oath and this covenant:

2. To hold him who has taught me this art as equal to my parents and to live my life in partnership with him, and if he is in need of money to give him a share of mine, and to regard his offspring as equal to my brothers in male lineage and to teach them this art—if they desire to learn it—without fee and covenant; to give a share of precepts and oral instruction and all the other learning to my sons and to the sons of him who has instructed me and to pupils who have signed the covenant and have taken an oath according to the medical law, but to no one else.

3. I will apply dietetic measures for the benefit of the sick according to my ability and judgment; I will keep them from harm and injustice.

4. I will neither give a deadly drug to anybody if asked for it, nor will I make a suggestion to this effect. Similarly I will not give to a woman an abortive remedy. In purity and holiness I will guard my life and my art.

5. I will not use the knife, not even on sufferers from stone, but will withdraw in favor of such men as are engaged in this work.

6. Whatever houses I may visit, I will come for the benefit of the sick, remaining free of all intentional injustice, of all mischief and in particular of sexual relations with both female and male persons, be they free or slaves.

7. What I may see or hear in the course of the treatment or even outside of the treatment in regard to the life of men, which on no account one must spread abroad, I will keep to myself holding such things shameful to be spoken about.
8. If I fulfill this oath and do not violate it, may it be granted to me to enjoy life and art, being honored with fame among all men for all time to come; if I transgress it and swear falsely, may the opposite of all this be my lot.

1.1.1 Self-Test   The following self-test can help explore how well you understand the Oath and some of its implications for concrete issues. The answers, with some explanation, are in the following section, but do not consult them until you have grappled with the self-test.

True/False Questions

1. *True/False*   The Hippocratic Oath is an ancient Egyptian document.

2. *True/False*   In the Hippocratic Oath, a physician promises never to perform an abortion.

3. *True/False*   It is a violation of the Hippocratic Oath for medical school faculty to accept salaries.

4. *True/False*   The Hippocratic Oath is a pagan pledge.

5. *True/False*   In the Hippocratic Oath, a physician promises to keep information about patients in confidence unless disclosure of this information is required by law.

6. *True/False*   In the Hippocratic Oath, a physician promises never to perform surgery.

7. *True/False*   In the Hippocratic Oath, a physician promises never to have sexual relations with patients.

8. *True/False*   In the Hippocratic Oath, a physician promises never to administer any drug that has potentially lethal effects.

9. *True/False*   The Hippocratic Oath implies that treatment might be forced upon patients if they unwisely refuse to consent to it.

10. *True/False*   The Hippocratic Oath forbids homosexual practices by physicians.

11. *True/False*   The Hippocratic Oath condones the institution of slavery.

12. *True/False*   The Hippocratic Oath states that a physician may choose whom to serve as patients.

Multiple-Choice Questions

A. You are a medical student. Your physiology professor is a nice guy—for example, he regularly goes to the local pub with his students on Friday afternoons. The only problem is that he never has any money on these occasions, so the students must always pick up the check. He always promises to pay the students back but to date has made no move to do so. What should you and your fellow students do about this?

   a. Confront him about this annoying practice, pointing out that he promised (when he took the Hippocratic Oath) to conduct his life, as well as his art, in "purity and holiness."

   b. Choose another pub to frequent, without telling him where you will be. This kind of freeloader you can best do without.

   c. Resolve to keep picking up the check for his drinks. After all, the code requires that you will give your teachers a share of your money when they are in need.

   d. Confront him and tell him honestly that you find this practice annoying. The code requires, after all, that you "deal honestly with colleagues."

Answer the remaining questions as if *you* were the physician involved in the case.

B. Mrs. V. brought her young granddaughter along when she came for her appointment. You notice bruises on the child's neck that seem very likely the result of child abuse. What (if anything) should you do?

   a. Ignore what you have seen, since the requirement of confidentiality forbids you from reporting this to anyone even if you had proof to back up your suspicions.

   b. Report your suspicions to the authorities, since you are required by law to report anything you observe "which is of such a nature as to reasonably indicate that it has been caused by brutality, abuse, or neglect."

   c. Point out the bruises to the grandmother and give her a chance to explain them before you decide whether to report them to the authorities.

   d. The code offers no guidance on this matter.

C. A patient in the final stages of a terminal illness tells you openly that he plans to kill himself by taking a deliberate overdose of a certain one of his medicines. You realize that this amount of this medicine will not kill him, but he would succeed if he took the rest of the bottle of another of the drugs he is on. What (if anything) should you do?

   a. Inform him that the other drug would be effective in achieving his purpose, since you owe your primary loyalty to helping the patient carry out choices he has made.

   b. Actively intervene to prevent the patient from attempting to kill himself, since the life of your patient is your first concern.

   c. The code forbids you from informing him that the other drug would be effective in ending his life.

   d. The code offers no guidance on this matter.

D. You have been treating Mr. Z. for two years in your office for severe back and leg pain that you have diagnosed as sciatica. You learn by chance that recently Mr. Z. slipped and fell while getting out of a taxicab, and, claiming he never had a backache for a day in his life before the accident, he is suing the cabdriver for injuries. What (if anything) should you do?

   a. Do not report your experience with this patient to the cabdriver's lawyer, since doing so would violate the patient's confidentiality.

   b. Report your experience with this patient to the cabdriver's lawyer, since Mr. Z. is suing him unjustly and you have pledged to protect against injustice.

   c. Make no contact with the cabdriver's lawyer, but be prepared to testify if they learn that you have been treating Mr. Z. in the past. At that point, you will be required by law to reveal information about treatment.

   d. The code offers no guidance on this matter.

E. From a friend at a party you learn that a physician in your community is doing a flourishing business administering vitamin shots, at high prices, for all sorts of maladies ranging from colds to ''tiredness'' to more serious illnesses. What (if anything) should you do?

   a. Expose this improper practice and have the physician reprimanded, since you have pledged to promote the honor of the profession.

   b. The code forbids you to intervene in any way, since this friend is not a patient of yours.

c. The code forbids you to say anything to your friend about the inappropriateness of this treatment, since you must preserve confidentiality toward the other physician.

d. The code offers no guidance on this matter.

1.1.2 Answers

1. *False.* The Oath *is* ancient, dating from about the fourth century B.C. However, it was *not* Egyptian in origin. It comes from ancient Greece. It was probably not written by Hippocrates himself (although he was the founder of the school from which it derives). [See Temkin and Temkin (1967) and Reich (1978), "Codes of Medical Ethics."] The Oath was not initially acknowledged by all physicians. The Hippocratic school was only one of several "schools" of physicians in Greece at the time, and the Oath was not accepted by the other schools.

2. *True.* This is one of several surprising provisions of the Oath, given the historical context in which it was written. Abortion was not generally frowned upon in Greek culture (although the primitive nature of the methods available made it dangerous to the mother). Not only was abortion available, but many Greeks practiced infanticide, exposing babies to die if they were born with defects. (There was a strong cultural ideal of having one's firstborn child to be a son; as a result, being *female* was considered a defect in the firstborn child and thus was sufficient reason for exposure.) Suicide was also accepted with approval by many Greek citizens and thinkers.

3. *False.* The provision this relates to is the promise to teach the art of medicine "without fee or covenant," but it applies only to *the offspring of one's teachers.* Other students are required to sign the covenant (i.e., the first paragraph of the Oath), and presumably they may be required to pay a fee for instruction as well. The only application this provision could have to present-day medical education might be to forbid charging tuition for the children of faculty members.

4. *True.* If by "pagan" is meant "non-Christian," then it surely is a pagan pledge. The deities invoked are those of the Greek pantheon. This element of the Oath was a source of discomfort to early Christian physicians who rediscovered it several centuries after it was written. In the second century A.D., one early Father of the Christian Church changed this reference in the Oath and retitled it "The Hippocratic Oath Insofar as a Christian May Swear To It."

5. *False.*This is a "trick" question. The statement of the principle of confidentiality in the question comes not from the Hippocratic Oath, but from Section 9 of the 1957 AMA Principles of Medical Ethics. The confidentiality provision in the Oath is stronger than this. It mentions no exception for legal reporting requirements or the like, stating categorically that "I will keep to myself" confidential information about patients.

One basis for tempering the strength of the Oath's confidentiality principle is its application only to that "which on no account one must spread abroad." However, it is left to the discretion of the individual physician to determine what falls inside this scope, so it would still not mandate revealing information just because the law requires it.

6. *True.* This provision (paragraph 5) must be an embarrassment to those medical students who take this Oath at their graduation ceremonies just prior to reporting for a residency training program in surgery. The origin of this provision is a mystery to scholars. Surgery was hazardous in the fourth century B.C. but was performed in desperate cases; some physicians of the Hippocratic School are even on record as having performed surgeries. There was no sharp division between internal medicine physicians and surgeons in Greek culture (as there is in British medicine, for example). Several explanations for this provision have been debated, but it may be most satisfactory to accept it as an idiosyncrasy of its authors—one of several ways in which the Hippocratic Oath is a product of its time and place and may need to be revised to provide a satisfactory basis for contemporary medical practice.

7. *True.* This is the clear implication of paragraph 6 of the Oath. The issue of sexual relationships with patients has received much attention in recent years, especially in the psychiatric community. Some psychiatrists today defend the sexual liaison as a therapeutic tool, but most medical groups agree with the strong provision of the Hippocratic Oath on this topic.

8. *False.* The pledge is made (in paragraph 4 of the Oath) not to give "a deadly drug," but this is most plausibly interpreted to refer only to drugs *designed* to produce death (e.g., poisons). Any drug has the potential of lethal side effects (at least in the rare patient who is sensitive to the particular substance contained in the drug), but the Oath's provision was not meant to rule out treatment by drugs altogether. (NOTE: This distinction between "direct effects" and "side effects" will appear again later in the book. It is central to a principle known as "the doctrine of the double effect," an important doctrine of Roman Catholic moral theology with implications for abortion, euthanasia, and other issues discussed below. For further discussion of the principle see Appendix I, Section 2.1.3.)

9. *True*. This may be put a bit strongly, but the Oath clearly makes no provision for seeking informed consent from patients prior to treatment. The physician pledges to apply therapies "in accordance with *my* ability and judgment," not in terms of the patient's judgment or preferences.

This paternalistic orientation becomes even clearer with the next sentence of the Oath (especially in light of scholarly comments based on a study of the references to it in other parts of the *Hippocratic Corpus*). The "harm and injustice" refers to harms the patient might *bring upon themselves* through improper diet and life-style, not to things *others* might do to the patient.

10. *False*. Homosexuality was practiced openly in Greek culture, and the Hippocratic Oath does not demand any especially restrictive sexual ethics in general for physicians. What it does rule out (in paragraph 6) is sexual relations of any type with one's patients or members of patients' households.

11. *False*. The reference to slaves in paragraph 6 might constitute a tacit endorsement of the institution. However, the *content* of the reference suggests a quiet opposition to slavery. Virtually every society that has had an institution of slavery has had a "double standard," in which sexual exploitation of slaves was acceptable. Thus, by applying the same standards against sexual exploitation of both slaves and freepersons, the Hippocratic medical community plants seeds of doubt about the institution of slavery.

12. *False*. This is another "trick" question. This provision is found in Section 5 of the 1957 AMA Principles, not in the Hippocratic Oath.

A. *c*. It looks as though you are stuck with the check, according to the Hippocratic Oath. Confronting him about his annoying habit (option *a* or *d*) would hardly be consistent with the demand to treat one's teachers as "equal to my parents," especially considering the deference with which Greek sons and daughters were expected to treat their parents. The quote in option *d* is not from the Hippocratic Oath.

B. *a* or *c*. As pointed out by question 5, the Hippocratic Oath does not recognize a legal demand to reveal information as sufficient basis for abridging confidentiality, so option *b* is ruled out. (The phrase quoted in this option is from the Tennessee statute requiring reporting of suspected child abuse.)

The Oath forbids the physician from reporting confidential information gained "in the course of treatment or even outside of treatment" (as specified by option *a*). However, nothing in the Oath forbids the physician from making inquiries of the patient, or (if suspicions of abuse are strengthened on the basis of the grandmother's answers) even initiating counseling with the patient. This in no way is a violation of confidentiality; and indeed, it might be seen as a laudable attempt to "keep [one's patients] from harm and injustice."

C. *c*. Paragraph 4 of the Oath clearly implies this option. On option *a*, see the comments on true/false question 9. The Hippocratic Oath recognizes no loyalty to patient self-determination, but only to the patient's best interests *as determined by the physician*.

   The Oath might require active intervention to prevent the patient from carrying out his plan (option *b*) if this were judged to be an instance of "harm and injustice." The issue of classifying and evaluating patients' requests will be discussed at length in Chapter 4.

D. *a*. This falls within the province of confidentiality, which is inviolable. The attempt to justify an abridgment of confidentiality on ground of "protecting against injustice" (option *b*) will not do, since this principle applies to injustices patients do *to themselves*, not those they do to others. The Oath makes no allowance for legal demands to reveal information (option *c*).

E. *d*. The phraseology in option *a* is taken from the 1957 AMA Principles. The Oath does not demand that practitioners monitor the practices of their colleagues. It does provide for a duty to uphold the honor of the profession in two ways: 1) by upholding the highest standards in *one's own practice* and 2) by developing a sense of "brotherhood" with other members of the profession.

   Confidentiality governs only information gained in connection with relationships with patients, not those with other physicians, so you would not be *forbidden* from expressing your view on this form of treatment to your friend (option *c*). Nor would you be forbidden to discuss this with your friend merely because she is not your patient (option *b*). However, although it would *permit* such discussions, nothing in the Oath implies that it is the physician's duty to warn persons of the improper practices of fellow professionals.

1.2 AMA Principles of Medical Ethics

The Hippocratic Oath is centuries old. The process of formulating codes of ethics, however, continues. As recently as 1980 the American Medical Association adopted a new code, presented below. (Compare this to the 1957 version of the AMA Principles, which can be found many places, including the Appendix in Volume 4 of *The Encyclopedia of Bioethics*.)

American Medical Association
PRINCIPLES OF MEDICAL ETHICS (1980)

PREAMBLE: The medical profession has long subscribed to a body of ethical statements developed primarily for the benefit of the patient. As a member of this profession, a physician must recognize responsibility not only to patients, but also to society, to other health professionals, and to self. The following Principles adopted by the American Medical Association are not laws, but standards of conduct which define the essentials of honorable behavior for the physician.

I. A physician shall be dedicated to providing competent medical service with compassion and respect for human dignity.

II. A physician shall deal honestly with patients and colleagues, and strive to expose those physicians deficient in character or competence, or who engage in fraud or deception.

III. A physician shall respect the law and also recognize a responsibility to seek changes in those requirements which are contrary to the best interests of the patient.

IV. A physician shall respect the rights of patients, of colleagues, and of other health professionals, and shall safeguard patient confidences within the constraints of the law.

V. A physician shall continue to study, apply and advance scientific knowledge, make relevant information available to patients, colleagues, and the public, obtain consultation, and use the talents of other health professionals when indicated.

VI. A physician shall, in the provision of appropriate patient care, except in emergencies, be free to choose whom to serve, with whom to associate, and the environment in which to provide medical services.

VII. A physician shall recognize a responsibility to participate in activities contributing to an improved community. (Judicial Council of the AMA 1984, ix)

1.2.1 Self-Test

True/False Questions

1. *True/False* Principles of medical ethics are developed primarily to uphold the dignity and honor of the profession.

2. *True/False* A physician has a special responsibility to seek changes in laws or other requirements contrary to the best interests of the patient.

3. *True/False* The Principles expressly prohibit receiving a commission for the referral of patients.

4. *True/False* A physician who considers responsibilities to self is unethical, for all that counts ethically is the duty to patients.

5. *True/False* The Principles explicitly acknowledge that other health professionals have rights the physician must respect.

6. *True/False* The Principles explicitly prohibit secret, proprietary remedies.

7. *True/False* A physician should never tell a patient an outright lie, not even when anything other than a lie would undoubtedly cause the patient to refuse the recommended treatment.

8. *True/False* The Principles explicitly acknowledge that a physician shall be free to choose whom to serve.

9. *True/False* A physician shall reveal confidential information whenever it becomes necessary in order to protect the welfare of the community.

10. *True/False* A physician has no responsibility to be active in politics.

11. *True/False* A physician has a duty to use the talents of other health professionals whenever the patient requests it.

12. *True/False* A physician has a responsibility to inform patients about the latest medical advances relating to their condition.

13. *True/False* A physician should respect the right of society to arrange the environment in which medical services are provided.

14. *True/False* A physician has no responsibility to society beyond rendering competent medical service to the patient.

15. *True/False* Claims of ''patients' rights'' are not given any acknowledgment in the Principles.

Multiple-Choice Questions   From the multiple-choice questions in the self-test on the Hippocratic Oath, choose the option implied by the 1980 AMA Principles. 1) In which cases would the 1980 code lead to a different choice than the Oath? 2) In what cases would it lead one to choose the same action but for a *different reason?* 3) In each case in which there is a difference between the two codes, which do you think is more satisfactory as an ethical guide?

1.2.2 Answers

1. *False*. The Preamble to the Principles states their primary purpose as "for the benefit of the patient."

2. *True*. Section III states this reponsibility explicitly.

3. *False*. This is not *stated* in the Principles, as it was in Section 7 of the 1957 version. However, it may still be implied in provisions such as that in Section II, which requires the physician to "deal honestly with patients."[1]

4. *False*. The Preamble acknowledges the propriety of recognizing responsibility to self. Ethics need not be *totally* selfless.

5. *True*. Section IV states this explicitly, although it does not delineate what these rights are.

6. *True*. The duty to "make relevant information available to patients, colleagues, and the public" (Section V) amounts to a prohibition on secret remedies.

7. *True*. Section II of the Principles says: "A physician shall deal honestly with patients." Chapter 1 described the Judicial Council's interpretation that this rules out lying.

8. *True*. This is explicitly stated in Section VI. The only acknowledged exception to this freedom is in emergency situations when no time for "choosiness" is available.

9. *False*. The stated exception to the principle of confidentiality comes from the 1957 form of the Principles. The 1980 form acknowledges only one exception: "the constraints of the law" (Section IV). Presumably this means the physician will reveal information whenever required to do so by law.

---

1. Interpreting the Principles and applying them to specific situations is delegated to a five-member body of the AMA known as the Judicial Council. Key policy statements drafted by this body are contained in a booklet entitled *Current Opinions*. Quotations from this body of professional ethical thinking are found throughout this text. With regard to the present question, the Judicial Council considers a commission for referral to be prohibited. [See *Current Opinions*, Section 6.03: "Fee Splitting" (Judicial Council 1984).]

10. *False*. Both Sections III and VII entail such a responsibility. The only effective means "to seek changes in those requirements which are contrary to the best interests of the patient" is through the political process, the most direct means to "contribute to an improved community" in many situations.

11. *False*. The obligation is to make use of such talents "when indicated" (Section V). Thus the physician must evaluate the medical indications underlying the patient's request before deciding whether to comply with it.

12. *False*. Here again, the responsibility is to "make relevant information available to patients" (Section V). But some recent medical advances may not offer promise for this particular patient, even if they do relate to the patient's general condition. Clinical discretion and judgment are required to decide what information to share and how to impart it.

13. *False*. In Section VI the Principles insist that the physician shall "be free to choose . . . the environment in which to provide medical services."

14. *False*. Additional responsibilities are described throughout the Principles, especially in the Preamble and Sections III, V, and VII.

15. *False*. Section IV acknowledges "the rights of patients," although the content of these rights is not specified. This is the first time a professional code claims the responsibility of honoring the rights of clientele.

A. *d*. Section II contains the phrase quoted in this option. There is nothing in this code to rule out the harsher action of option *b*, nor to demand the generosity of option *c*, so both of these would be *permissible*. The appeal of option *a* is to the Hippocratic Oath, so it would also not be available here.

B. *b*. Section IV of the Principles clearly indicates that confidentiality should be abridged when required by law, and the law in many states (as in Tennessee, whose statute is quoted in this item) requires reporting indications of child abuse.

   If there is genuine ambiguity about the nature of the bruises, it might be proper to offer the grandmother a chance to explain how they occurred (option *c*); but unless her explanation is compelling enough to remove any "reasonable indication" of child abuse, you must report your suspicions to the appropriate authorities. The law does not give physicians the authority to make a final determination as to whether child abuse has occurred. This authority is delegated to child protective services agencies.

C. *a*. This is a controversial answer that can be supported with reference to the 1980 Principles. Several sections can be interpreted in a way that leads to this conclusion, although in each case the interpretation may be challenged. Section I of the Principles speaks of showing "respect for human dignity"; this can be taken to include helping the patient carry out a considered choice. (This issue is discussed at length in Chapter 4.) Section II is also relevant here: to "deal honestly with patients" would surely include providing information of this nature. (Truth telling is dealt with at length in Chapter 1). Section V speaks of a duty to "make relevant information available to patients," and this can be interpreted as requiring the physician to provide the information about the other drug, since that is relevant to the patient's considered choice.

D. c. The *only* grounds specified for revealing confidential information is when it is required by law, so it would be improper to reveal anything to the lawyer now, as option *b* suggests. It may be frustrating to stand helplessly and watch an obvious injustice occur, but the principle of confidentiality stated here offers no alternative as long as there is no legal requirement that applies to the situation. However, if the cabdriver's lawyer should happen to find out that you had treated Mr. Z. and called you to testify, then you would be expected to reveal the information.

E. a. Section II clearly imposes a duty to expose these practices. It is advisable, however, to investigate this friend's charges further before taking drastic action with regard to them.

1.3 American College of Physicians Ethics Manual

A committee appointed by the American College of Physicians (ACP) developed an Ethics Manual in 1984. Too extensive to reproduce here, it can be found in the *Annals of Internal Medicine* (American College of Physicians 1984b). The Manual is also available in booklet form from the American College of Physicians (1984a).

The following questions analyze this code in the same way the previous ones did the other codes. Use the Manual if possible. Otherwise, speculate about the answers and read the "Answer" section, which contains extensive quotations from the Manual.[2]

1.3.1 Self-Test

True/False Questions

1. *True/False* In the last analysis, the patient, not the physician, determines what medical treatment is right for him.

2. *True/False* A physician who refers patients for participation in clinical investigations need not independently assess whether the

---

2. For the reader's convenience, quotations from the Manual will be followed by page citations from both the original booklet [ACP 1984a *(Manual)*] and from *Annals of Internal Medicine* [1984b *(Annals)*].

study provides adequate protection of human subjects. This is the responsibility of the institutional review board.

3. *True/False*   A physician's assessment of a patient's quality of life should never figure in clinical decisions.

4. *True/False*   The patient's diagnosis, prognosis, or treatment should not be discussed with the patient's family without the patient's express consent.

5. *True/False*   A physician ought to keep information about patients in confidence unless its disclosure is required by law.

6. *True/False*   It may be ethically proper to continue to support the body, even when clinical death of the brain has occurred.

7. *True/False*   When families oppose decisions to withhold supportive therapy for religious or other reasons, their wishes should be followed.

8. *True/False*   Resuscitation should be initiated when—and only when—there is a prospect of restoring the patient to a state of reasonable comfort and function.

9. *True/False*   Active voluntary euthanasia is never ethically justified.

10. *True/False*   When a patient faces a terminal event, the decision to resuscitate should be made by the patient himself.

11. *True/False*   A physician is not free to choose which patients he will serve if no other physician is available, as in some isolated communities.

12. *True/False*   Even if a patient indicates he prefers to have his physician make all the decisions, the physician should persist in efforts to keep the patient informed of what is being done.

13. *True/False*   If the patient elects to try a nonscientific remedy, the physician is ethically justified in severing all relationship with him.

14. *True/False*   Society has a right to control and regulate professional activities according to its own best interests.

15. *True/False*   Delegation of treatment or technical procedures to nonphysician practitioners relieves the physician of ultimate responsibility for these aspects of the patient's management, since these professionals are independently licensed and regulated by the state.

Multiple-Choice Questions From the multiple-choice questions in the self-test on the Hippocratic Oath, choose the option that is implied by the ACP Ethics Manual. 1) In which cases would the ACP Manual lead to a different choice than the Oath? 2) In what cases would it lead to a different choice than the 1980 AMA Principles of Medical Ethics? 3) In what cases would it lead one to choose the same action as one or both of these codes, but for a *different reason?* 4) In each case in which there is a difference between any two of the codes, comment on which you think is more satisfactory as an ethical guide.

1.3.2 Answers In connection with these answers, relevant sections of the Manual are quoted with the key statements in italics (all emphasis added).

1. *True.*

Patient Autonomy

Each patient is a free agent entitled to full explanation and full decision-making authority with regard to his medical care. John Stuart Mill expressed it as: "Over himself, his own body and mind, the individual is sovereign." The legal counterpart of patient autonomy is self-determination. Both principles deny legitimacy to paternalism by stating unequivocally that, *in the last analysis, the patient determines what is right for him.* Because physicians invest so much in acquiring the necessary knowledge for making the best diagnostic/therapeutic decisions, it is often difficult for them to accept the fact that what is the "best" decision for a particular patient (in the opinion of the patient) may not be the "right" decision for the patient (in the opinion of the physician). [ACP 1984a *(Manual),* 25–26; 1984b *(Annals),* 264]

2. *False.*

Clinical Investigation

. . . the premise on which all ethical research is based is mutual trust and respect between research subjects and physicians. This premise requires that physician-investigators involved in designing or carrying out research plans, or both, have primary concern for the potential subjects of these investigations. *Also, those physicians who refer patients for such studies must be satisfied that the research plans provide adequate protection of human subjects.*

. . . *Physicians referring their patients for participation must satisfy themselves that the research plans provide for informed consent, adequate assurance of safety, and an acceptably low risk/benefit ratio.*

. . . Further, in drug trials, physicians must feel free to advise their patients to withdraw from the trial and return to a standard mode of therapy or additional treatment, if such actions seem indicated." [ACP 1984a *(Manual),* 22–23; 1984b *(Annals),* 263–264]

3. *False.*

Quality of Life

Quality of life is the subjective satisfaction expressed or experienced by an individual with his current physical, mental or social situation. *Assessment by a physician of a patient's quality of life can feature prominently in making clinical decisions.* It is wise for physicians to be aware of the personal and subjective values that may contribute to such evaluations. Thus, the assessment may vary according to a physician's age, present health, history of personal illness, cultural background, and long-standing knowledge of the patient as a person. Clinical decisions that hinge on assessing the quality of life should be undertaken with great care and with full cognizance of the subjectivity of the assessment, with full patient participation, or, if that is not possible, with participation of knowledgeable and concerned relatives or guardian. Under ordinary circumstances, a physician's judgment about the quality of life of a patient should not be unilateral. [ACP 1984a *(Manual)*, 26; 1984b *(Annals)* 264–265]

4. *True.*

Care of the Hopelessly Ill

. . . The problem should not be discussed with his family unless the patient authorizes such a discussion.

. . . Physicians should not breach the confidential nature of the physician/ patient relationship by discussing the patient's care with persons who are not authorized by the patient to be made aware of the patient's diagnosis, prognosis, or treatment. [ACP 1984a *(Manual)*, 28; 1984b *(Annals)*, 265]

5. *False.*

Confidentiality

The patient's right to confidentiality of his medical record is a fundamental tenet of medical care. The physician must keep secret all that he knows about the patient and release no information without the patient's consent, unless required by the law *or unless resulting harm to others outweighs his duty to the patient.* If the physician thinks that his commitment to the patient's welfare overrides his duty to obey a court order, he may ethically refuse to give to the courts information not released by the patient but must be prepared to accept the legal consequences of his actions. [ACP 1984a *(Manual)*, 9; 1984b *(Annals)*, 132]

6. *True.*

Care of the Hopelessly Ill

The physician has a responsibility to ensure that his hopelessly ill patient dies with dignity and with as little suffering as possible. The preference of the patient in regard to use of life-support measures should be given the highest priority. *There may be circumstances in which the physician may elect to support the body when clinical death of the brain has occurred, but there is no ethical standard that dictates he must prolong physical viability in such a patient by unusual or heroic means.* [ACP 1984a *(Manual)*, 26–27; 1984b *(Annals)*, 265]

7. *False.*

Care of the Hopelessly Ill

If the patient's preference is contrary to the desires of his spouse or others, *the latter have no legal, ethical, or moral standing to enforce their desires unless a court declares the patient to be legally incompetent and appoints a guardian to make treatment decisions for the patient.*

When a do-not-resuscitate order has been written the physician must ensure that the patient is as comfortable as possible. *A decision to withhold supportive therapy, while ethically sound, may not be acceptable to some families for religious or other reasons. Their wishes must be considered but not necessarily followed.* The physician must be the final arbiter in decisions related to a patient, placing the wishes of the patient above all other considerations. [ACP 1984a *(Manual)*, 28–29; 1984b *(Annals)*, 265–266]

8. *True.*

Care of the Hopelessly Ill

Having reviewed the data on the clinical status of the patient, the physician must make a judgment as to *whether any known treatment can restore the patient to a state of reasonable comfort and function.* When treatment is judged useless, writing or giving a verbal order not to resuscitate such a patient is ethical.

A corollary observation: If a physician decides that the disease process or other medical condition that the patient has would not positively be affected by the initiation of resuscitative efforts—in other words, if resuscitative efforts would only prolong the dying process—then a decision to write a do-not-resuscitate order is ethically proper. [ACP 1984a *(Manual)*, 27–28; 1984b *(Annals)*, 265]

9. *False.*

Care of the Hopelessly Ill

Euthanasia: Active voluntary euthanasia is legally prohibited. However, *euthanasia is a classic ethical dilemma* that occurs when the ethical responsibility of the physician to preserve life, maintain the quality of life, or both, conflicts with his covenant with the patient who desires an end to pain and suffering that he considers no longer endurable or when immediate family members request termination of life for patients who are comatose or otherwise unable to exercise intellectual control.

The social, religious, and political implications of euthanasia have been discussed exhaustively. They remain controversial and will not be discussed here. While *there is no resolution of the problem on ethical grounds,* there are major legal prohibitions against euthanasia in the United States today. [ACP 1984a *(Manual)*, 30; 1984b *(Annals)*, 266]

10. *True.*

Care of the Hopelessly Ill

If the patient is a mentally competent adult, he has the legal right to accept or refuse any form of treatment, and his wishes must be recognized and honored by his physician. *He can decide whether he wishes to be resuscitated when faced with a terminal event.* [ACP 1984a *(Manual),* 28; 1984b *(Annals),* 265]

11. *True.*

A physician is free to accept or refuse to see a patient unless:
1) *no other physician is available, as in some isolated communities;*
2) emergency treatment is required under which circumstances the physician is morally bound to provide care, and, if necessary, to arrange for proper follow-up; and
3) the patient and the physician are assigned to each other under a closed-system arrangement. [ACP 1984a *(Manual),* 8; 1984b *(Annals),* 132]

12. *True.*

Informed Consent

Despite our best efforts genuine informed consent may elude us. Physician bias may be difficult to erase. There may be misunderstandings on both sides; scientific medical words often have different meanings to the patient and to the physician, and patients may use folk medical terms unintelligible to physicians. The complexities of the illness may be beyond the patient's comprehension, or he may be too frightened or sick to make a responsible decision. Also, some patients prefer to have their physicians make all the decisions. Under these circumstances the physician must assume responsibility for the patient's welfare and proceed to do what he thinks is best for the patient, but always in terms of what he thinks the patient would want for himself. *The physician should persist in his efforts to keep the patient informed about what is being done.* [ACP 1984a *(Manual),* 11–12; 1984b *(Annals),* 133]

13. *False.*

The Physician and Non-Scientific Medical Systems

Requests by patients for care outside the orthodox medical system pit the physician's commitment to provide optimal medical care against the patient's acknowledged right to choose what care he will get and from whom. Such a request warrants the physician's considerate attention. Before advising a patient the physician should determine the reason for the change: dissatisfaction with current care or merely inducement by claims for the non-scientific treatment. Next, the physician should be sure that the patient understands, in the spirit of informed consent, his condition, treatment, and outlook. He and the patient can then discuss realistically and dispassionately what the patient can expect from the two methods of care. *The physician should not abandon the patient if he should elect to try a non-scientific remedy and should accept his decision with grace and compassion.* The physician should not participate in such treatment. [ACP 1984a *(Manual),* 14–15; 1984b *(Annals),* 134]

14. *False.*

The Physician and Society

. . . Society has a vested interest in the professional activities of physicians and others in the health care field and *will seek to control* and regulate such professional activities to its own best interests as it perceives them. Society has conferred great authority on medicine in the belief that physicians will use such power for the benefit of patients. *Society has the right to require that physicians be competent and knowledgeable and that they practice with consideration for the patient as a person.* [ACP 1984a *(Manual),* 18; 1984b *(Annals),* 135–136]

15. *False.*

The Relationship of the Physician to Other Health Professionals

The interests of the patient have primacy in all aspects of the patient-physician relationship. The physician should act as an advocate and coordinator of care for his patient and should assume appropriate responsibility, especially when utilizing the help of other health professionals. The physician should deal only with competent health professionals when sharing the care of the patient. Delegation of treatment or technical procedures must be limited to persons who are known to be competent to conduct them with skill and thoughtfulness; *the physician who is primarily in charge of the patient's care must retain ultimate responsibility for all aspects of the patient's management.* Society has identified the physician as possessing the necessary training to undertake this responsibility and has granted a specific license to exercise this authority and responsibility. This relationship is implied between patient and physician. [ACP 1984a *(Manual),* 19; 1984b *(Annals),* 136]

A. *b.* Unlike the Hippocratic oath (from which the quote in *c* is taken), the ACP Ethics Manual has no special demand for respect for one's teachers. Unlike the 1980 AMA Code (from which the quote in *d* is taken), no special duty of honesty toward colleagues is explicitly demanded. Thus, you should act toward this fellow as you would anyone else who engaged in behavior you find objectionable.

B. *c.*

Medicine and the Law

Disclosure: In several areas of this manual we have discussed the physician's responsibility to the patient vis-a-vis his responsibility to society. The basic premise is that a physician bears primary responsibility to his patient, *except in those rare instances in which the societal need heavily outweighs all other considerations.* When the law specifies that a physician must inform others concerning an illness or a request for medical help, and such revelations could cause serious distress or disability to the patient, the situation is even more difficult. If the problem cannot be resolved by convincing the patient about the advisability of complying with the law, the physician must make a very difficult choice; he must decide if he is willing to violate the law for the sake of his covenant with the patient or make the decision to obey the law and jeopardize the trust of the patient. Either course of action carries significant consequences. [ACP 1984a *(Manual)*, 31–32; 1984b *(Annals)*, 267]

C. *a*. See the passage quoted under true/false question 1 for the weight given to patient autonomy in this code.

D. *b* or *c*. See the passages quoted under true/false question 5 and multiple-choice question B. The choice between *b* and *c* hinges on your judgment of the relative weights of the moral factors.

E. *a*.

Inadequate or Incompetent Colleague

It is unethical and harmful to the entire process of medical care for a physician to disparage for malicious reasons the professional skill, knowledge, qualifications, or services of another physician or to imply by word, gesture, or deed that a patient has been poorly managed or mistreated by a colleague. Use of such improper disparagement as a means of inducing a person to become one's patient is unethical. Care to avoid such improper inducement is especially necessary for the physician who has been called into consultation by another physician.

Of equal importance, it is unethical for a physician not to disclose fraud, professional misconduct, incompetence, or abandonment of a patient by another physician. The trust invested in physicians by patients and the public requires such disclosure to appropriate authorities. [ACP 1984a *(Manual)*, 16–17; 1984b *(Annals)*, 135]

1.4 Limitations of Professional Codes

Examination of these three medical codes reveals their limitations as guides to decision making in professional practice. Codes can be a helpful starting point in decision, and these shall be cited throughout this book. They are not, however, sufficient by themselves to guide decision. There are a number of difficulties.

1.4.1 Conflicts Between Codes   In the case involving suspected child abuse, different codes may yield conflicting directives. The Hippocratic Oath regards confidentiality as important enough to forbid revealing this information, even if society has determined it has a compelling need to know this sort of information and has established a legal reporting requirement. The 1980 AMA Principles, on the other hand, place the obligation to obey the law above the principle of confidentiality. The ACP Ethics Manual differs from both of the others, allowing both for revealing information not required by law (when required by a compelling social purpose) and refusal to reveal information that the law requires (on occasions in which loyalty to one's patient is judged more important than honoring the law). Which of these codes is one to follow?

1.4.2 Conflicts Within Codes   There are similar conflicts between provisions of the same code. For example, the 1980 AMA Principles contains injunctions to "deal honestly with patients" (Section II) and to show "compassion" (Section I). But what does this say about a situation in which the physician judges that to tell a patient the truth about his diagnosis would be an act of cruelty? Should one be honest and compromise the standard of compassion, or be compassionate and compromise the standard of honesty? (This issue is discussed at length in Chapter 1.) The code leaves one caught in its conflict.

1.4.3 Vague Provisions   Sometimes provisions in a code require interpretation before they can be applied to a situation. Consider, for example, the Hippocratic Oath prohibition against "giving any deadly drug." What *counts* as a "deadly drug" for purposes of this provision: any medicine with potentially lethal effects (which would include virtually all chemical substances), or only one whose primary and intended purpose is to kill (i.e., a poison)? Even more vague is the phrase in the Oath's confidentiality provision specifying that the physician ought to protect those pieces of information "which on no account one must spread abroad." What does this include, and what does it exclude? Additional interpretation is needed to apply this provision to concrete situations.

The 1980 AMA Principles have similar vague statements. Regarding the question about the suicidal patient, the phrases "respect for human dignity," "deal honestly with patients," and "make relevant information available" are all subject to interpretation. The same applies to the provision in Section IV that "a physician shall respect the rights of patients." *What* rights? Furthermore, patients may *claim* many rights that practitioners do not acknowledge as genuine. The code provision does nothing to arbitrate these sorts of disputes.

1.4.4 Unacceptable Implications   Sometimes the code provisions are clear, but some physicians may find them unacceptable on moral grounds. The most obvious example is the prohibition on surgery in the Hippocratic Oath. Perhaps that was justified in ancient Greece, when the lack of not only asepsis but also elementary anatomy made surgery a highly dangerous enterprise. But given today's sophisticated knowledge, skill, and techniques, prohibiting surgery would deprive patients of lifesaving and palliative possibilities.

More controversial are the absolute prohibitions in the Oath against abortion and mercy killing by means of drugs. As discussed in Chapter 4, many have come to conclusions at odds with the Oath. Should these people ignore their convictions and follow the code provision? Or ought the code be regarded as advisory, as a provisional guide to action, to be amended on certain occasions?

The American College of Physicians insists, with regard to diagnoses of terminal illness, that "the problem should not be discussed with his family unless the patient authorizes such a discussion" [ACP 1984a *(Manual),* 28]. However, some regions of the country and social groups expect a greater degree of openness with the family than is provided for here. The family is regarded in these areas as the unit of intimacy; free exchange of information within the unit is therefore a natural expectation. In this situation a patient would be astonished (and perhaps offended) at being asked his permission to have his medical case discussed with other members of his family; the family might be offended at having information exchange delayed while permission was sought from the patient. Furthermore, this approach may conflict with the practical necessity of talking with the family in order to corroborate the patient's history.

1.4.5 Incompleteness Finally, there are many ethical decisions on which the codes offer no advice at all. The Hippocratic Oath speaks of three sorts of therapies: diet (paragraph 3), drugs (paragraph 4), and surgery (paragraph 5). What of ethical issues arising in connection with radiation therapy? By what standard are they to be resolved? What of the issues posed by the newly developing techniques of genetic manipulation? Nothing in the Oath can guide decisions in these areas in a direct way. (Even the ACP Ethics Manual, though far more up-to-date than the Hippocratic Oath, leaves some questions unanswered—and new questions daily challenge its limits.)

Professional codes can be neither the final court of appeal nor the whole basis of decision making in health care practice. Although they are an important tool in deciding what to do (and they are used in other chapters in connection with specific cases and issues), they must be supplemented by more general, fundamental principles of ethical theory. A preliminary examination of these follows.

2 Fundamentals of Ethical Theory

2.1 Ethical Judgments

At least three judgments are associated with ethical issues.

2.1.1 Evaluative Judgments Judgments governing what is worthwhile or valuable to have or to do are evaluative judgments. For example, one might say, "That is a good car because it gets excellent gas mileage" (or "because it is comfortable to drive" or "because it looks pretty"). Or one might say, "A career in medicine is a worthwhile goal because you have the satisfaction of helping people" (or "because you can make lots of money" or "because you will find this sort of work absorbing"). In more general terms, one might judge that "the only thing that really matters is how much pleasure you get out of life. Even if you learned all there is to know, your life would not be satisfying unless you had lots of enjoyment from your knowledge.''

All these are evaluative judgments. They state goals people set in their lives (e.g., career), or they furnish the basis for choices one makes along the way (e.g., car).

2.1.2 Judgments of Moral Obligation   These are the judgments that come to mind when one thinks of ethics. They concern the choice of actions to be taken or not in a given situation. One might say, ''You really ought to write him a letter. He has written you several times, and you promised to reply if he wrote.'' Or one might say, ''You have a duty to attend the concert. Your sister is performing, and she will be disappointed if you are not present.'' Or one might speak of ''obligations,'' ''rights,'' ''the right thing to do,'' ''what one should do,'' etc.

These are obligation judgments. They embody insights about the proper choice and basis of choice of actions or omissions.

One set of obligation judgments is often singled out for special attention: claims of *rights*. As shown later in this chapter, rights claims have some special features. For one thing, the demand for action falls not on the person who *possesses* the right, but on the party or parties *against whom* the right is possessed. For example, if I have a right to be paid five dollars by you on Friday (because I loaned five dollars to you yesterday and you promised to pay me back on Friday), then the duty involved (i.e., to repay me) falls upon you, although I am the one who possesses the right. However, in spite of these distinctive features, it is most plausible to treat rights as a subclass of obligation judgments, since their focus is on the proper choice of actions and omissions.

2.1.3 Character Judgments or Judgments of Moral Evaluation   These concern evaluation of *persons* in their capacity as moral agents and assigning praise and blame to them for what they have done or have failed to do. Evaluations of agents' motives and character are central to these judgments. One might say, ''I think he is reprehensible for having done that.'' Or one might say, ''I admire her for having the courage to do a thing like that.''

Character judgments embody insights about the kind of person one ought to be, the kinds of motives one ought to develop, and the kind of character one ought to cultivate.

2.1.4 Self-Test   Examine each passage below and indicate whether it expresses an evaluative judgment (*E*), an obligation judgment (*O*), or a character judgment (*C*).

   1. *E/O/C*   ''A jug of wine, a loaf of bread—and Thou beside me singing in the wilderness. Oh, Wilderness were Paradise enow!'' (Omar Khayyam, *Rubaiyat*)

2. *E/O/C* "Brutus was an honorable man." (William Shakespeare, *The Tragedy of Julius Caesar*)

3. *E/O/C* "Thou shalt not kill." (Ten Commandments)

4. *E/O/C* "Is life so dear, or peace so sweet, as to be purchased at the price of chains and slavery? Forbid it, Almighty God! I know not what course others may take, but as for me, give me liberty or give me death!" (Nathan Hale)

5. *E/O/C* "I should not hold it desirable that either a man or a woman should enter upon the serious business of a marriage intended to lead to children without having had previous sexual experience." (Bertrand Russell, *Marriage and Morals*)

6. *E/O/C* "Man must live for his own sake, neither sacrificing himself to others nor sacrificing others to himself." (Ayn Rand)

7. *E/O/C* "Everyone who receives the protection of society owes a return for the benefit, and the fact of living in society renders it indispensable that each should be found to observe a certain line of conduct toward the rest." (John Stuart Mill, *On Liberty*)

8. *E/O/C* "It is desirable that in things which do not primarily concern others, individuality should assert itself. Where, not the person's own character, but the traditions or customs of other people are the rule of conduct, there is wanting one of the principal ingredients of human happiness." (Mill, *On Liberty*)

9. *E/O/C* "The sole end for which mankind are warranted, individually or collectively, in interfering with the liberty of action of any of their number, is self-protection. The only purpose for which power can be rightfully exercised over any member of a civilized community, against his will, is to prevent harm to others. His own good, either physical or moral, is not a sufficient warrant." (Mill, *On Liberty*)

10. *E/O/C* "It is not by wearing down into uniformity all that is individual in themselves, but by cultivating it and calling it forth, within the limits imposed by the rights and interests of others, that human beings become a noble and beautiful object of contemplation." (Mill, *On Liberty*).

11. *E/O/C* "A person whose desires and impulses are his own—are the expressions of his own nature, as it has been developed and modified by his own culture—is said to have character. One whose desires and impulses are not his own, has no character, no more than a steam-engine has a character." (Mill, *On Liberty*)

2.1.5 Answers

1. *E*. One's concept of a "paradise" is clearly an evaluative issue. Nothing is said about whether one *ought* to try to attain this state (the obligation issue) or what sort of person one is for regarding this as so important (the character issue).

2. *C*. The moral quality of Brutus' character or achievements is addressed here (by Mark Antony, in the famous funeral oration), not specifics about the rightness or wrongness of any particular actions he took (the obligation issue), nor anything about things he valued or the value he contributed to others (the evaluative issues).

3. *O*. This is a clear case of an obligation judgment. A demand is made that one refrain from certain actions. Preserving the life of others is valuable (the evaluative issue), and a person of high moral character would honor this demand (the character issue). However, although both of these judgments are *closely related* to the demand being made, they are not *directly* the subject at issue at this point.

4. *E*. This passage is harder to classify, but its primary thrust insists on the *value* of liberty. Liberty, Nathan Hale is saying, is more valuable than life itself—something worth dying for, something such that life without it is "not worth living."

5. *E*. The key word in this passage is "desirable," which gives the clue that an evaluative judgment is being made. The author is not claiming any *duty* or *laudable motive* or *trait of character*, but states merely that this would, in his judgment, be a good thing for one to do.

6. *O*. The key word here is "must," which indicates an obligation judgment.

7. *O*. The clue is the word "owes." Things we owe we have the *duty* to repay.

8. *E*. Key words are "desirable" and "human happiness." Individuality is claimed to be a good thing to develop.

9. *O*. The clues are words less common in obligation contexts than others you have encountered, but they indicate that duty is the subject. The words are "warranted" and "rightfully."

10. *C*. The clue to classification is in the last phrase. The claim that humans can "become a noble and beautiful object of contemplation" involves an evaluation of their *moral* qualities. [NOTE: Not *all* value judgments of persons are necessarily character judgments. One may consider persons and relationships with them (e.g., friendship) to be goals worth pursuing— an evaluative judgment.] However, more than that is going on here. The judgment made deals directly with the evaluation of persons from a *moral* viewpoint.

11. *C*. The word "character" is the clue that an evaluation of moral qualities is being offered.

2.2 Some Points About Ethical Theory

One way of showing the distinction between these judgments is to recognize that contrasting judgments can be made about an issue. One might say, for example, that a certain action was the *best* thing you could do (evaluative judgment), and perhaps it was even the *right* thing to do (obligation judgment), but it was *not* the *admirable* thing to do (character judgment). Suppose for example, you notice a wallet fall from a person's pocket. You go to considerable trouble to return it intact, but analysis of your motives reveals that your reason for doing so was your expectation of a large reward. (The wallet was expensive looking, and you saw the person get into a limousine after dropping it.) You may not be admired for what you did, although everyone would agree that your action was right and good.

Alternatively, one might say that a certain action was the *right* thing to do (obligation judgment) and an *admirable* thing to do (character judgment), but it was *not* the *best* thing to do (evaluative judgment). This might apply to some of the tragic choices faced daily in medical care. A patient with a terminal illness requests to be kept alive as long as possible, and the health providers comply. The suffering of the patient, family, friends, and caregivers may lead one to say it would have been best for all if the patient had not lingered so long, but honoring the patient's request seems to be the right thing to do, and the respect for the patient this decision embodies prompts admiration.

Further examples that vary the combinations of these three forms of judgment could be given, but these two should establish that these three types of judgments are distinct.

These three sorts of judgments vary in their *strength* or *weight*. The strongest of all these judgments are generally *rights claims*. If one has a right to some thing, that certain values could be promoted by violating it does not justify overriding that right. For example, if I have a right to be repaid the five dollars you borrowed from me, it is not acceptable for you to explain to me that you found a better use for the money. (See Appendix I, Section 2.1.1 for discussion of this example.) No clear-cut principles of ranking can be stated, but in general, obligation judgments are the most stringent or weighty. Character-judgments rank next, and evaluative judgments are least weighty.

2.3 Key Concepts

2.3.1 Autonomy

A. Concept of Autonomy   The notion of autonomy or self-determination was central to the discussion of informed consent, information exchange, and confidentiality in Chapter 1. It will be cited frequently in discussions throughout the book, so it is important to appreciate what it involves. The most helpful definition of autonomy comes from *Principles of Biomedical Ethics* (Beauchamp and Childress 1983, 59–60):

> "Autonomy" is a term derived from the Greek *autos* (self) and *nomos* (rule, governance, or law) and was first used to refer to self-rule or self-governance in Greek city-states. The most general idea of personal autonomy is still that of self-governance: being one's own person, without constraints either by another's action or by psychological or physical limitations. The autonomous person determines his or her course of action in accordance with a plan chosen by himself or herself. Such a person deliberates about and chooses plans and is capable of acting on the basis of such deliberations, just as a truly independent government is capable of controlling its territories and policies. A person of diminished autonomy, by contrast, is controlled by or highly dependent on others and is in at least some respect incapable of deliberating or acting on the basis of such deliberations.

This definition suggests that autonomy is multifaceted. There are a number of parameters along which autonomy may vary in degree.

Some people have gone further than others in *formulating life plans,* and the extent of applicability and coherence of sets of life plans may differ. Albert, for example, may have chosen one life goal: to practice medicine. He may be uncertain about or indifferent at present to other life issues, such as whether to marry and have a family. In contrast, Benita may have decided on two goals: medicine and motherhood. This means that, other things being equal, Benita will be more autonomous than Albert with respect to relevant specific choices, since she has two lodestars to guide her deliberations; Albert may face uncertainty. For example, Benita will find the unpredictable hours characteristic of obstetrics a consideration against pursuing this specialty and the regular hours characteristic of pathology an argument in its favor, whereas Albert may have no basis for preference on this choice at present.

This apparent advantage may vanish, however, if there are *inherent conflicts* between the multiple goals. Thus, someone who has chosen as life goals *both* 1) to avoid risk *and* 2) to experience the thrill of death-defying feats will have far less of a basis for deliberation about specific choices than one who has chosen either of these goals without the other.

There also may be variations (even between persons with equivalent sets of life plans) in the *degree* to which life plans are referred to when specific choices are being made. Thus, for example, Albert will be more autonomous than Benita with regard to choosing college courses if he makes his selections with an eye toward medical school admission requirements and strategies, whereas she chooses largely on the basis of the convenience of the time and place the courses are offered.

Another element of autonomy the definition emphasizes is the matter of *acting* on the basis of one's deliberations. For example, Albert and Benita may have calculated correctly that high grades in organic chemistry are requisite to achieving their goals of practicing medicine; but if Benita translates this realization into action through hours of diligent study, and Albert spends his evenings at the campus pub lamenting his low scores in the subject, then Benita is in this respect more autonomous than Albert. (Some may object that Albert merely exercised his autonomy differently than Benita. However, given the inconsistency of his choice with his life goal of a career in medicine, Albert's choice amounts to diminution of autonomy on his part. This would be true even if another of his life goals were to enjoy himself as much as possible, since that goal conflicts with his career goal.)

Since "a person's autonomy is his or her independence, self-reliance, and self-contained ability to decide" (Beauchamp and Childress 1979, 56), it is paradoxical to suggest that some elements of autonomy depend on the actions of others; but such is the case. For example, young children may find it difficult (if not impossible) to be autonomous unless their parents provide the *opportunity* for them to make decisions on their own. The rare, unusually rebellious child may achieve autonomy in some decisions in spite of parental opposition, but this will be the exception.

Another key example, discussed in Chapter 1, is the provision of *information* to the agent by others, which can greatly affect the agent's autonomy. Information is a central component in the process of deliberation, and thus one will be less effective in applying life goals to a situation if relevant information is lacking. For example, suppose that Carlos and Diane develop end-stage renal failure. If Carlos is never informed of the existence of one possible treatment modality (e.g., kidney transplantation) and Diane is told of all the options, she will be more autonomous than Carlos with respect to this choice, for she will be able to deliberate more effectively about which option is best in terms of her life goals. The same implication about degrees of autonomy applies to other types of information. If Diane is not told about material risks or discomforts of some of the modes of therapy, the effectiveness of her deliberations would be diminished and so would autonomy with respect to the choice.

Mental status may make a difference in degree of autonomy. Two people may be presented with identical information, but mental incapacity (e.g., mental retardation, senility, some forms of mental illness) may make one of them incapable of effectively using the information in deliberation. Something similar may happen, to a lesser degree, when a person is in a highly emotional state. Severe depression, for example, may impair one's deliberation: one may simply not *care* about the information given to him.

The actions of others also can interfere with autonomy through *constraint*. Others may limit a person's range of choices through coercion, e.g., threatening unpleasant consequences. The person who gives his wallet to the armed robber threatening "Your money or your life!" does not make a fully autonomous decision. Less drastic forms of coercion, manipulation, or constraint also diminish autonomy.

There is at least one more parameter of variance with respect to autonomy. *Uncertainties* in the situation can influence the degree of autonomy with respect to choice. If Elmer is deliberating between two familiar routes from his house to his office and Frieda is choosing between two unexplored routes from her base camp to the site of an exploratory archeological dig (selected by aerial surveys), then Elmer's choice is more autonomous than Frieda's, since he does (and can) know more about his choice than she does (or can) about hers.

This understanding of autonomy makes its achievement an ideal goal unlikely to be fully attained in practice. To be completely autonomous would require a fully articulated set of life goals that is coherent and comprehensive. One must also make *all* life decisions on the basis of deliberation by reference to these goals. This leaves no room, for example, for action based on the whims of the moment. It is an impossible goal in practice and indeed, there might be questions about whether so fully rational an approach to life is desirable.

Since complete autonomy is a practical impossibility, one must be content to make comparisons of partial autonomy, and even these are not without difficulties. Ranking the relative importance of these various sources of differences in autonomy is a puzzling task. For example, does lack of information diminish autonomy *more* than a state of depression that interferes with use of this information in deliberation? No general answer to these types of questions is possible. A case-by-case and feature-by-feature comparison is the most that can be given.

In general, individuals are "autonomous" if they are mentally competent and otherwise capable of exercising autonomy; a person "exercises autonomy" with respect to a particular choice if her decision exhibits enough features cited above to make the decision deliberative.

B. Importance of Autonomy   The importance of an autonomous state can be considered in different ways in ethical theory. At this point, some will be listed and explained. Which is *most appropriate* will be discussed in later chapters as each relates to specific issues.

Autonomy can be regarded as a positive *value*, something worth having or pursuing. Thus, each person is urged to see the development and exercise of autonomy as a personal goal, and one should recognize it as a goal for others. But there are many worthy goals, and how autonomy ranks in relation to the others would have to be determined before one could know how it ought to influence our choices.

Also in the realm of evaluative judgments, autonomy might be regarded in part as a *disvalue*. This kind of independence and freedom might be seen not as a benefit but as a *burden*. Making one's own decisions can take considerable effort, and taking personal responsibility for decisions and their consequences can stir considerable anxiety. This feature of autonomy might affect the way it is weighted against other goals. It might suggest, for example, that autonomy sometimes conflicts with the goal of happiness, and thus we have to sacrifice one of these to obtain full measure of the other.

In the realm of obligation judgments, several variations are possible. It might be regarded as merely *morally acceptable* to respect autonomy in others. It would not be morally wrong to consult others to determine their autonomous wishes and honor them in one's actions, but there would be no obligation to do this.

A stronger claim is that individuals have a *moral obligation* to respect autonomy in others: this is not only a nice and acceptable thing to do, but it would be *wrong not to*.

A different but related claim is that each person has a moral obligation to develop and practice autonomy in *his own actions*. The implication is that failing to do so is morally wrong.

It is probably most common to speak of autonomy as a moral right of the individual. The implications of this claim are examined in Section 2.3.3.

In the realm of character judgments, one might regard autonomy in the agent herself and/or the tendency to respect autonomy in others as *virtues*, that is, as traits to be admired and praised.

These possibilities are explored in later chapters. For now, the point is to understand the differences between these claims.

C. Professional Autonomy Related to personal autonomy is the notion of autonomy of professional practice. The central point is the agent's self-directed deliberation, action, and independence from external influences. The opposite of professional autonomy is social control of professional practice, which, as you saw in Chapter 1, Section 1.2.5, is widespread. Keep in mind the value—to both the practitioner and the patient(s)—of this dimension of autonomy.

2.3.2 Paternalism The concept of paternalism arises from the image of the benevolent but stern sort of father who makes decisions for his children without giving them any say in the matter. He always "has their best interests at heart," and his decisions often may be in their best interests (although they may be based on incorrect judgments about what their best interests are). His choices may be what they would choose themselves if given the opportunity, but he fails to give them the chance to participate in the decision making. (*How much* of a difference this makes and *why* are questions examined at length throughout this book.)

A comment on terminology here: Some authors use the term "parentalism" instead of "paternalism" on the grounds that the latter is sexist. The image of a dominant father, however, with its sexist overtones, is an important element of the notion's meaning, so we use the traditional term "paternalism."

Generalizing from the image of the dominant father, one can say that a person is acting paternalistically whenever he or she does something for or to another person 1) without that person's consent and 2) on the basis of the justification that "this is for your own good." Thus parents are acting paternalistically toward a small child when they yank away a bottle of poison the child is about to drink. Surely this instance of paternalism is fully justified. More controversial, though, would be for a parent to yank a bottle of beer away from her adult child "because you have had enough," yet this would still be an act of paternalism.

That paternalism involves acting without the person's consent puts it directly at odds with autonomy. To act paternalistically toward a person is *ipso facto* to deny, or to fail to respect, his or her capacity for independent deliberative choice. Thus the considerations given above *in favor* of autonomy would all count automatically as considerations *against* paternalism. If exercising autonomy is a value, then paternalism is thereby a disvalue (since it counters an exercise that is valuable). If autonomy is a duty, then paternalism is morally wrong insofar as it interferes with carrying out one's duty. If autonomy is a right, then acting paternalistically violates that right.

2.3.3 Rights   Claims of rights abound nowadays. Indeed, recent years have seen several "Bill of Rights" documents issued on behalf of patients. However, few who make these claims are aware of the philosophical complexities and questions raised by rights claims.

Rights demarcate a sphere of action within the discretion of the agent. Typically, it is within the power of the possessor of a right to choose whether to exercise the right or waive it. For example, if you have a right to be paid five dollars on Friday by someone (because he borrowed that amount from you and promised to pay it back), it is always within your power to release him from the obligation by saying: "Forget about paying it back. Let's call it a gift." In doing this, you would *waive* your right to be repaid.

One person's rights are another person's obligations. In the preceding example, your right to be paid five dollars is related to an obligation on your debtor's part to pay you the five dollars. In other examples the number of people who have obligations correlative to your rights may be much larger. Your right to freedom of speech, for example, is related to an obligation on the part of *everyone else* not to interfere with your speaking.

Some rights impose duties on others that require them only *not to interfere* with certain actions of the right-holder. (An example of this is the right to free speech.) These are called *negative* rights. Others, called *positive* rights, demand *action* by the other party. (An example of a positive right is the right to be paid back five dollars.)

The strongest and clearest rights claims are those established on a *firm basis*, e.g., by the law of the land. One serious difficulty with claims of *moral* rights is that their basis is much less clear. A related point is that the strongest rights are backed by mechanisms of enforcement that add "bite" to the individual claims made by the rights-holders. Again, the best example is in legal rights, such as the right to security of private property, which is protected by criminal penalties for theft.

In the following discussion, keep these points in mind. Variations in the basis of rights, in mechanisms of enforcement, and/or in the scope of the correlative group obligated to grant the right can make a significant difference to the strength of such claims.

Look back at the discussion of confidentiality in the previous chapter, especially the professional code principles (Chapter 1, Section 4.3). All these principles take the form of obligation judgments. Terms employed to express the principle include "should," "must," "shall," "owes," and "a right." Protecting confidentiality is something required (and failing to protect it would be wrong) and not merely a good thing to do (an evaluative judgment) or an admirable thing to do (a character judgment).

The principle of confidentiality is most naturally interpreted as stating a *right* of the patient. It has all the features of typical rights: 1) The obligation falls on someone other than the possessor of the right. In the case of confidentiality, action to preserve confidentiality is the responsibility of the health professional. 2) The patient can choose to waive this performance by the other party. In the case of confidentiality, this occurs when the patient authorizes release of information to others. 3) Since protecting confidentiality requires measures beyond mere non-interference, this is classified as a *positive* right. 4) The promulgation of this principle in professional codes such as those cited furnishes one *basis* for the right, and 5) mechanisms for professional discipline underwrite it with a certain "bite."

If autonomy is spoken of as a *right*, the chief question is whether it is a *negative* right, i.e., the obligation of others is limited to refraining from interfering with one's attempts to exercise autonomy, or whether it is a *positive* right, i.e., others have a duty to take positive steps to promote the development and exercise of autonomy. In turn, what of the scope of the group with the corresponding obligation? It may not be excessively burdensome to ascribe a duty of non-interference to everyone who comes into contact with the patient, but a duty of active assistance may amount to a considerable burden, and thus it is less plausible to impose it on everyone involved. In particular, what is the responsibility of physicians here? These issues underlie the discussion in Chapter 1 about the nature of the doctor-patient accommodation and the physician's responsibility in information exchange and informed consent.

3 Review Exercise

3.1 Instructions

The parts of this exercise make use of the following case. Read the case carefully and answer the questions with reference to it.

3.2 Case: "To Make the Parents Happy"

This case was taken from Brody (1981, 25).

> You are a pediatrician in a private practice. A mother and father bring in their four-year-old daughter, who has been complaining for three days of slight fever, runny nose, and irritability. Some of the irritability has rubbed off on the parents, and they demand rather abruptly that you prescribe an antibiotic for the child.
>
> According to your diagnosis, the child, with high probability, has a viral infection. At any rate, the infection seems to be self-limiting and you feel that no medication is required. You know that antibiotics can do no good in viral conditions and that the indiscriminate use of antibiotics is considered poor medical practice.
>
> Your first inclination, therefore, is to explain this to the parents and prescribe no medication, while encouraging them to call back if the child gets worse.
>
> However, you see that the parents have a hostile attitude, and you are aware that it is standard practice among many pediatricians to prescribe antibiotics just to save themselves the explanation and to "make the parents happy."
>
> You are certainly not looking forward to taking the time to give the parents a full explanation, and even so they might call another doctor or go to an emergency room.
>
> What should you do?

3.3 Questions

1. What is the central ethical issue in this case?

2. What *kind* of issue is it: evaluative, obligation, or character? Defend your answer. (See Section 2.1 for this distinction.)

3. Is the *patient* in this case (i.e., the child) an autonomous individual? Explain why or why not, by reference to our discussion of the concept of autonomy in Section 2.3.1.

4. Are the *child's parents* exercising autonomy in this situation? Why or why not? (Be sure to comment on the variety of factors that influence autonomy—in particular, the issues of rationality, information, and constraint.)

5. Identify at least one *factual* issue central to a decision in this case. Can you identify one *conceptual* issue that is central here?

3.4 Options for Action

The author of this case (Brody 1981, 26) identified the following alternatives for action by the pediatrician:

1. Prescribe a mild antibiotic; no explanation.
2. Try to explain why an antibiotic would not be indicated, without committing yourself to any action. If, after a few minutes, it seems that the parents do not understand or are still dissatisfied, give up and prescribe a mild antibiotic.
3. Explain to the parents the pros and cons of prescribing an antibiotic, ask them what they want, and follow their wish.
4. Same as above, but in addition to giving the pros and cons, add that you strongly recommend against prescribing. However, you will do it if they desire.
5. State, "I am not going to give your daughter an antibiotic because . . . " and then explain, taking as long as required to answer all the parents' questions.
6. State, "I am not going to give your daughter an antibiotic because in my professional judgment it can't do any good and may do some harm." Answer a few questions, but if they are dissatisfied after you have spent a few minutes with them, end the conversation by saying that if they don't like it they can see another doctor.

3.5 Additional Questions

1. Can you think of other options? Describe them.

2. Would any of these options (those presented in the text or those you suggested) embody *paternalism?* Defend your answer by reference to the discussion of paternalism in Section 2.3.2.

3. Is the pediatrician professionally autonomous in this situation? To what extent (if any) is professional autonomy compromised by the social setting of practice, the structure of prescription laws, and other factors in the context?

4. Look over any one of the medical codes discussed earlier—the Hippocratic Oath, the 1980 AMA Principles of Medical Ethics, the ACP Ethics Manual. Does this code offer guidance for the situation in this case? Defend your answer by drawing on the key provisions of the code.

5. What do *you* think the health practitioner should do? Defend your answer.

References

ACP: *See* American College of Physicians.
American College of Physicians: *Ethics Manual*. American College of Physicians, Philadelphia, 1984a.
————: American College of Physicians Ethics Manual. *Ann. Intern. Med.* 101:129–137, 263–274, 1984b.
Beauchamp TL, Childress JF: *Principles of Biomedical Ethics*, ed 1. Oxford University Press, New York, 1979.
————: *Principles of Biomedical Ethics*, ed 2. Oxford University Press, New York, Chapters 3 and 5, 1983.
Brody H: *Ethical Decisions in Medicine*, ed 2. Little, Brown & Company, Boston, 1981.

Judicial Council of the American Medical Association: *Current Opinions of the Judicial Council of the American Medical Association–1984*. American Medical Association, Chicago, 1984.
Reich WT (ed-in-chief): *Encyclopedia of Bioethics*. Macmillan and the Free Press, New York, 1978.
Codes of Medical Ethics
  I. History (Konold D)
  II. Ethical Analysis (Veatch RM)
Temkin O, Temkin CL: *Ancient Medicine: Selected Papers of Ludwig Edelstein*. Johns Hopkins University Press, Baltimore, 1967.

Further Reading

Beasley AD, Graber GC: The range of autonomy. *Theor. Med.* 5:31–41, 1984.
Childress JF: *Who Should Decide? Paternalism in Health Care*. Oxford University Press, New York, 1982.
Dworkin G: Moral autonomy. *In* Engelhardt HT Jr, Callahan D (eds): *Morals, Science, and Sociality*. The Hastings Center, Hastings-on-Hudson NY, 1978.
————: Autonomy and informed consent. *In* President's Commission for the Study of Ethical Problems in Medicine and Biomedical and Behavioral Research: *Making Health Care Decisions: The Ethical and Legal Implications of Informed Consent in the Patient-Practitioner Relationship. Vol. 3: Appendices: Studies on the Foundations of Informed Consent*. US Government Printing Office, Washington DC, 1982.
Graber GC: On paternalism and health care. *In* Davis JW, Hoffmaster B, Shorten S: *Contemporary Issues in Biomedical Ethics*. Humana Press, Clifton NJ, 233–244, 1979.
A discussion of autonomy and paternalism (including a Kantian defense of the limits of justified paternalism).

Pellegrino ED: *Humanism and the Physician*. University of Tennessee Press, Knoxville, 95–116, 1979.
A thoughtful critique of the Hippocratic tradition and exploration of issues to be included in a professional ethic adequate to today's issues.
Reich WT (ed-in-chief): *Encyclopedia of Bioethics*. Macmillan and the Free Press, New York, 1978.
Medical Profession
  I. Medical Professionalism (Pernick MS)
  II. Organized Medicine (Burrow JG)
Paternalism (Beauchamp TL)
Patients' Rights Movement (Annas GJ)
Rights
  I. Systematic Analysis (Feinberg J)
  II. Rights in Bioethics (Macklin R)
Appendix: Codes and Statements Related to Medical Ethics (Introduction by RS Gass)
Veatch RM: *A Theory of Medical Ethics*. Basic Books, New York, 1981.
Especially Chapter 1: "The Hippocratic Tradition"; Chapter 2: "The Dominant Western Competitors"; and Chapter 8: "The Principle of Autonomy."

Chapter Three

The Scope of Professional Responsibility

In Chapter 1, several important aspects of the physician-patient relationship were examined: expectations, information exchange, informed consent, and confidentiality. Drawing an analogy to a nation, one could say that most of the chapter was concerned with "domestic relations," since these topics (especially the second and third) deal with issues wholly internal to the physician-patient relationship. However, the topic of confidentiality introduces issues of "foreign relations," that is, matters that reach beyond the domain of the professional relationship and involve other persons (else who would there be to breach confidentiality *to*?).

In the present chapter this focus on "foreign relations" will continue. First, the boundaries of the professional relationship will be explored (to determine, one might say, the "national boundaries" as a reference point for border disputes with neighboring territories). Second, other loyalties will be explored that could conflict with loyalty, as a physician, to your patient.

1 The Scope of Medical Service

The 1980 AMA Principles of Medical Ethics indicate the goal of professional practice in these terms:

I. A physician shall be dedicated to providing competent medical service with compassion and respect for human dignity.

Because of the position of respect and authority physicians occupy in society, they are asked by their patients (and sometimes by the society at large) to perform many services, some of which are not obviously medical in nature. Because of their compassion for patients, physicians may try to help them out in a variety of ways, not all of which are forms of "medical services." How can you, as a physician, determine which of these are appropriate? In the following cases, try to determine:

1. which (if any) such opportunities for helping patients you have a professional *duty* to respond to, even if you are not particularly enthusiastic about getting involved,

113

2. which (if any) are a matter of your own discretion, such that you would be *warranted* in getting involved if you chose to do so, but have no obligation to address if you are not so inclined; and
3. which (if any) are really "none of your business" as a physician, such that you would be stepping outside the scope of medical practice if you became involved.

Let us explore this issue by examining a clinical situation that raises these questions in a concrete form. The scene is a family medicine practice. You are the physician. You have a full schedule of patients this afternoon.

1.1 Case: Joyce and Brent Blackspott

Your first patient is Joyce Blackspott.

Joyce (52 years old) and her husband Brent (who is 53) have been your patients for more than ten years, but you have not seen them often during that time. Joyce comes in yearly for a Pap test. Brent follows your recommendation for males in his age group and schedules a complete physical examination every three years. (His last physical was 18 months ago.) One or the other of them has seen you once a year or so for a stubborn sore throat or other minor ailment, but neither has had any major illness. You do not have any social contacts with them, so you do not know them particularly well.

Today, Joyce is here for her annual Pap test. She seems distraught, so you ask if something is troubling her.

She hesitates, but then she summons courage and says, "Oh, Doctor, I don't know whether there is anything you can do to help; but I don't know where else to turn.

"*The problem is that Brent has this black mole on his back that has been increasing in size over the past several months. I am afraid that it might be cancer. Both his father and his older sister died of cancer, and he has often expressed a fear that he will get cancer. But when I first pointed out to him that this mole seemed to be growing and urged him to have you examine it, he said I must be imagining things. I have tried to talk with him about it several times since, as the mole got larger and larger, but he gets angry and denies that it is a problem. I can tell he is concerned about it himself, though. I suspect he is thinking "What you don't know can't hurt you," but that is not correct at all in this sort of case. There is no way to get him to seek help on his own as long as he refuses to acknowledge this as a problem.*

"But he respects you, and I think he would listen to you. Would you contact him and ask him to come in to see you? Then you and I together could try to get him to face his problem and to seek help for it."

This case raises a number of questions. (Give these questions some thought on your own before reading the next section.)

1. Are there indications that Brent may have a *disease*?

2. Do you have a professional *right* to initiate contact with Brent about this matter, since he has not raised the issue himself? To what extent does the answer to question 1 influence your answer here? What *other* factors influence your answer here?

3. Do you have a professional *obligation* to get involved with Joyce and Brent's situation? To what extent does the answer to question 1 influence your answer here? What *other* factors influence your answer here?

4. a) If you decide to approach Brent, as Joyce requests, specify exactly what you would *say* to him. b) If you decide that you would *not* approach Brent, specify exactly how you would explain this decision to Joyce.

5. Suppose you contact Brent, and he angrily denies that he has a problem and refuses to come see you about it. Should you pursue the matter further? a) If *so*, what should be your next step? *b)* If *not*, specify what you would tell Joyce at this stage.

1.2 Analysis: Physician Responsibility for Health and Disease

1. *Are there indications that Brent Blackspott may have a* disease?

The answer to this question is clearly "Yes." If the "mole" is a melanoma, it represents a life-threatening disease.

Of course, it is possible that Joyce is mistaken in her perception that the mole has grown in size. Perhaps a morbid fear of cancer is leading her to imagine or exaggerate what she has observed.

But, all things considered, there seems to be adequate indication of the possibility of a serious disease to justify further investigation. If Brent came in himself with this history, you would certainly want to examine the lesion, and unless it looked obviously benign, you would probably want to biopsy.

2. *Do you have a professional* right *to initiate contact with Brent about this matter, since he has not raised the issue himself?*

The problem, of course, is that Brent himself did *not* come to see you. The awkwardness created by his wife bringing this problem to your attention confirms the point made in Chapter 1, Section 3.1.1 about the way elements of informed consent are built into the social structure of health care. If Brent had come in, his initiative would have indicated willingness to gain awareness of potential threats to his life or sense of well-being and thus could be considered tacit consent to initial steps in diagnosis and treatment.

The existence of an established physician-patient relationship may have some-what the same effect. Think back to the ideals and expectations for relationships with patients you expressed in the exercises in Chapter 1. Is it compatible with the sort of relationship you seek to establish with patients for you to take this kind of initiative in serving their health needs?

Furthermore, that Brent has seen you regularly over the years—indeed, has fully followed your recommendations for the frequency of visits—may indicate that he considers himself to have "placed his health in your hands." Surely, then, you would be justified in contacting him with regard to any and all information relevant to his health needs that comes to your attention. Tacit consent to this level of initiative on your part would seem to be implied in his practice of continuing to maintain a physician-patient relationship with you.

Suppose strong evidence came to your attention that suggested Brent generally should undergo certain screening exams more often than you had previously recommended. For example, suppose some element of his occupational setting became implicated as a risk factor for a certain life-threatening disease.[1] If you were satisfied with the level of reliability of such information, surely it would be appropriate to contact him (hopefully in a manner that would not unduly arouse his anxiety) and suggest a modification in your previous recommendations. Further-more, one would expect a positive reaction from Brent at being contacted, for he would be pleased to recognize your concern and thoroughness.

The current situation is not different in principle from this. New information has been brought to your attention that is relevant to Brent's health status, and it seems perfectly appropriate to follow this up by contacting Brent.

If Brent failed to welcome your making contact with him in this way, the reason would probably be either 1) that he is disturbed that his wife brought this information to you and/or 2) that he does not want to face the danger these symptoms represent. But both these factors can be dealt with. The first suggests that caution be exercised in the way he is approached (see item 4 for discussion of this); the second indicates that a part of the task involved is helping him come to grips with the matter.

3. *Do you have a professional obligation to get involved with the Blackspotts' situation?*

We contend that the long-standing professional relationship you have with Brent creates a responsibility for you to take any initiatives necessary to protect and

---

1. One important question that arises here is to determine the threshold of reliability that would prompt action on your part. A single case report in the literature suggesting such a connection as a bare possibility may not be enough to prompt contacting Brent. Uncertainty about data reliability has created a dilemma in connection with the results that arrive at physicians' offices from commercial multifactorial screening tests their patients have arranged independently. What is the responsibility of the physician to act upon an abnormal value on such a test?

promote his health, including contacting him to follow up on the information his wife has brought to you If this sort of action is not now standard medical practice, perhaps it *ought* to be.

> 4. a) *If you decide to approach Brent, as Joyce requests, specify exactly what you would say to him.*

This is where the caution mentioned earlier comes into play. Since there is a possibility that Brent will be disturbed by the fact that his wife brought this information to you, it is important to approach him in a way that would obviate or minimize this reaction. One possible approach is to say, "Brent, your wife has expressed some anxiety that I have been unable to dispel. Help me deal with her worries by coming in and letting me take a look at that mole on your back." By characterizing it as doing something *for his wife*, Brent may be persuaded to act whereas he would not admit (perhaps even to himself) that *he* is worried about the mole.

> 4. b) *If you decide that you would* not *approach Brent, specify exactly how you would explain your decision to Joyce.*

Since this is not the option we recommend, we leave it to those who choose this route to find their own way to deal with this chore that attaches to their choice. Good luck!

> 5. *Suppose you contact Brent, and he angrily denies that he has a problem and refuses to come see you about it. Should you pursue the matter further?*

Here again, the justification for any further action on your part would be rooted in your established professional relationship with Brent. There could still be a general question as to whether Brent's refusal is an *informed* one.[2] Unfortunately, even if his refusal is *not* adequately informed, you have no basis (absent an established professional relationship) for intervening. However, given an established relationship, we contend that you would be warranted to take *some* further steps to 1) urge him to see you for examination of the mole and/or 2) inform him about the risks he is running in refusing to do so.

Perhaps it would amplify this discussion of Joyce and Brent Blackspott to step away from this specific case for a moment and relate their situation to some general points about medical practice.

---

2. The law does not appear to recognize a requirement on the patient's part to base refusals of treatment on as much information as decisions to accept treatment. However, an argument that there is a *moral* requirement to this effect will be presented and discussed in Chapter 4, Section 2.2.1.D.

2 The "Moral Center" of Medicine

Our understanding of a subject is often heavily influenced by an image of its "heart" or "center." This core example (or "paradigm case" as it is sometimes called) plays an important role in definition and analysis of concepts; it also has a function in determining our sense of values or our judgments of right and wrong. The paradigm case is regarded as "real medicine" in a conceptual sense, and it seems more obviously *justified* as a field of action for the practitioner. Situations that depart from this paradigm are not only less fully deserving of the conceptual label "medicine" but they also require some justification for being included within professional practice. (There may be an inclination to ask: "What is a nice professional like you doing engaged in an activity like this?") It may appear that the professionals have, perhaps inadvertently, stepped across the border of their home territory and begun to encroach on foreign soil.

Edmund Pellegrino (1979, 222–230) has called this paradigm situation the "moral center" of medicine. The discussion of expectations in Chapter 1 (and, we would venture to guess, your responses to the exercise in Chapter 1, Section 1.1) points toward a particular conception of this paradigm, which is examined in the present section. As you read, locate your fantasies and reflections about expectations within the spectrum of medical activities described. Also, evaluate your claims. Do you agree that there is one specific type of activity with the central place we describe? Do you agree that the one we identify occupies this position? What implications do these claims have for the expectations of all parties involved? What are specific implications about the situation of Joyce and Brent Blackspott?

2.1 Content of the Moral Center

One pair of authors (Jonsen and Jameton 1977) describes the content of the medical paradigm as follows:

a. diagnosis and treatment
b. of an illness or injury
c. for an individual
d. who presents a complaint
e. within the context of an established therapeutic relationship.

An interaction with all these features clearly present is *real* medicine. An individual patient presents to a physician with whom a relationship has been previously established, bringing a specific complaint that points toward a clearly defined illness or injury. The physician diagnoses and treats the condition.

(*Thought exercise:* Are all these elements *equally important*? If not, rank them in order of their importance to your decision making in specific cases. Keep this ranking in mind in the discussions that follow.)

Pellegrino and Thomasma clearly presuppose something very close to this description throughout their book, but in the following passage, they state the *goals* of the paradigm medical interaction: "The end of medicine . . . is therefore a right and good healing action taken in the interest of a particular patient" (Pellegrino and Thomasma 1981, 211).

2.2 Importance of the Moral Center

Why is this situation the center of our thinking about medicine? What is so important about it? Several suggestions have been offered.

Jonsen and Jameton (1977, 388–389) point to two factors that give special importance to the relationship: First, there is the fact that the relationship was established through deliberate acts of both patient and physician. Thus it is a relationship that both parties *took upon themselves*, an especially personal relationship. Second, there is the fact of the proximity of the patient. Here one is dealing with "actual and present persons, not statistical and future persons." This serves to heighten the physician's obligations.

Pellegrino and Thomasma (1981, 207–212) also stress two (somewhat different) factors: First, there is the vulnerability of the patient as a result of his illness. The special *needs* the patient has give rise to an especially gripping obligation for the physician to attempt to meet them. Second, there is the content of the "profession" or pledge made by the physician upon entering the profession of medicine that he or she "can and will help" the patient. By entering the professional field, the physician has made a promise to address the needs of patients.

Charles Fried (1974, 67–78) subordinates all of these more general moral considerations to something much more specific and intrinsic to the relationship:

. . . the relationship of assisting a person in need is an action and a relationship which have a special integrity of their own. They form a unit, a unit of value . . . . (p. 69)

. . . the notion is one of doing unstintingly what it is that one does, though choosing with care the occasions on which one will do it. (p. 75)

. . . this ideal implies an interest and a right on the part of the doctor as well to maintain the integrity of his activity, to work not as a tool or as the bureaucratic agent of a social system, but as one whose professional activity is a personal expression of his own nature, the relationships he enters into being freely chosen, the obligations freely assumed, not imposed. (p. 77)

2.3 The Blackspotts and the Moral Center

In your interaction with Joyce Blackspott, the element of the moral center most obviously missing is item *c*: the one-on-one relationship between the practitioner and the patient who has the illness. Instead, you are confronted with three entities: the wife's concern that prompts her to bring the information to your attention; the danger to the husband that the information suggests (although the presence of item *b* cannot be confirmed until after analysis of a biopsy); and the long-standing relationship of each person to you.

In considering Brent Blackspott as the patient, the chief element of the moral center that is lacking is item *d*. He refrains from presenting any complaint, although you learn from his wife that he may have reason to come to you.

As indicated earlier, we contend that given 1) the seriousness of the disease and 2) the on-going relationship between you and Brent, intervention is appropriate.

2.4 Additional Cases

What are the *limits* of this justification? Examine each of the following situations, asking yourself the same questions you did in the situation of Joyce and Brent Blackspott. If you are *not* willing to draw the same conclusion in each of these cases, try to identify what it is about the situation that makes the difference. [NOTE: The only parts of the case described are the elements that *differ* from the case of the Blackspotts. Look back at the full statement of that case (Section 1.1) and replace the section in italic with the information given for each case.] Your day in the office continues . . . .

2.4.1 Joyce and Brent Phthisis   Your next patient is Joyce Phthisis.[3]

"The problem is that I am afraid Brent has developed tuberculosis. He had a negative skin test a year ago, shortly after his father developed TB and came to live with us; but in the past few months, he has had a chronic cough, and I have noticed lately that he has coughed up blood several times (although he has tried to keep me from seeing this). I have tried to talk with him about this several times, as the cough seemed to get worse and worse, but he gets angry and denies he has a chronic cough or that he has coughed up blood. I can tell he is concerned about it himself, though. There is no way to get him to seek help on his own as long as he refuses to acknowledge this as a problem."

Consider these additional questions about Brent Phthisis:

1. Does the risk of exposure to Brent Phthisis' wife and children justify action on the part of the physician in this case?

2. Should the possibility of disease be reported to the area TB control officer?

---

3. If this name is unfamiliar, look it up in your medical dictionary!

3. Is there an obligation to warn others? If so, who: Brent's family, his co-workers, other associates, his clients?

2.4.2 Joyce and Brent Enditt   Your next patient is Joyce Enditt.

"The problem is that I am afraid Brent is going to kill himself. He has been getting more and more depressed over the past year, since he was passed over for promotion at work. He has talked about suicide several times in the last few months; now he has bought a shotgun, although he never had any interest in guns before. I have tried to talk with him about it several times, as his depression increased, but he gets angry and denies he has any problem. There is no way to get him to seek help on his own as long as he refuses to acknowledge this as a problem."

Consider these additional questions about Brent Enditt:

1. Is depression a *disease*?
   a. If not, how does it *differ* from conditions you would be willing to call diseases? Is this degree of depression obviously less *dangerous* (i.e., less likely to lead to harm to Brent and others) than, for example, tuberculosis?
   b. If you are willing to call it a disease, on what basis do you do so? Compare and contrast it with other diseases and nondiseases.
2. Should your decision be influenced by the possibility that approaching Brent Enditt might *provoke* him to carry out his threat? Is this a real danger?
3. What influence is contributed by your close relationship with Brent?
4. What is the influence of medicolegal considerations on your decision whether to intervene?

2.4.3 Joyce and Brent Martini   Your next patient is Joyce Martini.

"The problem is that I am afraid Brent is becoming an alcoholic. He has always had two or three martinis in the evening, but over the past year or so, his drinking has steadily increased to the point that he now drinks himself into a stupor every evening. He often stops by his club on the way home, and he is drunk by the time he gets here. I have tried to talk with him about it several times, as the problem has progressed, but he gets angry and denies he has any problem with drinking. There is no way to get him to seek help on his own as long as he refuses to acknowledge this as a problem."

Consider these additional questions about Brent Martini:

1. Is alcoholism a *disease*?
   a. If not, how does it *differ* from conditions you would be willing to call diseases? Is this level of alcoholism obviously less *dangerous* (i.e., less likely to lead to harm to Brent and others) than, for example tuberculosis?

    b. If you are willing to call it a disease, on what basis do you do so? Compare and contrast it with other diseases and nondiseases.

2. What influence should the unpleasant nature of treating alcoholics have on your decision whether to approach Brent Martini? Would you react in the same way if Brent's problem were increasing obesity, for example?

3. What influence on your decision is contributed by the recognition that there is a high probability of failure in overcoming the condition without a strong personal commitment on the part of the patient to change?

4. What difference does it make to your thinking here that the most successful approach for this problem is not a medical treatment but a support group of laypeople who formerly suffered from this condition themselves (i.e., Alcoholics Anonymous)?

2.4.4 Joyce and Brent Kant   Your next patient is Joyce Kant.

"The problem is that over the past year or so, Brent has gradually lost the ability to maintain an erection. We have always had an active sexual relationship, and I have always (well, *almost* always) been a willing and eager partner. But he has been avoiding sex lately; obviously his problem distresses him. I have read that worrying about this sort of thing often aggravates the problem. I have tried to talk with him about this several times, as the problem has progressed, but he gets angry and denies he has any problem. He just says, "Sex isn't everything, you know" as if *I* were the one who has the problem. I can tell he is concerned about it himself, though. There is no way to get him to seek help on his own as long as he refuses to acknowledge this as a problem."

Consider these additional questions about Brent Kant:

1. Is impotence a *disease*?

    a. If not, how does it *differ* from conditions you would be willing to call diseases? (Must a condition pose a threat to *life* in order to classify as a disease, or is it sufficient that it involves disability in some normal human functioning?)

    b. If you are willing to call it a disease, on what basis do you do so? Compare and contrast it with other diseases and nondiseases.

2. What difference does it make to your decision that you might find such a discussion with Brent Kant personally uncomfortable?

2.4.5 Additional Questions: General

1. For each of these cases, list some key ways in which the situation illustrated exemplifies the "moral center of medicine." List some key ways in which it departs from the moral center.

2. Rank the cases from strongest to weakest in terms of the strength of the professional right to initiate contact with the husband.

a. To what extent does a high index of suspicion that a *disease* is present influence your answer here?

b. You were asked earlier to rank the elements of the moral center of medicine in order of their importance to your decision making. What influence did this ranking have on your reaction to these cases? To what extent might a reordering of these priorities change your answer in these cases?

3 Beyond the Moral Center

Medicine extends beyond the core defined by the moral center in a variety of ways. (In terms of the geographical metaphors with which this chapter began, we might say that some exploring is done beyond the borders of the central territory—and perhaps even some homesteading takes place if the territory is found to be hospitable.) However, each step away from the paradigm requires some justification (and even then it may retain a flavor of not quite being real medicine). Let us look at some of these expansion areas.

3.1 Research

3.1.1 Day-to-Day Learning in Clinical Practice The descriptions of the moral center given earlier are incomplete in an important way. The fact is that benefiting this specific patient is not the *entire* goal in typical clinical interchanges. At the same time the physician is figuring out the "right and good healing action taken in the interest of a particular patient," she is working to strengthen her own clinical skills and increase her general knowledge of specific disease processes. (You can see this goal at work when the physician reads an article that comes across her desk the day *after* the patient for whom it would be relevant has died or been discharged from the hospital. Preparation for the *next* patient is suggested.)

This is a research and/or learning component in everyday clinical medicine. You try a new antibiotic with an eye *both* to aiding this patient and to testing its usefulness for future patients. If the dosage you tried this time appears insufficient, you may increase the dosage for your next patient and see whether effectiveness is improved. If not, you may try a still different antibiotic, or a new combination of them, with future patients.

At least this much of a research orientation is implied in the Section V of the 1980 AMA Principles of Medical Ethics: "A physician shall continue to study, apply and advance scientific knowledge. . . ."

This focus may create conflicts of loyalty within clinical practice. Invasive and expensive diagnostic tests sometimes may be employed in search of a remotely possible "zebra" or "fascinoma"—often to the exclusion of more likely approaches far more effective in addressing *this patient's* complaint. This fascination with knowledge for its own sake is a self-indulgence. It may have beneficial effects in keeping one's knowledge up to date and one's intellectual skills fresh, but it can interfere with the process of reaching the "right and good healing action" for this particular patient.

Think back to the ideals and expectations for the physician-patient relationship you expressed in the exercises in Chapter 1. Consider whether, and to what extent, the pursuit of knowledge for its own sake is compatible with the sort of relationship you want to develop with patients.

3.1.2 Clinical Research   Clinical research is in spirit an extension and formalization of this learning component of clinical practice. As such, it is clearly different in important respects from the moral center of medicine. For the researcher, the goals of the interaction with the patient are not limited to benefiting the individual patient being treated. Rather, there is a coordinate goal of gaining knowledge that will benefit a whole group of future patients. Hence, virtually all of the elements of the paradigm, moral center case are either absent or altered in significant ways. The focus is on gaining knowledge rather than exclusively on diagnosis and treatment (item *a*) of this specific patient's complaint (items *b* and *d*), although helping this patient certainly may be a central goal as well. The intended beneficiary is the group of future patients rather than (or in addition to) this individual patient (item *c*). And the nature of the relationship (see item *e*) is changed as a result of this altered focus.

3.1.3 Rationale   The rationale for including clinical research as a part of the mission of medicine is that acquiring new knowledge is necessary to enhance effectiveness of the central activity. It will be possible to provide the sort of help patients seek only if we continue to broaden our understanding of the nature of disease and human response to illness and, on this basis, develop new modalities of treatment. Hence research is closely related to the central purposes of medicine, even though it is also to be distinguished from paradigm activities.

3.1.4 Conflicts of Loyalities   The danger here of course is that a conflict may arise between one's loyalty to the present patient and the goal of acquiring knowledge that may benefit future patients. Personal motives of eagerness to establish or maintain a professional reputation (e.g., relentless pursuit of the reportable case) may lead to a violation of the loyalty owed to specific patients (i.e., to the comparative neglect of less "interesting" cases). The popular press has offered "exposés" of several instances of alleged wanton disregard for the welfare of patients in the interest of gaining medical knowledge or statistical significance.

However, even with the best motives in the world, it is not easy to avoid difficulties in this area. Complex and difficult judgments must be made, balancing the value of the knowledge to be gained against the risk to the patient/subject present before you. These judgments are made even more difficult by the inevitable elements of uncertainty attending the situation. (After all, if there were not uncertainty, there would be no reason to do *research* in the area.)

3.1.5 Federal Regulation of Research   In recognition of the complexity of these decisions, the federal government has taken action to review and regulate research involving human subjects. The structure for this review comes from the Code of Federal Regulations (CFR), Title 45, Part 46—Protection of Human Subjects (revised as of March 8, 1983). This was devised over a number of years by the National Commission for the Protection of Human Subjects, and has some features worth noting.

A. Decentralization   The application of regulatory standards to specific cases is thoroughly decentralized, rather than being assigned to some central bureaucratic office at the state or federal level. The regulations require that each institution in the nation receiving federal funds for research establish an Institutional Review Board (IRB); this body has the responsibility to evaluate specific research protocols.

B. Diversity of Viewpoint   Membership on the IRB must be diverse in order "to promote respect for its advice and counsel in safeguarding the rights and welfare of human subjects." The research sciences must be represented to provide expertise needed to understand the issues involved in the research project under review, but there also must be representatives of other groups within the institution and from the community.

C. Elements to be Evaluated   Requirements that must be satisfied in order to approve a research project include:

1. minimization of risks to the subjects
2. reasonable risks to subjects in relation to the anticipated benefits (if any) to them and the importance of the knowledge reasonably expected to result
3. equitable selection of subjects
4. acquisition of informed consent from each prospective subject or the subject's legally authorized representative [A detailed list of the basic elements of informed consent is included in the regulations (45 CFR 46.116).]
5. appropriate documentation of informed consent
6. provision for monitoring the data collected to ensure the safety of subjects
7. provisions to protect the privacy of subjects and to maintain the confidentiality of data
8. appropriate additional safeguards to protect the rights and welfare of especially vulnerable subject populations (45 CFR 46.111).

However, it is left to the local IRB to determine, in terms of its own understanding of the elements involved, whether a given research protocol satisfies these requirements.

D. Expedited Review   Procedures that involve "no more than minimal risk" may be subjected to expedited review by a subcommittee or representative of the IRB, rather than having to await full-scale review by the entire IRB.

E. Wide-Ranging Authority   The IRB has authority to monitor the informed consent process and the conduct of the research, and to engage consultants and advisors to assist in evaluating the project proposal or activities involved in its execution.

The goal of this review process is to assist investigators, with a minimum of bureaucratic hassles, in resolving the complex loyalty conflicts that arise in designing research. (Some researchers may dispute this analysis, seeing plenty of "red tape" involved in the process as it stands—but this is a matter of perspective.)

3.2 Other Potential Conflicts of Loyalties

Parallel issues occur in other areas in which loyalties that develop for the physician may conflict with loyalty to the immediate patient.

3.2.1 Clinical Training   Here again, goals other than the healing action for this individual patient are important—in particular, training future practitioners who can aid future patients. The clinical teacher deals with the immediate patient indirectly, through the clinical interaction of the student practitioner; the trainee deals with the immediate patient, with the twin goals of rendering care and developing personal skills for future use. The rationale for this enterprise is clearly the need to provide skilled health care for other patients now and in the future.

The notion of the moral center implies some important guidelines for teaching activities. (1) Students should not initiate procedures on patients until they are sufficiently skilled to render "the right and good healing action for a particular patient." This core value must not be compromised in the interests of training. (2) Clinical teachers must convey the other elements of the moral center in their own interactions with patients (and with students, insofar as similar norms are applicable) to provide a role model for their students.

3.2.2 Company Physician   The physician employed by an industry promotes the health of workers. This may be accomplished through a variety of activities, including:

1. Monitoring the health effects of the work environment and perhaps establishing a baseline for potentially hazardous elements in the environment.

2. Preemployment physical examinations to determine the fitness of a person for working in that environment. (This may necessitate a detailed individual health history to assess its relevance to conditions in that environment. For example, the risk of lung damage for workers in a uranium mine is apparently greatly increased if they smoke. Hence, a physician must inquire about this risk factor in a preemployment physical.)
3. Physical examinations to determine the safety to the employee and others of having that employee return to work at a certain stage of recovery from a job-related injury.
4. Physical examinations to determine the safety to the employee and others of having that employee return to work at a certain stage of recovery from illness or non-job-related injury.

However, these goals may conflict in several ways with loyalties to the individual patient. These conflicts are addressed by the Judicial Council of the AMA (1984, 23):

> *5.09 Confidentiality: Physicians in Industry.* Where a physician's services are limited to pre-employment physical examinations or examinations to determine if an employee who has been ill or injured is able to return to work, no physician-patient relationship exists between the physician and those individuals. Nevertheless, the information obtained by the physician as a result of such examinations is confidential and should not be communicated to a third party without the individual's prior written consent, unless it is required by law. If the individual authorizes the release of medical information to an employer or a potential employer, the physician should release only that information which is reasonably relevant to the employer's decision regarding that individual's ability to perform the work required by the job.
>
> A physician-patient relationship does exist when a physician renders treatment to an employee, even though the physician is paid by the employer. If the employee's illness or injury is work-related, the release of medical information as to the treatment provided to the employee may be subject to the provisions of workers compensation laws. The physician must comply with the requirements of such laws, if applicable. However, the physician may not otherwise discuss the employee's health condition with the employer without the employee's consent or, in the event of the employee's incapacity, the family's consent.
>
> Whenever statistical information about employee's health is released, all employee identities should be deleted. (IV)

One interesting aspect of the foregoing statement is the insistence, even in the situations in which no physician-patient relationship is in force, that the duties of confidentiality still must be carried out. One would expect parallel judgments about other loyalties inherent in the physician-patient relationship.

3.2.3 Military Physician The physician in the military faces a similar sort of dual loyalty. If the absolute best interests of the patient were the sole consideration in the military physician's mind, the prime advice to be given to every patient would undoubtedly be "Go home. You can get hurt here." Service in battle is obviously fraught with hazards, and even military training carries considerably more risk of injury than almost any civilian occupation.

However, as a military employee, the physician is committed to the goal of preserving and enhancing the patient's capacities to serve in the organization. If the physician accepts the premise that maintenance of a military force has a social value, then he may not have special difficulties of conscience about promoting this goal. However, even then there is still the problem that this goal may sometimes conflict with what is felt to be in the best interests of the patient's health.

One step toward reconciling these dual loyalties is to recognize that another aspect of one's goal is an attempt to *minimize* the risk to the individual patient. This can be accomplished through careful monitoring of the health status of individuals, as well as evaluating the risks inherent in proposed activities.

The physician also is obligated, by virtue of a pledge made upon joining the armed forces, to follow detailed regulations concerning the practice of medicine. On occasion this may conflict with specific professional judgments; thus the individual will have to consider whether to abide by the regulations in the situation at hand. (For examples, watch any episode of "M*A*S*H*.")

3.3 Conflicts of Loyalties: Toward a Policy Solution

How can the conflicts of loyalties arising in these and other situations be avoided and/or resolved? Several proposed policy solutions will be discussed in the present section.

3.3.1 Absolute Priority to the Patient's Welfare The traditional way of dealing with this sort of situation is to insist that the patient's welfare take absolute priority in any situation of conflict. This, for example, is the spirit of the following provision from the Declaration of Geneva: "The health of my patient will be my first consideration."[4] However, this sort of statement is extremely vague and thus may not be easy to apply in concrete situations.

Furthermore, it seems unrealistic in the extreme form in which it is stated. Surely it is not unreasonable to increase the cost (or even the risk) to a given patient by a small amount (say, by ordering an additional blood study that may not be absolutely necessary for effective management of this patient's case) in the interest of gaining knowledge that could provide considerable benefit to future patients. After all, it can be argued that patients have some *obligation* to contribute to medical knowledge, since they are beneficiaries of past research in the care they have received.

4. World Medical Association, 1948.

This standard can serve usefully, nevertheless, as a focus for self-examination: which loyalities have primacy in your own decisions? But more concrete guidelines are needed to structure evaluation of choices and motives.

3.3.2 The Golden Rule Another guideline that has been appealed to is the Golden Rule: "Do unto others as you would have them do unto you." However, this may have problems, especially in the research context. Stated without restrictions, the Golden Rule can serve as an invitation to impose our own personal value choices on other people. The clinical researcher, for example, is likely to strongly favor research values and thus would probably be willing to be used as a subject of clinical research, if appropriate. (Witness the many researchers who have volunteered as subjects in their own or colleagues' projects.) But the fruits of clinical research may not be valued as highly by other patients, and thus it would be a violation of their own value priorities to apply the Golden Rule to them in this way.

3.3.3 Informed Consent "The best way to tell whether the shoe pinches is to ask its wearer." Similarly, the best way to determine whether a given step to promote knowledge would be acceptable to the patient is to ask the patient. More generally, informing the patient of possible conflicts of interest can put the individual on guard so that later choices can be monitored from that perspective. For example, with regard to one specific area of possible conflict, the Judicial Council of the AMA (1984, 14–15) relies on disclosure as a primary patient protection:

> *4.04 Health Facility Ownership by Physician.* A physician may own or have a financial interest in a for-profit hospital, nursing home or other health facility, such as a free-standing surgical center or emergency clinic. However, the physician has an affirmative ethical obligation to disclose his ownership of a health facility to his patient, prior to admission or utilization.
>
> Under no circumstances may the physician place his own financial interest above the welfare of his patients. The prime objective of the medical profession is to render service to humanity; reward or financial gain is a subordinate consideration. For a physician to unnecessarily hospitalize a patient or prolong a patient's stay in the health facility for the physician's financial benefit would be unethical.
>
> If a conflict develops between the physician's financial interest and the physician's responsibilities to the patient, the conflict must be resolved to the patient's benefit. (II)

A parallel procedure could be helpful in other areas of possible conflict, such as clinical teaching, clinical research, company employment, or military status. In each case, revealing to the patient the potential conflict is a first step. This should be followed by a thorough provision for informed consent for each specific element of the interaction. A willingness to share with patients the *basis* for recommendations being made is essential to allow them to resolve for themselves any questions about the influence of external loyalties. When a given procedure serves primarily an external goal (e.g., the blood study for clinical research purposes), this could be explained to the patient. If the patient is convinced of the value of this purpose, he will agree to the procedure. If the patient cannot be made to see the point, perhaps it should not be done.

3.3.4 Peer Review   Traditionally, one powerful safeguard against overzealous pursuit of loyalties that conflict with the welfare of patients has been various formal and informal mechanisms of peer review. The most formal variety of peer review takes place in hospital practice, through tissue review, death review, and quality-assurance review procedures.

The cooperative nature of hospital practice (which will be discussed in some detail in Section 3.5) also provides additional peer review. The consultants called in to assist with aspects of a patient's care will review the entire chart and thus have an opportunity to evaluate the decisions being made by the primary physician and by other consultants involved in the case.

The teaching hospital intensifies this element of peer review still further. Cases are discussed in depth by a variety of faculty physicians, even without formally requested consultations; in addition, the questioning and intellectual exploration of the issues by physicians-in-training may prompt rethinking of all elements of decision making.

Less formally, the medical community's "standard of care" has an influence on the decisions of individual physicians. The effect of this via its possible use in legal proceedings is perhaps the most obvious basis of its appeal, but this is far from the whole story. A consensus reached by the professional community on an issue is to be taken seriously in one's own decision making on the matter.

Trends are developing that may establish national norms by specialties, and perhaps even lead to the formation of algorithms for clinical decisions. If these continue to gain acceptance, they may become the basis for evaluation in much of the peer review process. This development would be regrettable, in our judgment, if it resulted in the application of these algorithms in a mechanical way. Much to be preferred are case-by-case judgments based on interpretation of the particulars of the individual situation and on standards that have gained understanding and acceptance through thorough debate among those who apply them.

Another mechanism that can serve as a safeguard against gross violations of professional ethics is the possibility of professional sanctions for improper practice.

One issue for discussion is the extent to which peer review and other "checks and balances" are likely to be preserved in the forms of medical practice likely to predominate over the next few decades.

3.3.5 Legal Liability The spectre of a malpractice suit can also serve as a safeguard against improper choices among conflicting loyalties. One is likely to think through a choice especially carefully if he realizes that it might have to be explained and defended in a courtroom. (This is not to say that the current increase in the number of malpractice suits is wholly benign in its effects. Our claim here is only that the possibility for legal redress by the patient may have *some* good effects, even though other effects may be far from beneficial to anyone concerned.)

3.3.6 Other Safeguards Additional mechanisms may help to guard against conflict of interest. For example, the American Heart Association has considered a policy stipulating that the cardiologist who determines the need for coronary arteriography ought *not* be the person who does the procedure (and thereby profits from it). This is intended to remove any temptation of making such a decision on the basis of profit motives.

Similarly, the following guideline might be proposed as a device for checking your motives in connection with a decision you face: Consider whether you would still regard the procedure as necessary if it were to be carried out by (and thereby profit) the specialist you most *dislike* personally. If you are sufficiently convinced of the clinical value of the procedure to answer affirmatively, then the procedure is probably needed.

3.4 Family Medicine

As the goal of family medicine is to take the *family* as the unit of care, it departs from item *c* of the paradigm. This may create problems in practice when the interests of the individual appear to conflict with those of the family unit. [For one example of this sort of case, see Eaddy and Graber, (1982).]

The rationale for this step beyond the paradigm is that this wider focus is adjuvant to the central, individually-oriented practice, since the roots of an individual patient's problem and/or the means to alleviate it may lie in family dynamics and home environment.

3.5 Team Care

Just as focus on more than one patient is a step away from the moral center, so is involvement of more than one health practitioner. The "established therapeutic relationship" referred to in item *e* of the paradigm is clearly a one-on-one relationship.

The rationale for this step away from the paradigm is to enhance the effectiveness of treatment. The burgeoning complexity and technical sophistication of today's medicine make it impossible for the primary physician to master all the skills required to render ideal medical care for all patients at all times. This has led to specialization and differentiation of roles in the health professions and to cooperative team efforts in dealing with individual patients.

These developments present three especially important challenges:

1. To preserve the strengths of the traditional physician-patient relationship with the primary physician in an atmosphere of diversified (fragmented?) treatment.
2. To foster appropriate features of the physician-patient relationship (notably trust, honesty, and candor) with other members of the health care team.
3. To develop cooperative working relationships among members of the health care team for the benefit of the patient.

3.5.1 Expectations in Interprofessional Relationships   The following exercise is designed to help you think about these issues *before* reading the guidelines offered in the following sections. Think of specific examples from your own experience in dealing with consultants. Answer the following questions by generalizing from elements of these situations that you found especially satisfactory and elements you found frustrating. The first exercise focuses on relationships with physician consultants; the second focuses on dealing with nurses, technicians, and other nonphysicians involved in cooperative efforts in the care of patients.

A. Physicians

1. Spell out what you expect from consultant physicians in each of the following areas:

   a. trust in professional integrity and competence
      —truthfulness
      —dedication to the moral center
      —shared commitment to the best interests of the patient
      —upholding your relationship with the patient
      —providing *your* standard of care
      —courtesy and mutual respect
   b. communication with you, as primary physician
   c. communication with the patient
   d. communication with others involved in the patient's care
   e. independence (initiative?) in planning and carrying out elements of patient care
   f. other (specify): _____
      _____

2. In what areas of expectations do you think physicians are likely to *disagree*?

3. Where you perceive discrepancies between your expectations and those of others, what steps could be taken to resolve or prevent misunderstandings and/or conflicts?

4. What expectations do other physicians involved in consultation rightfully have *of you* as the primary physician?

5. Where there are expectations you are unwilling to satisfy, what steps could be taken to resolve this discrepancy?

6. What obligation does the primary care physician have to evaluate the competency of the consultant? What are the limits of his capabilities to do this?

B. Nonphysician Practitioners

1. Spell out what you expect from nonphysician cooperative practitioners in each of the following areas:
   a. level of competence
   b. professional integrity:
      —truthfulness
      —dedication to the moral center
      —shared commitment to the best interests of the patient
      —upholding your relationship with the patient
      —providing *your* standard of care
      —courtesy and mutual respect
   c. communication with you, as physician
   d. communication with the patient
   e. communication with others involved in the patient's care
   f. independence (initiative?) in planning and carrying out elements of patient care
   g. other: _____
   _____

2. What expectations in these areas do you think nonphysician practitioners have *for themselves*?

3. Where you perceive discrepancies between your expectations and those of others, what steps could be taken to resolve these?

4. What expectations do other practitioners rightfully have *of you* as physician?

5. Where there are expectations of you that you are unwilling to satisfy, what steps could be taken to resolve this discrepancy?

6. In general, what key *differences* do you see between interactions among physicians and interactions with nonphysician practitioners?

Difficulties in interprofessional relationships are illustrated in the following case. As you read it, compare the relationships illustrated with the expectations you just outlined.

3.5.2 "The Compazine Incident"

Background

I was a second-year resident on an ICU service, functioning as an intern once again. It was a rough service with very ill patients, long intensive hours, and, unfortunately, an attending physician who was not very supportive. This attending frequently relied on the information given by the ICU nurses (whom he knew well) rather than the information given by the "interns" and the supervising resident.

This incident began with the admission of a patient who had just been discharged from another hospital, two weeks after a massive infarction of the anterior myocardium, giving rise to an early ventricular aneurysm. He had been doing well at home until he developed some angina-like chest pain and took a nitroglycerin. He promptly passed out and was brought by [the Emergency Medical Squad] to the emergency room, where he began to vomit. His vital signs were stable, but since he had ST segment elevations across the precordium on EKG, he was admitted to rule out extension of the previous myocardial infarction.

The Incident

The incident was precipitated by the supervising resident insisting that I give this elderly gentleman an intravenous bolus of 100 mg of lidocaine. I felt this was too large a bolus for an older person. However, the resident insisted. The large bolus was given and the patient promptly began vomiting and developed paresthesias. We finally stabilized the patient and admitted him to the ICU with an intravenous drip of lidocaine at 2 mg per minute. He was still nauseated, so we were allowing him only clear liquids by mouth. At approximately 2:00 AM, I received a call from an ICU nurse saying that the patient was nauseated and had just vomited. I ordered that the patient be restricted to nothing by mouth and be watched closely. The nurse asked if I would order Compazine to be given for the nausea and I said no.

Fifteen minutes later I received a frantic call from the same nurse saying that the supervising resident had ordered IM Compazine to be given seven minutes ago and now the patient's blood pressure was 60/0 and he was comatose.

After a quick burst of profanity on my part, I said that I would be right down and raced to the ICU. The patient was as the nurse described him. Fortunately, he quickly responded to IV fluids and Trendelenburg positioning. After the patient's vital signs stabilized, I notified the supervising resident, who rushed over to the patient and began giving orders to increase the IV rate. I told him that I thought that the Compazine may have been responsible for the hypotensive episode. He naturally disagreed with me, but I let the matter drop since there was a lot of emotion involved at that time.

The patient recovered uneventfully, but I was furious with both the supervising resident and the nurse who had deliberately circumvented my order. (It turned out that she had been unhappy with my refusal to order Compazine and had sought out the supervising resident and asked if he would order Compazine, not telling him what I had said.) The next morning I sought out the head nurse of the ICU. After I told her my side of the story, she began to lash out at me, claiming that I was not interested in my patients and that the nurse in question had to actually ask me to come down and take care of the patient when his blood pressure dropped. In addition, she began to tell me that she was not comfortable with a "non-cardiologist" (meaning me) taking care of a cardiac patient in the ICU. At this point, I went from angry to livid. With poorly concealed rage, I informed her that I was very angry with nurses circumventing our (the interns') orders on a regular basis and that if they have doubts about our orders, they should bring them up with us directly or with the attending on rounds. I also told her that the nurse on duty the preceding night was lying outright when she stated that she had to insist that I come down to see my hypotensive patient.

Gradually we both calmed down. It turned out that the nurses felt that they should be more involved in the treatment of patients. I agreed to try to involve the nurses more in the treatment plans for the patients. However, I added the reservation that I didn't feel that the nurses should be managing the care of the patients. The head nurse didn't answer; she pursed her lips and turned away.

Discussion

The issue raised in my mind surrounds what to do when a nurse feels that she should manage the patient's care and deliberately circumvents your orders. To what extent should you involve the nurses in the treatment plan for the patient? Was I as negligent of my patient's care as the head nurse claimed? I felt that I was being very diligent in the care of my patients and that my patients were doing very well in general. How do you deal with the resentment you feel when everybody begins to treat you like an intern again? More specifically, what do you do when your supervising resident (who is also a second-year resident with less ICU experience than yourself) insists on your doing things that you feel are inadvisable? How big a fuss should you raise regarding the Compazine incident and the subsequent behavior of the nurse when it is going to put you in conflict with your supervising resident, the nurse on duty, and the head nurse as well? (Kushner et al. 1982, 128–130)

NOTE: If you are a *medical student*, for whom the status of intern is a goal to which you aspire, you may have difficulty appreciating the author's feeling that it is demeaning to be "functioning as an intern once again." But take our word for it: once having endured their prescribed sentence in that status, residents are not eager to be thrust back into the role. If you are a *practitioner* who is confident that days of functioning as an intern are firmly behind you, you may also escape the grip of the emotions conveyed in this story. In this case, translate the character of the supervising resident into a specialist you have consulted whose demeanor toward you makes you *feel* like an intern again.

3.5.3 Case Analysis   This case situation illustrates virtually everything that could go wrong with interprofessional interactions. Communication was inadequate on all sides, roles were ill-defined, and personal feelings interfered with careful judgment serving the interests of the patient. Let us examine these problems in detail.

A. Resentment   To begin, the author of the case carries into the situation considerable resentment, which undoubtedly influences his perception of events. Some of the sources of these feelings are:

1. "the resentment you feel when everybody treats you like an intern again"
2. being subordinated to a supervising resident no further advanced in training than the author, and with "less ICU experience"
3. "an attending physician who was not very supportive." In particular, he "frequently relied on the information given by the ICU nurses (whom he knew well) rather than the information given by the [house staff]." (This remark also suggests underlying negative feelings toward the ICU nursing staff in advance of the events recounted.)
4. anxieties about the ICU setting, suggested when it is described as "a rough service with very ill patients [and] long intensive hours."

Some of these elements point toward conditions that ought to have been addressed in advance either by the author or by those supervising this training program. If the roles of the attending physician, the supervising resident, and the ICU nursing staff had been clarified, perhaps a good deal of this resentment would have been avoided and the incident would have featured more cooperation and negotiation and less emotional confrontation.

B. Supervising Resident   In addition to the general underlying resentment at the supervising resident's role, two specific incidents cause difficulties for our author:

1. his insistence on a dosage of lidocaine that the author felt was "inadvisable"
2. his responding to the nurse's request for Compazine without checking this out with the author.

Both of these problems stem, in part, from circumstances of the training setting. The author of the case appears to have primary responsibility for the care of the patient, but his training status limits his authority. (However, it would be unrealistic to ascribe the whole problem to the training setting. Sometimes consultants act in similar ways with regard to primary care physicians when called in to consult on a case.) Furthermore, even in the context of training, key elements of the ideal procedure for consultation should be observed (see Section 3.5.4). This would not only have the educational function of preparing the participants for interactions in which they will engage in the "real world" of practice, but it could have the practical benefit of heading off resentment, such as the author felt at the way things were handled.

For example, the supervising resident should have explained the reasoning behind the initial lidocaine order, thus gaining willing agreement by negotiation and persuasion instead of relying on an authoritative order. If the two could not agree, a third professional should have been brought into the discussion to arbitrate the disagreement. (In this setting, the third person probably would be the attending physician; in a practice setting, it could be an additional consultant.) When the nurse called asking for Compazine, the resident should at the very least have contacted the author to discuss the matter before giving the order.

C. Nurse   Several elements of the interaction with the staff nurses (and one of them in particular) introduce difficulties:

1. The author is troubled, in general, by the desire on the part of the ICU nurses for a greater role in patient management.
2. He is disturbed further by the extent to which the attending physician appears to validate these desires by taking seriously the nurses' evaluations of the patients' conditions.
3. The telephone call at 2:00 AM may have been regarded by the author as no more than a routine minor nuisance. However, there are indications that it had greater significance than this for the nurse involved. Although she did not explicitly ask him to come down to assess the patient and give her guidelines for managing his continuing nausea, this is probably what she really *wanted* and *expected*. (It is likely that his failure to meet her expectation here is the basis of her later charge that he neglected his patient and did not come down until asked.)
4. When the author refused to order a medicine the nurse judged was needed, she contacted the supervising resident—and did not tell him the whole story about the situation.
5. She accused the author of failure to respond to her need for help with the patient until asked.

These problems could have been greatly minimized (if not avoided entirely) by acknowledging the contributions and concerns of the nursing profession and, in particular, an explicit definition of the role of the staff nurses on this unit. The particular disagreements could have been resolved by negotiation and discussion on the basis of this general understanding (see Section 3.5.5).

3.5.4 Consultation with Other Physicians

8.03 Consultation. Physicians should obtain consultation whenever they believe that it would be helpful in the care of the patient or when requested by the patient or the patient's representative. When a patient is referred to a consultant, the referring physician should provide a history of the case and such other information as the consultant may need and the consultant should advise the referring physician of the results of the consultant's examination and recommendations relating to the management of the case. A physician selected by a patient for the purpose of obtaining a second opinion on an elective procedure is not obligated to advise the patient's regular physician of the findings or recommendations. (V)[5] (Judicial Council of the AMA 1984, 28)

Using this statement as a basis, William Kammerer and Richard Gross (1983, 1) developed a list of nine ethical principles of consultation:

1. Consultations are indicated
   a. "upon request"
   b. in doubtful or difficult cases
   c. when they enhance the quality of medical care.
2. Consultations are primarily for the patient's benefit.
3. A case summary should be sent to the consulting physician unless a verbal description of the case has been given.
4. *One* physician should be in charge of the patient's care.
5. Overall responsibility for the treatment of the patient remains with the attending physician.
6. The consultant should not assume primary care of the patient without consent of the referring physician.
7. Prompt response should be made to consultation requests.
8. Discussions in consultation should be with the referring physician, and only with the patient with the prior consent of the referring physician.
9. Conflicts of opinion should be resolved by a second consultation or withdrawal of the consultant; however, the consultant has the right to give his opinion to the patient in the presence of the referring physician.

Two themes in these guidelines especially raise questions. First, the provision for consultation upon request invites attention to your personal reaction when a patient requests a consult. The right of patients to choose their physicians (including consultants) is firmly established in law and professional ethics, but this does not make it easy to take at an emotional level. Are you able to accept this request graciously, without viewing it as a sign of a lack of confidence in your abilities?

Some physicians find a patient request for a consult most difficult to accept when they themselves are unsure of their management of the case, since it may show that the patient has detected the physician's uncertainties. Other physicians, in contrast, are most disturbed by a patient request for a consult when they are most confident in their handling of the case, since it may show that their self-confidence has not been communicated to the patient.

In fact, the patients' reasons for requesting a consult may not be due to either of these factors. It may stem from something else entirely. Sometimes such a request is an expression of psychological denial ("Maybe the next doctor will not tell me

---

5. We assume the consultant *would* be obligated to communicate with the patient's regular physician about the case *if* the patient requested this be done.

this disturbing news'') or unrealistic expectations (''Surely a *specialist* can rescue me from this fate''). It is always wise to explore the reasons for such a request with the patient (in a nonthreatening and nonjudgmental manner, of course). By this means, they can be guided to the consultant who can best meet their realistic expectations, and unrealistic expectations can begin to be dealt with.

Second, the guidelines dictate that the primary physician remain in control of all aspects of care (especially items 4–6). These guidelines appear to have been developed with only the inpatient situation in mind. In the hospital a consultant might come by the patient's room to do an examination, order diagnostic tests, etc., and leave the room without explaining any of his conclusions to the patient. After all, reporting to the primary physician can be direct and prompt, and the primary physician will be coming by to convey these reports to the patient in a short while. However, it would be too much to expect an outpatient to keep an appointment with a referral specialist, pay for the visit, and leave the office without learning anything about the consultant's impressions, the results of tests, or advice for management of the case. The patient's next appointment with the referring physician may not be for several days, a long time to wait for information from the consultation.

Furthermore, in today's highly technical era, it is not uncommon (even with a hospitalized patient) for a physician to request ''consult and manage,'' which in effect turns over an aspect of the patient's care to the consultant. However, the guidelines previously cited appear to recognize the legitimacy only of the ''consult and advise'' category of consultation.

The development of a consult-and-manage form of consultation is an attempt to capitalize on unique or special skills. As such, it involves trade-offs among myriad important values, including notably the sacrifice of the coherence and continuity of care provided by having one primary physician making the final decisions for all aspects of care, to gain the increased technical sophistication that a highly trained subspecialist can bring to management of the case. However, it is not enough to strike a temporary compromise between these values covering only this particular case. There should be an attempt to establish permanent procedures that would preserve *both* these sets of values to the highest degree possible.

Thus, for example, it is imperative that mechanisms be developed to enhance communication between physicians. Even if the primary physician cannot personally make the final decision on every aspect of care, he or she ought to be kept *well-informed* about on-going developments—and in a more timely fashion than a dictated note appearing on the chart a day or more later (or, in the outpatient situation, a letter that may take several days to arrive at the referring physician's office). Furthermore, a burden is created for both the primary physician and the patient when multiple consultants present the patient with an uncoordinated array of information.. This can create even more confusion when timely communication with the primary physician is lacking. In this situation the primary physician may be left to question the patient about what the consultant said and to piece together the picture from the patient's possibly fragmented and confused recollections.

We do not propose a set of rigid rules of consultation etiquette as an alternative to the set quoted earlier. In our view no set of rules left to interpretation by each practitioner involved would be adequate to resolve the problems arising in this area. What is needed most urgently is face-to-face accommodation of expectations on both sides by the parties involved. (If a face-to-face encounter is not feasible, an ear-to-ear telephone contact may be equally effective. Communication by letter does not allow the same give-and-take, but it can be effective if it includes the elements being discussed here.) Just as we earlier stressed the important role of an individually negotiated doctor-patient accommodation (Chapter 1, Section 1.2.4.B.2), we urge negotiation of a parallel "doctor-doctor accommodation."

There may be several ways to structure cooperative working relationships to accomplish these goals, although coordination is unlikely to develop without an explicit effort to bring it about. All parties involved must communicate their expectations to the others, and a mutually satisfactory working relationship must be negotiated. The exercise in Section 3.5.1.A—in which you stated your expectations of collaborators—is a first step toward this goal.

A distinction was drawn in Chapter 1 between a doctor-patient *accommodation*, worked out with regard to a specific set of interactions, and a doctor-patient *relationship*, which includes a relatively permanent set of mutually accepted groundrules for interaction. Similarly, a parallel distinction is applicable between referring physician and consultant. The initial dealings with a new consultant may require explicit and detailed discussion about mutual expectations. However, after working together on a case or two, expectations should be clarified sufficiently that repeatable patterns of interaction will have become established.

New situations may, of course, alter expectations and thus require fresh discussion and accommodation. For example, a consultation request entered on the Friday afternoon before a big football game at the local university may invite a more independent role by the consultant in patient management than one entered on a typical Tuesday morning. For their part, however, consultants may be *less* eager to offer on-going management in these Friday afternoon cases than in Tuesday morning ones. These variances in expectations ought to be settled in advance on the basis of discussion, lest management of the patient's case be subject to harmful delays.

More serious, physicians sometimes develop doubts about their competence (either generally or in certain areas), and they may deal with them by increasing the frequency of consultation requests and/or expecting a more active management of the case by consultants. (This response from physicians is admirable in that it shows an overriding concern for the welfare of the patient as well as an absence of vanity.) This may also make physicians reluctant to engage in face-to-face discussions of the case with the consultant for fear that the gaps in their knowledge will become manifest. The skillful and compassionate consultant will respond to these requests in a way that minimizes embarrassment to the referring physician and, ideally, will help him restore self-confidence (perhaps through the consultant's continuing education function,[6] by increasing his knowledge base in the area).

Related to this is the thorny question of whether a consultant can work effectively with a referring physician whose competence she doubts. On one hand the assistance of a consultant may result in better care for the patient than if the incompetent practitioner handled the case alone. However, for the consultant to "bail out" the physician on one occasion may contribute to the continuance of substandard practice with other patients, and obviously the consultant cannot monitor every aspect of every decision. Here again, the educational role of the consultant may be a partial remedy. But in cases of extreme incompetence, the consultant has an obligation both to patients and the profession to initiate stronger remedial action. Section II of the 1980 AMA Principles says firmly: "A physician shall . . . strive to expose those physicians deficient in character or competence, or who engage in fraud or deception." The consulting physician may be in an especially appropriate position to carry out this mandate.

In short, physicians involved in consultation need to be as sensitive to the variations and complexities of interactions with other physicians as they are to the individual needs of each patient. Just as physicians maintain distinctive patterns of interactions with different patients, they must develop individualized patterns for working with professional colleagues.

Different ways of enlisting other physicians include:

1. *Consult and advise.* The primary physician retains most fully the management of the case. The consultant's expertise is sought, but only as one element taken into account in the decision to be made by patient and referring physician. The only doctor-patient accommodation in this situation is between patient and primary physician. The consultant is represented only by means of a doctor-doctor accommodation with the referring physician.

2. *Consult and manage.* The primary physician will continue to assist the patient in making decisions, thereby providing coordination and a certain amount of continuity of care. However, much more of the decision making (especially with regard to technical details of care) is transferred to the specialist. Each physician will need to work out an individual doctor-patient accommodation with the patient, as well as a doctor-doctor accommodation with each other.

3. *Referral, but continuing to follow.* The referring physician seeks to maintain the doctor-patient relationship, perhaps because it is a relationship of long

6. On this role of the consultant, see Howard Brody's description of the "good clinical consultant" (Brody, in press).

standing and is expected to continue with regard to other of the patient's health care needs. However, decision making with regard to specific aspects of care *in this situation* is turned over almost entirely to the specialist. One way of stating this point is to say that the doctor-patient *accommodation* in this situation is worked out between specialist and patient, with little if any participation by the referring physician. He will be represented through a general, on-going doctor-patient *relationship* (and perhaps by doctor-patient accommodations with regard to other aspects of treatment), but he will have little involvement in the accommodation concerning this aspect of treatment. The doctor-doctor accommodation is also altered in this situation. The specialist has no duty to confer with the referring physician about specific treatment decisions prior to initiating doctor-patient accommodations with the patient.

4. *Referral.* The management of the patient's condition is turned over entirely to the specialist, and day-to-day coordination of treatment decisions with the referring physician is unnecessary. The doctor-patient accommodation is worked out entirely between the patient and the specialist. The doctor-patient relationship with the referring physician is temporarily suspended, and a deeper relationship may begin to be established with the specialist. Doctor-doctor accommodation takes a different form as well. The only necessary contact may be communication with the referring physician upon discharge of the patient, to inform him what treatment was carried out and, especially, its implications for the patient's continuing health-care needs.

Doctor-doctor accommodation is especially important in the face of recent changes in organizational structures in medicine. In the past, primary-care physicians exercised some control over subspecialists indirectly through their selection of consultants. If dissatisfied with aspects of the interaction with a consultant, the primary-care physician could stop referring patients to that doctor and choose another practitioner of the same subspecialty. However, organizational structures such as HMOs, mixed-specialty group practices, PPOs, and the like may significantly limit the primary-care practitioner's range of freedom here. But this makes it even more imperative that satisfactory working relationships be established through explicit negotiations.

We have stressed the importance of the working relationship between the referring physician and the consultant, but we do not suggest this is the *only* basis for selection of a consultant, nor that it is always the decisive consideration. Indeed, we believe that technical competence is of primary importance. If you are convinced that a particular specialist possesses unique skills that would contribute to the best possible treatment for your patient, you have an obligation to refer the patient to him or her—even if your working relationship with this physician is far from ideal.

3.5.5 Relationships with Nonphysician Practitioners A similar accommodation is necessary to develop working relationships with nurses and the variety of other nonphysician practitioners involved in patient care. We might speak of still another sort of informal working agreement: the doctor/limited-practitioner accommodation. However, this gives an air of simplicity and unity to what necessarily must be myriad individual negotiations with many different practitioners. The diversity here is likely to be even greater than in doctor-doctor accommodations.

A great many nonphysician practitioners in the health-care setting covet the respect, economic standing, and traditional independence of action of the physician. For example, in "The Compazine Incident," there was mention of the interest of ICU nurses in "more involvement in treatment plans for patients."

Ironically, these campaigns by limited practitioners to gain the privileges and power of physicians are based largely on a mythical view of what that status involves. Physicians' responsibilities and liabilities are often ignored. Furthermore, current "social developments" are altering the prerogatives of the physician in a direction even further away from the mythic ideal pictured by these groups. Such developments as direct federal regulation of medical practice (e.g., the proposed "Baby Doe rules"), federal programs that have a strong indirect impact on physician decision making (e.g., mandatory prospective payment for hospital expenses), and social changes (e.g., the increase in malpractice litigation) are discussed in Chapter 5.

There is a significant grain of truth in the arguments of these groups, however, that must be acknowledged in day-to-day practice. This is that today's nonphysician practitioners are expert and highly skilled in their area of practice. Once it may have been the case that the physician knew everything there was to know about health care, and other practitioners functioned merely to carry out procedures that were ordered (and often taught to them on the job) by the physician with whom they worked. But today the amount of knowledge is so vast and the details of technical procedures are so complex that no one person can presume to be master of them all. Formal and extensive training programs have been developed for allied health professionals that incorporate large amounts of this material in special areas.

The result is that, for example, physical therapists may have an understanding of certain treatment modalities (and their physiological bases) surpassing that of the average physician. Similarly, dietitians may have a knowledge of principles of nutrition in health and illness, through their years of concentrated study, that is more extensive than that of the physician (whose study of this topic may be limited to a few lectures here and there within the medical curriculum). In other cases a level of practical knowledge may have been achieved through experience. For example, nurses who have worked for many years in an ICU may have acquired an understanding of certain aspects of acute, critical illness that could be instructive to the physician who has contact with this level of care only with an occasional patient. In other settings nurses may gain greater awareness of patient needs than the attending physician as a result of their more continuous contact with the patient.

Furthermore, these groups of practitioners each have a strong code of ethics in which they accept a distinct professional responsibility to promote the patient's welfare. [Codes of several health practitioner groups are contained in an appendix of the *Encyclopedia of Bioethics* (Reich 1978).] Consider, for example, the following excerpts from the International Council of Nurses Code:

> The fundamental responsibility of the nurse is fourfold: to promote health, to prevent illness, to restore health and to alleviate suffering.

> The nurse's primary responsibility is to those people who require nursing care.

> The nurse carries personal responsibility for nursing practice and for maintaining competence by continual learning.

> The nurse takes appropriate action to safeguard the individual when his care is endangered by a co-worker or any other person. [International Council of Nurses, "Ethical Concepts Applied to Nursing." Adopted by the ICN Council of National Representatives, Mexico City in May, 1973; see Reich (1978, 1788–1789)]

The best interests of the patient require that mechanisms be developed to incorporate this expertise and skill into patient care as efficiently and thoroughly as possible. A physician who fails to draw upon these additional resources—who, for example, fails to consult the experienced clinical dietitian for advice and instead writes detailed orders for nutritional support in an uncommon situation on the basis of what he remembers from medical school lectures—does an extreme disservice to his patient.

The only real question is *how* to bring about this needed integration of expertise and skill. The push by many groups of nonphysician practitioners seems to be to demarcate zones of autonomous practice for each group, within which practitioners would have the full decision making authority traditionally possessed by the physician. The danger of this approach is that it could lead to fragmented and uncoordinated patient care—something that has already happened all too often as a result of medical specialization and multiple consultation. If the dietitian succeeds in having the task of nutritional planning placed on his shoulders, as an autonomous sphere of practice, it may be left *too much* to his responsibility. Thus, for example, the neurologist may not bother to pay sufficient attention to nutritional implications of the treatments she is administering—much less to their possible combined effects in association with the therapies ordered by, say, the rheumatologist (yet another consultant).

The solution we propose is not to create additional zones of autonomous practice, but rather to 1) encourage development of structures for cooperative decision making and practice involving all the practitioners whose expertise and skill are relevant to the patient at hand, and 2) provide for a coordinating function for the primary-care physician. But all this must be developed in face-to-face negotiations (or some suitable equivalent), in what we have labeled "doctor-doctor" and "doctor/limited-practitioner" accommodations and relationships.

3.5.6 Concept of the Health-Care "Team" The closest approximation to the ideal proposed here is found in institutional units in which the nature of the tasks has fostered close working relationships in a stable group of practitioners. Notable examples include intensive care nurseries and oncology units. Important questions arise when cooperative relationships of this sort develop within a team of practitioners.

First, to what extent can relationships characteristic of the moral center of medicine be developed and maintained with the several caregivers? Is it realistic to suppose that the patient can develop attitudes of trust and openness with each member of the team? Will the frequent presence of several team members at once inhibit openness of communication? Will it be a source of discomfort for the patient? What is the role of the institution in relationship to the team and to the patient?

Second, how is responsibility assigned in team decision making and action? The model of consultation in the professional literature suggests the only acceptable team structure is one with a clearly defined "captain" who bears primary responsibility for making the final decisions. However, in actual practice, decision making for certain areas of care is often delegated to specialists asked to consult and manage. Furthermore, some teams that have worked together for a considerable time may develop decentralized processes of decision making in which all team members make fundamental contributions to key decisions. In these cases can responsibility be said to be shared equally by all members of the team? Is this a viable model for team structure in other settings?

Third, one can see how crucial this delicate balance is and how severely it could be disturbed were decisions made on the basis of considerations other than the patient's best interests, e.g., economic factors, research values, teaching needs, etc.

Fourth, can a team approach to the patient preserve the patient's ability to appraise and criticize the care he or she has received? On whom is any criticism to be focused? How is it to be brought to bear on the decisions and actions of a team?

3.6 Institutional Delivery of Health Care

Alternative forms of organization for delivery of treatment influence many dimensions of professional practice. Some recent developments are examined in Chapter 5, but it is helpful to indicate here the relevance of these matters to the discussion of the moral center of medicine.

The presupposition of the moral center is one of undivided loyalty to the patient's interests. This is summed up well in the comment by Fried quoted in Section 2.2.

In particular, it is felt that medical decisions should not be influenced by financial considerations. This is underscored by the provision of the International Code of Medical Ethics: "A doctor must practice his profession uninfluenced by motives of profit."[7] The AMA Judicial Council makes a similar claim in the ruling on "Health Facility Ownership by Physician," quoted in Section 3.3.3.

Indeed, the image suggested by the moral center description is one of a physician who gives *no* consideration to the financial implications of choices that must be made. "My responsibility is to offer the most thorough work-up and treatment that I, and my institution, can provide—without consideration of cost." The hospital business office or the business function of a private practice office is viewed by many physicians as not centrally related to what they are about. These physicians may be unaware of the cost of a specific test they order, concentrating entirely on its scientific validity and usefulness.

In contrast to this ideal, health-care institutions have undergone in recent years a transformation that Eli Ginzberg (1983) terms "monetarization." This he describes as the "penetration" of the "money economy" into "all facets of the health-care system." In simpler terms, it means that financial considerations have come to influence, in various ways, the whole range of health-care decisions.

This obviously can produce a conflict of loyalties. The physician no longer bases decisions wholly on the comparison of probabilities of benefit versus harm to this specific patient. He now has to add into the calculus a consideration of economic factors. This influence is seen most dramatically when dealing with patients who lack health insurance but whose resources are sufficient that they are expected to pay for treatment. Physicians may become more sensitive to the economic implications of decisions in these circumstances. "Is this diagnostic test important *enough* to justify the cost to the patient? In these cases are found careful calculations of the most cost-efficient path to diagnosis and treatment decisions. The question, of course, is whether patients in this situation receive "the bare essentials" and patients who have insurance receive *excessive* levels of procedures, or whether insured patients receive the ideal arrangement of procedures and the level of care received by private-pay patients is *deficient*. (There is, of course, a third possibility: the insured patients receive *somewhat too many* procedures and that private-pay patients receive *somewhat too few* for ideal case management.)

The intrusion of economic considerations will contine to grow with changes such as the shift to prospective billing rather than cost reimbursement. Physicians will find it necessary to include in their deliberations considerations about how to

---

7. World Medical Association, 1949.

minimize the impact of concerns over general health-care expenditures, perhaps counting on the good will of the institution to balance and subsidize the costs of patient care.

3.6.1 Differences in Hospital Staffs   The description of the moral center does not include reference to the institutional affiliations of the physician and the influence these may have on doctor-patient accommodations. These affiliations may give rise to conflicts of loyalties, which are also undergoing change nowadays. New structures may not include some of the checks and balances on professional decision making embodied in traditional structures. For example, a tissue-review committee, which functions in connection with in-hospital surgeries to provide review of decisions by an economically disinterested group of peers, may not exist in free-standing, out-patient surgery facilities.

3.6.2 Filling Out Forms   Another element of practice not indicated in the description of the moral center of medicine—and, furthermore, that we venture to guess was rarely included in responses to the "Fantasies" exercise in Chapter 1, Section 1.1.—is the responsibility to fill out forms of various sorts on behalf of patients. Yet professional spokespersons clearly indicate that physicians can rightfully be expected to fulfill this task. The AMA Judicial Council insists that the physician's responsibilities to patients may include these sorts of certifications [Section 5.08: "Confidentiality: Insurance Company Representatives" (Judicial Council of the AMA 1984)].

To get at the issues that arise here, let us consider a case.

A. Case: Perry Payne

You are a primary-care physician in private practice in a small community. Perry Payne is a 46-year-old truck driver whom you have been following for the past several weeks for a back injury.

Today, Perry has struggled into your office for a follow-up appointment, and he asks you to write a note to his employer certifying that he is not able to work and indicating that the injury prevents his returning to work for an indefinite period.

The injury resulted when Perry fell from a ladder while he was painting a classroom in the educational building of the church his family attends. One of the other men who was also painting inadvertently bumped into the ladder on which Perry was standing, knocking him to the ground.

At the time of the injury, you hospitalized Perry and consulted the orthopedist who visits your small community hospital one day per week. After a thorough work-up, she reported back to you that the injury was relatively minor. She prescribed a regimen of exercises, to be administered by the staff physical therapist at the hospital, and she said she expected that the pain and disability would resolve over the next few days.

However, Perry's condition did not seem to improve. He moaned and groaned and begged constantly for a narcotic pain medication for "this agony." He refused to cooperate with the physical therapy—saying it hurt too much.

After a week of this reaction, on the occasion of the orthopedist's next weekly trip to your hospital, you asked her to examine Perry again. Her subsequent report reaffirmed her initial evaluation. "The organic pathology is not sufficient to account for the level of pain he reports," she said. "In my clinical judgment, his medical condition is stable and there is nothing physically wrong with him that is severe enough to interfere with his returning to work immediately. I am convinced that what is sustaining his symptoms is pent-up hostility and resentment relating to the frustrating nature of his job and elements of his life situation. I recommend psychological counseling."

But Perry resolutely refused any suggestion of counseling. You discharged him from the hospital after a few more days, but his wife reports that he remains confined to bed at home, complies poorly with the regimen of exercises he was taught by the physical therapist, and constantly begs her to persuade you to prescribe more potent pain medication.

And now here he is in your office, asking you to provide him with a medical excuse from work. "You gotta do this for me, Doc," he says. "My boss says that, unless I produce a note from you, he will not give me sick pay; without that, I won't be able to put food on the table for my family."

How should you respond to this request?

B. Options

1. Write the note, as requested.

2. Write a note certifying that you have been treating Perry, but word it in such a way that it conveys the message that his disability is not as serious as he claims.

3. Strike a bargain with Perry. Agree to write a note certifying disability until two weeks from today, but only if he promises to

   a. comply with the exercise regimen he was taught
   b. seek psychological counseling
   c. return to work when the two weeks are up
   d. other (specify): _____

4. Tell Perry the orthopedist ought to write the note, so he ought to make an appointment to see her the next day she is in town.

5. Refuse to write the note.

6. Refuse to write the note, and contact Perry's employers independently to tell them Perry is not as disabled as he claims.

7. Other: _____

C. Issues

1. Is it consistent with a proper role of the physician to be asked to make certifications of this kind?

   a. What are the implications of this sort of request for the physician-patient relationship?

   b. What are its implications for the physician's relationship to the employer and/or other social institutions?

2. What consideration should be uppermost in the physician's mind when handling certifications of this kind?

   a. the medical needs of the patient exclusively

   b. the welfare of the patient generally, including elements above and beyond medical needs

   c. the rights and welfare of the employer and/or other social institutions

   d. the Truth (with a capital "T")

   e. other: _____

3. What are the implications of certifications of this kind for the issue of medical confidentiality?

4. What other ethical issues are raised by requests for certifications of this kind?

D. Case Analysis   It is clear that to *refuse* to fill out this form (option 5) will disrupt the physician-patient relationship (issue 1a). Furthermore, in many situations, filling out such forms can have beneficial effects for your patients. Sometimes it directly serves their medical needs (issue 2a)—as when it allows a patient to delay returning to a work situation that would impair recuperation. At other times, such an authorization by the physician might not be strictly necessary for recuperation, but it might be justified on the grounds of serving elements of the patient's general welfare (issue 2b). This consideration might apply to the case of Perry Payne. A delay in returning to work—although apparently not strictly medically necessary—might provide the respite that would enable him to begin addressing his life problems.

Turning to the involvement of the employer and/or other social institutions (issue 1b), groups in society are only too ready to shift the burden of a variety of difficult determinations to physicians; the medical community should consider which of these tasks it is appropriate to undertake. Insisting on a "doctor's excuse" or a "medical certification" is a relatively easy way for an employer or manager to shunt aside a difficult decision. Physicians should not *always* be willing to take on these roles.

Once having accepted responsibility to assist employers or managers in this way, however, the physician acquires an obligation to consider the rights and welfare of the institution (issue 2c) in making such a determination. But above all, there is an obligation to be *honest* (issue 2d). Just as honesty is an obligation in the physician-patient relationship,[8] it is a central social norm. Thus to write the note [containing as it does a declaration that the physician believes to be false (option 1)] would be ethically wrong, and it also would be less than honest to write a note with a disguised message (option 2).

At the other extreme, it would be a violation of confidentiality to contact the employer independently to tell him of Perry's actual condition (option 6). Perry would be unlikely to authorize release of this information, and without his authorization, disclosure would violate his right of confidentiality.

Option 4 would remove the immediate burden from your shoulders, but only to impose it on someone else—and the orthopedist is likely to bring a new burden to bear on you for creating this difficult situation for her.

Thus, we would hold that the only viable choices are option 5: to refuse to write the note, explaining to Perry why it is not justified; or option 3: to certify disability on the basis of the overwhelming impact of his life problems, but to use the occasion as a bargaining tool to persuade him to begin dealing with these problems.

If the "bargaining" in option 3 is heavy-handed, it can amount to coercion and therefore is ethically suspect. However, accompanied with a supportive and understanding attitude, it can initiate a mutually negotiated doctor-patient accommodation without any objectionable coercive component.

3.6.3 Patient Nonpayment of Bills   Consideration of the monetary aspect of medical practice inevitably brings up the issue of the patient's responsibility for payment for services, and the appropriate response of the physician when this responsibility is not met. To illustrate this in concrete terms, the saga of the Perry Payne family continues.

A. Case: Perry Payne Revisited

Two weeks have passed since your last encounter with Perry Payne. Today, as you walk by your receptionist's desk, she looks up from a telephone conversation and says, "Doctor, Mrs. Payne is on the phone. She wants to make another appointment for Perry to see you. You realize, don't you, that they have not paid a cent on their bill since Perry's injury? I have pointed this out to Mrs. Payne repeatedly, and she always promises to send us a check for at least a few dollars towards the bill. But we have received nothing.

"What do you want me to do about this? Should I remind her again about the bill? Should I schedule the appointment?"

What should you tell the receptionist to do?

---

8. See Chapter 1, especially Sections 2.2 and 2.3, for a discussion of this norm in the physician-patient relationship.

B. Options

1. Refuse to schedule another appointment for Perry until the bill is paid in full.

2. Refuse to schedule another appointment for Perry until some payment is made on the bill.

3. Schedule the appointment, but tell Mrs. Payne that you will refuse to see Perry unless she brings with her when they come for the appointment
   a. some payment towards the bill
   b. full payment for the entire outstanding past balance
   c. full payment for the entire outstanding past balance plus full payment for this visit.

4. Schedule the appointment and remind her once again about the bill.

5. Schedule the appointment and do not mention the bill.

6. Other: _____

C. Questions

1. Would it make a difference to your decision if you learned that the Paynes' nonpayment had gone on for several months *before* Perry's injury? Why or why not?

2. Would it make a difference to your decision if you learned that Perry was receiving sick pay from his employer? Why or why not?

3. Would it make a difference to your decision if you learned that Perry had been reimbursed by his health insurance for your treatment of him? Why or why not?

D. Case Analysis   Physicians often find it uncomfortable to discuss with the patient the financial component of the physician-patient relationship. However, this is clearly a part of the physician's expectations from the relationship, and it ought to be dealt with in the doctor-patient accommodation along with other issues.

The patient has a clear responsibility to make serious efforts to pay the charges for professional services. Even if one questions the current private-enterprise form of medical services and views altenative financing arrangements as preferable on moral grounds (an issue discussed in Chapter 5), these beliefs about ideals do not nullify the responsibility to honor the financial commitment embodied in *current* doctor-patient accommodations.

If a given family is unable to pay, the physician should work out arrangements to allow responsibilities to be met to the extent possible. This has been done in the present situation by inviting the Paynes to pay a few dollars against their bill. Patients should accept this much responsibility, even if their finances are in dire straits. This does little more than acknowledge their financial responsbililty.

Thus, it clearly would be justified to call the Paynes' attention to their responsibility here in some way or other. The question is *how* best to do it.

Since the financial arrangement is part of the doctor-patient relationship, it is appropriate for the physician to deal with it directly (especially once it has gotten to the extreme point that it has with the Payne family). Repeated reminders of this issue from your receptionist have already been tried and found ineffective. Thus we recommend *against* options 1–4, since they involve ancillary personnel raising the issue with the Paynes.

Of the options listed, we recommend option 5, supplemented by the suggestion that the physician initiate a frank discussion of payment when the Paynes arrive for the appointment.

However, another possibility might be preferable to any of those listed. Since you, the physician, are right by the telephone, this might be the best time and place to raise the issue with them. You could get on the phone right now and discuss with Mrs. Payne arrangements about payment on the bill. (It would be best, we think, *not* to link payment with the up-coming appointment. They will undoubtedly get this message from the context, and one does not want to suggest they could avoid responsibility for this bill by not making future appointments.) Then give the phone back to your receptionist to make the appointment.

Nonpayment for services can serve as a means to communicate one's dissatisfaction with the nature of the services rendered. This may provide the patient with a valuable communication tool in a system in which barriers of social status, institutional structures, and custom inhibit other ways of conveying this message. Insurance reimbursement arrangements that make payment directly to the patient have the value of preserving this capability to communicate dissatisfaction. However, it seems clearly wrong for the patient to *profit* from such a communication. Thus a patient who plans to take such a step should refrain from filing for insurance reimbursement for the services in question. Furthermore, if the decision is made after the forms have already been filed, the patient should *return* the money to the insurance carrier.

E. Case: Perry Payne Revisited Yet Again

Two more weeks have passed since your last encounter with the Paynes. Today, your receptionist informs you that Perry has called to request his records be sent to another physician in your community. She reminds you that the Paynes have still not made any payment on their bill.

What should you tell her to do?

F. Options

1. Send the other physician all the records you have on Perry. Keep nothing for your own files except a brief note.

2. Make a photocopy of all Perry's records.

   a. Send the other physician the original records and keep the copy for your permanent files.

   b. Send the other physician the copy and keep the original records for your files.

3. Select items to copy and send to the other physician

   a. the consultant's interpretation of EKGs, x-rays, etc., but keep the items themselves for your files

   b. copies of records *you* have generated, but not the records sent to you by a previous physician when the Paynes first came to you

   c. all objective data, but keep "subjective" material—i.e., your personal impressions of Perry and his family, discussions of sensitive issues like sexuality and family violence—to yourself

4. Discuss with Perry what information in his file should be sent; e.g., if there are records of discussions you have had with the patient about sexual matters or family violence, remind him that these are referred to in the record and ask whether these should be sent to the new physician. Then send copies of the patient-approved items to the physician.

5. Dictate a brief "discharge summary" and send it to the other physician, but keep the full records for your files.

6. Dictate a note explaining your doubts about the organic basis of Perry's current complaint, and send it with whatever records you select.

7. Dictate a note explaining the Paynes' poor payment record, and send it with whatever records you select.

8. Telephone the other physician to explain

   a. your doubts about the organic basis of Perry's current complaint

   b. the Paynes' poor payment record.

9. Refuse to send any records to another physician until the Paynes' bill with you is paid in full.

10. Refuse to send any records to another physician until the Paynes have at least started to pay on their bill.

11. Other: _____

G. Case Analysis The physician's obligation to maintain records about patients is an aspect of the duty to render quality care. The assumption is that information about the patient's medical history is important for assessment of future health situations. The duty to make this information available to other physicians at the patient's request stems from the same basis: an obligation to provide *these physicians* with a basis for rendering the highest quality care.

However, this duty should not be made conditional on the patient's financial responsibility. Thus, options 9 and 10 must be rejected on the grounds that they improperly mix two morally independent issues.

The problem with options 5 and 3a is they provide too little information for effective management of care. If the underlying goal is to enable provision of quality care, these seem inadequate to the purpose.

Options 6–8 raise questions of confidentiality. To communicate this information to another physician—whether in written or verbal form—obviously goes beyond Perry's expectations when he authorized release of information. We contend that, at the very least, explicit authorization from Perry to communicate this information is required.

The response to option 3b depends, in part, on whether the records you received from the other physician were originals or copies. If they were originals, then you should forward them to the physician the patient has chosen. After all, it is possible that the originating physician did not retain copies and thus that there is no other source for this baseline material to be supplied to the new physician. On the other hand, if they are copies, then it might be advisable to suggest that the new physician contact the earlier physician to attempt to obtain the original data. You might also ask Perry his wishes about this choice.

Option 1 is probably inadvisable on personal, prudential grounds. Since questions about your past care of the Paynes might arise at a later date (e.g., in legal actions), it is wise to retain enough information to be able to defend yourself in detail regarding care rendered. This might also be essential to serve the best interests of the Paynes—for example, if Perry were to sue someone with regard to his back injury. Reference to the details of your records would be necessary to testify on his behalf.

Option 2a raises similar questions. If the original records are out of your hands, they are subject to alteration, and your possession of a copy may not be regarded in court as sufficient evidence of the original form of the record.

One problem with option 2b is that the copies may not be of good enough quality to provide needed information to the other practitioner. This can be especially true with attempts to copy x-rays, but the same thing can happen in making photocopies of handwritten notes. The obligation here is to provide the best quality copy that is feasible; if no copy is fully satisfactory, perhaps one ought to offer the other physician an opportunity to *study* the original in your office if you are unwilling to give up possession of it permanently.

An additional problem with option 2b is that the records might contain information that the Paynes would prefer *not* to have communicated to a new physician. If they had discussed with you sensitive issues they no longer regard as "live" issues, such as sexual problems or worries about family violence they now consider to have been overcome, they might prefer not to have their new physician made aware of these items from their history.

You might try to determine this on your own (option 3c), but clearly it would be more reliable to contact Perry and ask him what information to transmit. Thus our recommendation is option 4.

4 Expansions of the Scope of Responsibility

Recall that item *a* of the description of the moral center refers to "diagnosis and treatment," and item *b* focuses on "an illness or injury" (Section 2.1). A number of common and important medical activities go beyond the scope of medical services indicated in this description. Some of these have been seen in concrete examples in this chapter, but it is worthwhile to step back and view this in a general way.

4.1 Beyond Treatment

A number of clinical activities are aimed not at treatment of existing illness but at its prevention. Vaccination and patient education are two significant examples. The rationale for stepping beyond the paradigm is that this approach offers a more efficient means to achieve the same goal as the central activity. To prevent illness offers assistance to the patient no less valuable than removing the illness once it appears—indeed, prevention may significantly reduce the total amount of pain and suffering.

4.2 Beyond the Clinic

Similarly, addressing the remote, root causes of illness or injury through attention to occupational health and safety, environmental medicine, social medicine, etc., is justified by the efficiency of these approaches in achieving the same goal as paradigm practices.

4.3 Beyond Illness or Injury

A more dramatic step away from the paradigm is to shift the focus from preventing or relieving illness or injury to the broader focus of promoting positive states: 1) health promotion, 2) wellness promotion, and 3) well-being promotion. The ultimate extension along these lines is suggested in the following statement by renowned physician-educator Rudolf Virchow: "Should medicine ever fulfill its great ends, it must enter into the larger political and social life of our time, it must indicate the barriers which obstruct the normal completion of the life-cycle and remove them. Should this ever come to pass, medicine, whatever it may then be, will be the good of all" [quoted in Health Policy Committee (1982, 450)].

4.4 Palliation, Comforting, and Strengthening Coping Skills

This also represents a substantial departure from the core goal of diagnosis and treatment of the illness or injury. The rationale for including these tasks in the medical mandate is that these elements are, in many instances, adjuvant to the central task (and perhaps even continuous with it, in many respects). The most careful diagnosis and the most focused pharmacological or surgical treatment may be hampered in effectiveness if the patient is anxious, frightened, and mistrustful of their value.

However, this is not the *whole* justification for these elements of care. They also (especially?) seem to be called for when the condition has passed the limits of effective treatment. Here the rationale is that such activities embody a helping orientation parallel with, and a natural extension of, the central paradigm.

4.5 Conclusion

This discussion of the moral center and extensions from it is in no way intended to discount the importance of these ''off-center'' elements. Rather, the point is to call your attention to a character they may have in your priorities because of their distance from the moral center. You need to give thought to what importance they *should* have in your professional practice.

Clearly there are some things you will be asked to do by patients and/or society that will fall outside the scope of what you think is properly part of professional practice.[9] Consider, for example, one final case that raises these issues.

> The elderly woman explains to you that in the public housing project in which she and her husband live, two-bedroom apartments are assigned to couples without children only on the grounds of ''medical necessity.'' She asks you to certify that there is a medical necessity for a two-bedroom apartment in her case because her husband's snoring keeps her awake at night when they sleep in the same room.

How should you respond to this request? Do you have any obligation to assist the patient in this matter?

---

9. For an interesting discussion of one such issue, see Gillick (1984).

References

Brody H: Teaching clinical ethics: Models for consideration. In: Ackerman T, Graber GC, Thomasma DC, et al. (eds) *Clinical Medical Ethics: Exploration and Assessment*. University of Tennessee Inter-Campus Graduate Program in Medical Ethics, Knoxville, in press.

Eaddy JA, Graber GC: Confidentiality and the family physician. *Am Fam Physician* 25: 141–145, 1982.

Fried C: *Medical Experimentation: Personal Integrity and Social Policy*. American Elsevier, New York, 67–78, 1974.

Gillick MR: Is the care of the chronically ill a medical prerogative? *N. Engl. J. Med.* 310:190–193, 1984.

Ginzberg E: The monetarization of medical care. *N. Engl. J. Med.* 310:1162–1165, 1983.

Health Policy Committee, American College of Physicians: The medical consequences of radiation accidents and nuclear war. *Ann. Intern. Med.* 97:447–450, 1982.

Jonsen AR, Jameton AL: Social and political responsibilities of physicians. *J. Med. Philos.* 2:376–400, 1977.

Judicial Council of the American Medical Association: *Current Opinions of the Judicial Council of the American Medical Association–1984*. American Medical Association, Chicago, 1984.

Kammerer WS, Gross RJ (eds): *Medical Consultation: Role of the Internist on Surgical, Obstetric and Psychiatric Services*. Williams & Wilkins, Baltimore, 1983.

Kushner KP, Mayhew HE, Rodgers LA, et al: *Critical Issues in Family Practice: Cases and Commentaries*. Springer Publishing, New York, 1982.

Pellegrino E: *Humanism and the Physician*. University of Tennessee Press, Knoxville, 222–230, 1979.

Pellegrino ED, Thomasma DC: *A Philosophical Basis of Medical Practice*. Oxford University Press, New York, 1981.

Reich WT (ed-in-chief): *Encyclopedia of Bioethics*. Macmillan and the Free Press, New York, 1978.

Further Reading

Bayles M: *Professional Ethics*. Wadsworth Publishing, Belmont CA, 1981.

Caplan AL, Engelhardt HT Jr, McCartney JJ (eds): *Concepts of Health and Disease: Interdisciplinary Perspectives*. Addison-Wesley, 1981. Approaches the issue of the scope of medical responsibility in a more theoretical way than our chapter, through analysis of the central concepts of "health" and "disease."

Ducanis AJ, Golin AK: *The Interdisciplinary Health Care Team*. Aspen Systems, Rockville MD, 1979.

Judicial Council of the American Medical Association: *Current Opinions of the Judicial Council of the American Medical Association–1984*. American Medical Association, Chicago, 1984.
3.02 Nurses
3.04 Referral of Patients
3.05 Specialists

3.07 Teaching
4.04 Health Facility Ownership by Physician
6.01 Fees for Medical Services
6.03 Fee Splitting
7.00 OPINIONS ON PHYSICIAN RECORDS
8.00 OPINIONS ON PRACTICE MATTERS
9.00 OPINIONS ON PROFESSIONAL RIGHTS AND RESPONSIBILITIES

Kass L: Regarding the end of medicine and the pursuit of health. *The Public Interest* 40:11–42, 1975.

Kass L: Ethical dilemmas in the care of the ill: 1. What is the physician's service? *JAMA* 244:1811–1816, 1980.

Kass L: Ethical dilemmas in the care of the ill: 2. What is the patient's good? *JAMA* 244: 1946–1949, 1980.

Katz J (ed): *Experimentation with Human Beings*. Russell Sage, New York, 1972.

Levine RJ: *Ethics and Regulation of Clinical Research.* Urban & Schwarzenberg, Baltimore, 1981.

Mechanic D, Aiken LH: A cooperative agenda for medicine and nursing. *N. Engl. J. Med.* 307:747–750, 1982.

Reich WT (ed-in-chief): *Encyclopedia of Bioethics.* Macmillan and the Free Press, New York, 1978.

Advertising by Medical Professionals (Havighurst CC)

Civil Disobedience in Health Services (Madden EH, Hare PH)

Drug Industry and Medicine (Coulter HL)

Health and Disease
  I. History of the Concepts (Risse GB)
  II. Religious Concepts (DeGraeve F)
  III. A Sociological and Action Perspective (Parsons T)
  IV. Philosophical Perspectives (Engelhardt HT Jr)

Health Care,
  I. Health-Care System (Lee PR, Emmott C)
  II. Humanization and Dehumanization of Health Care (Howard J)
  III. Right to Health-Care Services (Jonsen AR)
  IV. Theories of Justice and Health Care (Branson R)

Health Insurance (Riesenfeld SA)

Health, International (Missett JR, Taylor CE)

Health Policy
  I. Evolution of Health Policy (Strickland SP)
  II. Health Policy in International Perspective (Anderson OW)

Hospitals (Williams KJ)

Human Experimentation
  I. History (Brieger GH)
  II. Basic Issues (Capron AM)
  III. Philosophical Aspects (Fried C)
  IV. Social and Professional Control (Frankel MS)

Informed Consent in Human Research
  I. Social Aspects (Gray BH)
  II. Ethical and Legal Aspects (Lebacqz K, Levine RJ)

Institutionalization (Wexler DB)

Mass Health Screening (Missett JR, Taylor CE)

Medical Education (Pellegrino ED)

Medical Malpractice (Hauck GH, Louisell DW)

Medical Profession
  I. Medical Professionalism (Pernick MS)
  II. Organized Medicine (Burrow JG)

Nursing (Stanley T)

Orthodoxy in Medicine (Kaufman M)

Pain and Suffering
  I. Psychobiological Principles (Robinson DN)
  II. Philosophical Perspectives (Shaffer JA)
  III. Religious Perspectives (Bowker JW)

Prisoners
  I. Medical Care of Prisoners (Sagan LA)
  II. Prisoner Experimentation (Branson R)
  III. Torture and the Health Professional (Sagan LA)

Research, Behavioral (Kelman HC)

Research, Biomedical (Levine RJ)

Research Policy, Biomedical (McCarthy CR)

Social Medicine (Silver GA)

Warfare
  I. Medicine and War (Vastyan EA)
  II. Biomedical Science and War (Sidel VW, Sidel M)

Relman A: The medical industrial complex. *N. Engl. J. Med.* 303:963–970, 1980.

Starr P: *The Social Transformation of American Medicine.* Basic Books, New York, 1982.

Chapter Four

Life and Death

For everything there is a season,
and a time for every matter under heaven:
a time to be born, and a time to die;
a time to plant, and a time to pluck up what is planted;
a time to kill, and a time to heal;
a time to break down, and a time to build up;
a time to weep, and a time to laugh;
a time to mourn, and a time to dance;
a time to cast away stones, and a time to gather stones together;
a time to embrace, and a time to refrain from embracing;
a time to seek, and a time to lose;
a time to keep, and a time to cast away;
a time to rend, and a time to sew;
a time to keep silence, and a time to speak;
a time to love, and a time to hate;
a time for war, and a time for peace.
[Ecclesiastes 3:1–9 (Revised Standard Version)]

The challenge is, of course, to discern just *when* the proper time for a given activity has arrived. The author of Ecclesiastes appears, in general, to be quite pessimistic about the capability of the human mind to fathom the details of cosmic purposes. The thematic refrain of that book is the lament: "Vanity of vanities, all is vanity!"

And yet physicians cannot avoid this challenge. Medical practices inevitably affect the determination of these "times," and hence physicians, once involved, cannot avoid influencing these "times"—by default, even if not by conscious design. Continuing intensive, life-prolonging efforts to refrain from "playing God" may amount to "playing God" in the other direction by dragging out the dying process with pain and anguish for all involved.[1] The proper "time to die" is *neither* too early *nor* too late.

---

1. It must be acknowledged that some do claim to find positive value in suffering: some strengthen character through enduring it courageously; others find meaning in suffering by regarding it as a sort of punishment. These belief systems explain why a minister counseling a patient to accept pain medications may be more influential than a physician who gives the same advice. The guidelines developed in this chapter provide for these belief and value systems, as well as for those that see no redeeming value in the suffering of terminal illness.

This, then is the issue explored in this chapter. What standards can be employed to help determine the appropriate limits for therapeutic efforts or life-sustaining treatment? What is the role of the patient in making these determinations? What is the role of the patient's family and friends? What legal guidelines bear on these decisions?

1 Determination of Death

One obvious limit to therapeutic efforts is death. There is clearly no point in continuing treatment after the patient has died, and indeed it might even be considered a desecration of the body to do so. However, the determination of even this boundary is not totally clear.

Some of the problematic dimensions of declarations of death are nicely illustrated in the film *The Wizard of Oz*. Dorothy and her house have just dropped into the Land of Oz, right on top of the Wicked Witch of the East. The Munchkins are dancing around celebrating their liberation from the witch's oppression when the voice of caution intervenes. The town officials emerge onto the steps of City Hall and interject the following:

Munchkinland
Town Council (unison):   "We've got to verify it legally,
                               to see
                               if she
                               is morally,
                               ethically,
                               spiritually,
                               physically,
                               positively,
                               absolutely,
                               undeniably,
                               and reliably,
                               DEAD."[2]

In response to this call, the coroner emerges from City Hall, ceremoniously walks over to the recently arrived house, and for a moment peers under it where the witch's feet are sticking out (still encased in the ruby slippers). Then he returns to the steps of City Hall and sings his report to the Mayor and the members of the Town Council gathered there:

Coroner: "As coroner,
          I must aver

---

2. "THE WIZARD OF OZ" by Harold Arlen and E.Y. Harburg © 1938, Renewed 1966 LEO FEIST, INC. Rights Assigned to CBS CATALOGUE PARTNERSHIP. All Rights Controlled and Administered by CBS FEIST CATALOG INC. All Rights Reserved. International Copyright Secured. Used by Permission.

I thoroughly examined her.
And she's not only merely dead;
She's really most sincerely dead."[3]

His claim to thoroughness would certainly be questioned by any pathologist, but in spite of that technical reservation, the incident illustrates the multifaceted nature of determinations of death. The parameters provided by the Town Council are especially illuminating here, for they recognize clearly that determination of death is not merely a medical issue, but also one of law, ethics, and religion. In the discussion that follows, we shall see how these myriad issues are involved in determinations of death.

At the most general level, death is defined as "the irreversible cessation of vital functions." But this definition leaves several important questions unanswered.

1.1 "Irreversible"

The determination that the cessation is *irreversible* requires a *prediction*, and no prediction about the future can be 100% certain. There is always some possibility (even if only one chance in a billion) that one more shock or a few more minutes of external cardiac massage would reinitiate vital functions.

Furthermore, the prediction of irreversibility may become a self-fulfilling prophecy. If further attempts to restore vital functions are abandoned on the basis of this judgment, then the likelihood of the judgment's being proven false decreases still further.[4]

It was this concern with predictive accuracy that prompted development of the modern medical operational definition of death. Until the eighteenth century, determination of death was not considered a medical matter. In most cases a physician would not be in attendance at the time of death. The family would determine on its own that death had occurred and would initiate the preparation of the body for funeral rituals and burial. One important step in the change from this pattern was an article, published in 1740 in a French medical journal by a young physician named Jean Jacques Winslow, entitled "The Uncertainty of the Signs of Death and the Danger of Precipitate Interments and Dissections" (see Alexander 1980, 25–31). Winslow urged that physicians be summoned for pronouncements of death and that medical science work to develop operational criteria for making these determinations. Winslow's interest in this issue was not entirely academic. As a child, he had been chronically ill and had awakened on at least two occasions to find himself in a coffin and at the center of a wake! (Fortunately for him, embalming was not done in those days; the body was merely washed. He was also

---

3. Ibid.
4. The component of irreversibility can also serve to distinguish death from those situations of reversed cardiac arrest or temporary hypoxia from which people have awakened and reported certain bizarre experiences. Whatever is going on in these situations (and we do not delve into this issue here), it is *not* that they have experienced death and returned to tell us about it, since by definition death involves *irreversible* cessation of function.

lucky to have regained consciousness before the burial.) No doubt partly as a result of his own experience, he proposed an extremely conservative operational criterion of death: putrefaction.

This operational test was not adopted, but the medical community did accept the general point that a medical criterion should be developed. After a good deal of discussion, tests related to respiration became the accepted medical means of determining death. (One such test still portrayed in movies is the placing of a mirror to the nose to check for breath, the moisture in which clouds the mirror.)

1.2 "Vital Functions"

Why was Winslow's proposal to make putrefaction the operational criterion of death not accepted? One reason may relate to public health considerations: it is *unhealthy* to leave corpses lying around until they begin to rot. Another reason was undoubtedly aesthetic: it is extremely *distasteful* to delay preparing a corpse for burial until after it has begun to rot. But there appears to be yet a deeper reason, which stems from a fundamental, philosophical understanding of what it is to be a human being. In our shared view of what constitutes the person, it seems that he or she has lost what is essential to be a *living human being* long before putrefaction of the flesh sets in. The core of being a human person has more to do with the *functioning* of the body than with the organic integrity of the flesh.[5]

The question of what human functions are "vital," then, is a *philosophical* one. The issue is to discern what traits are so fundamental to our understanding of what it is to be human that, once they have irreversibly ceased, we would say that the person no longer exists.

At an earlier stage of technological development, the philosophical niceties underlying this question may have been less important in practice. Cessations of any of a variety of bodily functions were operationally equivalent as indications of death. In those days it was beyond the capability of medical science to sustain other bodily processes when certain central processes had failed. For example, if the patient stopped breathing, an energetic bystander might shake her vigorously (perhaps shouting the patient's name) in hopes of "waking her up again," or the group might watch anxiously for a few moments to see if signs of breathing reemerged, but few other interventions were even attempted. Thus cessations of breath and heartbeat (which are the most readily observable of the central bodily functions) were plausible operational criteria of death.

Nowadays technology is more effective and selective, however. Medical science is capable of maintaining heart and lung function, for example, after the brain has irreversibly ceased to function. Thus, we must be correspondingly more precise in our understanding of what functions are fundamental or vital.

---

5. As it turns out, putrefaction is not even a sufficient condition for determining death, since it is possible for putrefaction to occur while significant life processes continue. Thus a patient may have a gangrenous foot while heart, lungs, and brain continue to function more or less normally.

If we consider a human being a fundamentally *physical organism,* for example, then we might favor retaining the traditional operational criteria of determining death that center on heart and lung function. In this view, a person is still alive as long as the key organic processes of respiration and circulation are maintained, even if conscious life is irreversibly lost and heart and lung processes are maintained artificially by a mechanical ventilator.

If we consider a human being as fundamentally a *consciousness,* then we might favor operational criteria of death in terms of *neocortical function.* (This involves, of course, acceptance of the physiological premise that the neocortex is the organic seat of these functions.) In this view, that heart and lung functions could be maintained (indeed, in rare cases, these might even exist spontaneously) is unimportant to the judgment that the person has died. Irreversible cessation of the functions of conscious awareness and the capability to interact with others marks the death of a person, even though certain processes of the body continue to function.

If we regard a human being as fundamentally an *integration of mental and physical processes,* then we might favor operational criteria of death in terms of *whole-brain function.* As long as any brain function remains, the sense of the person as that which enlivens the body is not entirely lost. However, as soon as brain function ceases altogether, that sense vanishes. Thus it is appropriate to declare the person dead even if other processes (i.e., respiration and circulation) are continuing with technological assistance.

1.3 Statutory Definitions of Death

Society has expressed strong preferences among these possibilities. For several centuries the determination of death has been left to professional medical judgment. However, a number of state legislatures recently have passed statutory definitions. The process began in 1970 when Kansas enacted the nation's first such law. Over the next ten years more than half of the 50 states enacted in one form or another statutes specifying what constitutes death.

All of these gave prominence to the operational criteria related to whole-brain function, although they dealt with them in some distinctly different ways. For example, the Kansas statute provided for determinations *both* in terms of "absence of spontaneous respiratory and cardiac functions" *and* "absence of spontaneous brain function," without any indication of when one is to be preferred to the other (presumably the choice is left to the individual physician's discretion). Several other states specified that brain criteria were to be applied "if artificial means of support preclude a determination that these functions have ceased." (This would appear to limit the physician's discretionary authority to employ them in other situations.) Several states required independent confirmation of death by a second physician. Others required such confirmation only when removing organs for transplantation. Others did not require that a physician be involved in making the determination at all, allowing the coroner to determine death in certain cases and not requring this official to be a physician.

In 1981 the President's Commission for the Study of Ethical Problems in Medicine and Biomedical and Behavioral Research proposed a model uniform statute, designed to resolve discrepancies between the various states' statutes. [See President's Commission (1981). This volume contains texts of the states' legislation as of 1980. It also contains "Guidelines for the Determination of Death," drawn up by a medical panel and originally appearing in *JAMA* 246 (1981):2184–2186.] It reads as follows:

> *Uniform Determination of Death Act*
>
> An individual who has sustained either:
> 1. irreversible cessation of circulatory and respiratory functions, or
> 2. irreversible cessation of all functions of the entire brain, including the brain stem,
>
> is dead. A determination of death must be made in accordance with accepted medical standards. (President's Commission 1981, 2)

This statute has already been adopted by a number of states (including the authors' home state of Tennessee), and other states are likely to follow suit in the next few years.

The practicing physician should be aware of the law on this matter in his own state. Even more important, these legislative developments ought to prompt reflection on the underlying issues and a reexamination of one's own attitude toward dealing with patients at the end of life.

Of course, one might question the appropriateness of a law that dictates medical practice in this area. However, this is a *fait accompli* in many states; thus ignoring it amounts to an act of civil disobedience. If the law says that patients lacking brain function are dead, then in legal terms it may be inappropriate to continue respiratory support, just as it obviously would be inappropriate to keep a patient in a hospital bed (and especially to bill for services rendered) long after the patient's cardiac and respiratory functions had ceased irreversibly.

In short, a translation of attitudes is required to honor the new operational criteria of death. Whatever was regarded as inappropriate with regard to "chest dead" patients under the old understanding is now inappropriate toward "brain dead" patients, and whatever was appropriate toward "chest dead" patients (e.g., autopsy, preparation for burial, etc.) is now appropriate toward "brain dead" patients. This extends even to language: a "brain dead" patient for whom cardiac and respiratory functions are restored following an arrest has *not* been "resuscitated" or "revived." She is still dead, even though those organic functions are continuing. More serious, of course, is the question of whether it is appropriate to take action to restore these functions when brain function is lost.

1.4 "Pronouncing" Death

The physician is called to "pronounce" death. This suggests an important social ritual (Peschel and Peschel 1983; Shem 1978, 71–72). The social role of pronouncing death goes beyond the technical act of diagnosing that death has occurred. In an important sense, the patient has not died until the physician certifies that he has.

One important aspect of this social ritual is its impact on the family and close friends of the patient. Pronouncement of death marks an end to "hoping" (i.e., a "time to dance"?) and initiates the grieving process (i.e., a "time to mourn"). The timing of this pronouncement, the style of communication with the family, and the preparation for it greatly influence the adjustment they will make. This is a situation in which the physician has an obligation to serve the interests of the survivors, in addition to his or her obligations to the (primary) patient.

Wherever there are *dual* loyalties, a *conflict* may arise. For example, the physician treating a comatose dying patient may conclude on the basis of his knowledge of the patient's fundamental values that this person would prefer *not* to be resuscitated and yet the family may not yet be prepared for the patient to die. Honoring the values of the patient would dictate nonresuscitation; serving the needs of the family would dictate maintaining artificial support for awhile to give the family more time to adjust to the inevitable outcome. You as the physician must determine which of these obligations takes priority in a given situation.

This may be part of what the American College of Physicians (ACP) Ethics Manual intends to convey when it says: "There may be circumstances in which the physician may elect to support the body when clinical death of the brain has occurred, but there is no ethical standard that dictates he must prolong physical viability in such a patient by unusual or heroic means" [ACP 1984a *(Manual)*, 26–27; 1984b *(Annals)*, 265]

Additional obligations may influence the decision in this case. A principle of reverence for life may be interpreted to dictate aggressive efforts to extend life as long as possible, or alternatively, it may be interpreted to prohibit extending life for the purpose of promoting the interests of others.

2 Other Limits to Treatment

Even more difficult decisions must be made in situations in which death may be near but has not yet occurred. Contemporary medical technology and skill provide physicians with the awesome power to postpone death, and with this power (as with any power) comes the burden to make responsible decisions about its use. Intensive life support measures are undoubtedly beneficial in certain situations, e.g., when they sustain the body as it recovers from a critical but reversible insult. However, the benefit of these measures is doubtful if they only prolong an inexorable downhill course. The challenge is, of course, to discern which of these you are presented with in a given case. Is this "a time to heal" or "a time to die"?

In the following pages you will be asked to consider the appropriate role of the various parties concerned with these decisions, and the standards to be used in the decision making. Three resources from which the discussion will draw heavily are included for your reference: 1) a summary of the recommendations from the President's Commission report *Deciding to Forego Life-Sustaining Treatment,* in Section 2 of Appendix II; 2) relevant sections from the ACP Ethics Manual, in Appendix III; and 3) the relevant statements from the AMA Judicial Council, in the following section.

2.1 AMA Policy Statements

2.14 Quality of Life. In the making of decisions for the treatment of seriously deformed newborns or persons who are severely deteriorated victims of injury, illness or advanced age, the primary consideration should be what is best for the individual patient and not the avoidance of a burden to the family or to society. Quality of life is a factor to be considered in determining what is best for the individual. Life should be cherished despite disabilities and handicaps, except when prolongation would be inhumane and unconscionable. Under these circumstances, withholding or removing life supporting means is ethical provided that the normal care given an individual who is ill is not discontinued.

In desperate situations involving newborns, the advice and judgment of the physician should be readily available, but the decision whether to exert maximal efforts to sustain life should be the choice of the parents. The parents should be told the options, expected benefits, risks and limits of any proposed care; how the potential for human relationships is affected by the infant's condition; and relevant information and answers to their questions. The presumption is that the love which parents usually have for their children will be dominant in the decisions which they make in determining what is in the best interest of their children. It is to be expected that parents will act unselfishly, particularly where life itself is at stake. Unless there is convincing evidence to the contrary, parental authority should be respected (I, III, IV, V)

2.15 Terminal Illness. The social commitment of the physician is to prolong life and relieve suffering. Where the observance of one conflicts with the other, the physician, patient, and/or family of the patient have discretion to resolve the conflict.

For humane reasons, with informed consent a physician may do what is medically necessary to alleviate severe pain, or cease or omit treatment to let a terminally ill patient die, but he should not intentionally cause death.[6] In determining whether the administration of potentially life-prolonging medical treatment is in the best interest of the patient, the physician should consider what

---

6. This contradicts—at least as applied to the medical situation—the claim of Ecclesiastes that there can be "a time to kill." This point is discussed further in Section 2.4.

the possibility is for extending life under humane and comfortable conditions and what are the wishes and attitudes of the family or those who have responsibility for the custody of the patient.

Where a terminally ill patient's coma is beyond doubt irreversible and there are adequate safeguards to confirm the accuracy of the diagnosis, all means of life support may be discontinued. If death does not occur when life support systems are discontinued, the comfort and dignity of the patient should be maintained. (I, III, IV, V) (Judicial Council of the AMA 1984, 10–11)

2.2 Limits Set by Patients

The term "patient-set limits" is used to refer to any of the several different ways in which patients may indicate preferences that amount to limiting medical treatment. The first task is to recognize the several forms this may take and to consider the appropriate response by the physician to each.

2.2.1 Varieties of Patient-Set Limits

A. Religious Constraints This is the sort of patient-set limit to treatment addressed most often by the courts and usually involves the Jehovah's Witnesses, who accept all forms of medical treatment except blood transfusions. This position will be discussed at some length in Section 2.2.2. It is not the most common form of patient limitation of treatment.

B. Not Seeking Treatment As discussed in Chapter 1 (Section 1.2.4.A.3), the vast majority (as much as 75–90%, by some estimates) of incidents the individual would describe as a state of illness are managed entirely without recourse to the medical system. People will merely "tough it out," apply home remedies or over-the-counter preparations, and/or seek assistance from nonmedical friends. This behavior can be viewed as a form of patient-set limit to medical treatment.

The social structure of informed consent prohibits overriding these decisions. If the situation is perceived as serious, friends may try to persuade the person to go to a medical facility for treatment, but except in the case of a public health danger, an incompetent patient, or a minor, the patient cannot justifiably be *forced* to submit to treatment.

These incidents most often involve fairly minor illnesses, and here no serious ethical problems arise. In a self-limiting condition, for example, self-treatment may be as effective and efficient as submitting to medical treatment. Chicken soup provided by Mama may be the treatment of choice.

However, the same behavior is sometimes manifested in life-or-death situations (although it usually is not perceived as such by the parties involved, as when a man insists that his chest pain is merely heartburn and takes an antacid and lies down to rest, only to die from a myocardial infarction as he lies there). Here, obviously, matters are more serious. Chicken soup is *not* the treatment of choice for a myocardial infarction.

In some cases the decision not to seek medical treatment is based upon a highly articulated theoretical understanding of the nature of health and illness (e.g., Christian Science), but this sort of rationale is not always present. Situations do occur in which the participants understand the seriousness of the condition and the benefits to be gained from medical treatment, but (accurately or not) they judge that they have no access to medical care, e.g., the case of a family with no money to pay for treatment and too much pride to accept "charity," or the family that has been judged to abuse medical institutions in the past and now believes that its members will not be admitted without an advance cash deposit.

Most often, however, the decision not to seek treatment hinges on some presuppositions (many of them misjudgments) about the nature of health and disease:

1. The condition is not serious.
2. Nonmedical remedies will be effective in overcoming it.
3. "What you don't know cannot hurt you" (and thus one is safe as long as no diagnosis is made).
4. Hospitals are places one goes to die (and thus one is somehow protected from death by staying away).

Obviously, many of these presuppositions are not rationally justified. However, it is difficult for physicians to counter these misconceptions head-on since those who hold them do not present themselves to the medical system. Thus one-on-one patient education cannot be begun.

One social obligation of physicians is to promote public health education that provides a more enlightened view of the nature of health and illness, to overcome resistance to treatment based on unfounded superstition.[7] Appropriate self-care should be encouraged, but the public needs to be educated to recognize situations in which it is unwise to attempt self-care.

C. Unheralded Noncompliance   The sort of patient-set limit to treatment that arises most frequently within the medical setting is *unheralded noncompliance*. Physicians become accustomed to having a certain proportion of patients who simply fail to return for recommended follow-up appointments. Some of these are

---

7. The construction of these educational materials also involves ethical elements. For example, in communicating the importance of seeking medical diagnosis and following treatment regimens for diseases such as hypertension, diabetes, etc., to those who have not yet sought treatment, care should be taken not to cause anxiety for those who are currently under treatment and yet still concerned about the long-term effects of a chronic disease. One measure that could mitigate this effect would be to include in all educational materials the assurance (to the extent appropriate) that careful medical management dramatically reduces the risks of catastrophic sequelae from the disease in question.

probably receiving medical care elsewhere, but some employ this tactic to avoid recommended treatment entirely.

Even more frustrating is the patient who simply ignores (wholly or in part) the treatment regimen recommended by her physician and allows the hypertension, diabetes, or other disease process to rage on unchecked. This may have life-threatening consequences, but generally these are not dramatically apparent immediately after ceasing the regimen. Thus noncompliance may continue for some time, much to the frustration of the health care professionals who detect it and try to persuade the patient to follow the treatment regimen. But eventually this may reach a life-threatening stage: the noncompliant diabetic patient may be brought to the hospital with diabetic ketoacidosis, or the hypertensive patient who ignores treatment may be admitted with a stroke. Once stabilized, such patients may continue their noncompliance.

In a way, medicine here is the victim of its own successes. Patients have such strong faith in the ability of medical professionals to rescue them from catastrophic situations that they underestimate the danger of their own irresponsible behavior. Indeed, the most difficult cases of this sort involve patients who themselves have been rescued from dire straits repeatedly in the past. They seem to assume that, no matter what they do to themselves in the future, the doctors can restore them to a relatively normal state.

This type of treatment refusal is difficult to deal with. The treatment regimen involved is an on-going process that cannot be monitored at every stage by health-care professionals. Home health-care visits might be used to provide periodic reminders, but constant monitoring ("handholding") is totally unfeasible.

The only hope for combating this behavior lies in aggressive patient education to impress upon the patient the dangers of nontreatment and the benefits of treatment. This may be especially difficult to accomplish in cases in which the patient receives secondary gains from illness. Here, at least in the short range, the loss of these secondary gains may outweigh the benefits from treatment. Even without this factor, it may be difficult to communicate to patients the importance of benefits that are remote and less visible in order to offset the disvalues of treatment that are close at hand and quite palpable.

D. Treatment Refusal   It is also not uncommon for patients to take the initiative by refusing recommended treatment explicitly when it is proposed. Some patients undergoing chemotherapy for tumors announce that they wish to suspend treatment; some on chronic dialysis announce that they want to withdraw from it; others for whom radical procedures such as amputation are seen as the only hope for cure or extension of life refuse to sign the consent form for surgery. It is a recurrent phenomenon in hospitals for a patient to refuse to continue all treatment being offered and to carry out this refusal by leaving the hospital "AMA" (against medical advice).

The ethical principle of autonomy is often taken to imply that any and all of these forms of refusal of treatment are to be respected equally. Also court reactions generally have not distinguished between one situation of refusal and another. This reaction by the legal system is heavily influenced by one of two foundations of the informed-consent principle: the criminal category of battery. To authorize touching requires an explicit consent, but *nontouching* does not require the same weight of justification—it is the "default" state of affairs. As Robert Veatch puts it:

> It makes no sense to talk about getting a patient's consent to nontreatment, whether that patient be terminally ill or not. . . . One does not consent to nontouching. Nontouching is the initial presumption of autonomous individuals barring any consent that establishes a medical relationship.
>
> Legally and morally, treatment without consent is assault and battery. Conversely, consenting to nontreatment is like consenting to not having assault and battery committed. (Veatch 1981, 207–208)

However, as explained in Chapter 1, informed consent is also grounded in a principle of autonomy or self-determination; this principle can form a basis for distinguishing forms of refusal that should be honored from those that perhaps should not. From the discussion of autonomy in Chapter 2 (Section 2.3.1), it should be clear that many of these acts of refusal are not sufficiently deliberative or grounded in core personal values to be considered autonomous. Rather, they are based on the whims of the moment or unexamined emotional reactions to some element of the treatment proposed. But, if this is so, then nothing about the principle of autonomy requires that these sorts of refusals be honored.

If physicians can be faulted for providing inadequate information and emotional support before enlisting consent to treatment (and they can, as indicated in Chapter 1), then patients can similarly be faulted for rejecting treatment without making every effort to gain and assimilate information and deliberate on the basis of it. Refusal of treatment is a choice no less than acceptance of treatment, and the same responsibilities of autonomy apply. Treatment refusal can be seen as a privilege that must be earned, not an automatic right to be exercised on any basis one chooses. Another way to express this point is to say that achieving autonomy is a *responsibility* both of caregivers and patients and not a *license* for the patient to choose on any basis whatsoever.

A method for achieving autonomous participation of patients in setting limits to treatment is sketched in the following paragraph and elaborated in Section 2.2.3ff.

E. Negotiated Limits The discussion of informed consent in Chapter 1 (Sections 2 and 3) developed the notion of shared decision making by negotiation with the patient. This approach is applicable throughout the clinical course, including life-threatening stages of illness. The patient must be provided with all relevant information if he is to share fully in decision-making about his care, and the emotional support stressed as a component of information exchange will assist him in coming to grips with the realities of his situation and will enable him to employ this information in rational deliberation. Indeed, at every stage of illness, one goal of the doctor-patient accommodation process (DPA) ought to be helping the patient clarify his personal values and relate them to the realities of his medical condition.

Through this process the patient may develop firm preferences regarding aspects of the management of his illness. These preferences may include a desire to set certain limits to medical treatment.

This is the form of patient-set limit to treatment addressed in Sections 2.2.3 and 2.2.4. However, before turning to the task of developing a policy for this sort of situation, let us examine in some depth one of these other varieties of treatment refusal.

2.2.2 Religious Constraints: Jehovah's Witnesses Refusal of blood transfusions by Jehovah's Witnesses is based on an interpretation of certain scriptural passages, such as

> Every creature that lives and moves shall be food for you; I give you them all, as once I gave you all green plants. But you must not eat the flesh with the life, which is the blood, still in it. (Genesis 9:3–4)

> If any Israelite or alien settled in Israel eats any blood, I will set my face against the eater and cut him off from his people, because the life of a creature is the blood, and I appoint it to make expiation on the altar for yourselves; it is the blood, that is the life, that makes expiation. Therefore I have told the Israelites that neither you, nor any alien settled among you, shall eat blood. Any Israelite or alien settled in Israel who hunts beasts or birds that may lawfully be eaten shall drain out the blood and cover it with earth, because the life of every living creature is the blood, and I have forbidden the Israelites to eat the blood of any creature, because the life of every creature is its blood: every man who eats it shall be cut off. (Leviticus 17:10–14)

> But you must strictly refrain from eating the blood, because the blood is the life; you must not eat the life with the flesh. You must not eat it, you must pour it on the ground like water. If you do not eat it, all will be well with you and your children after you; for you will be doing what is right in the eyes of the LORD. (Deuteronomy 12:23–25)

These passages cite not only the rule itself, but also the *reason* behind it: "because the life of a creature is the blood." In other words, their view is that the soul or individual identity is contained in the blood. Thus receiving someone else's blood "contaminates" one's individual integrity. An analogous situation that might strike us at a similar emotional level would be the prospect of a partial brain transplant: suppose an experimenter proposed to remove half of your brain and replace it with tissue from another person. Most people would react with revulsion and fear that they would no longer be the *same person* as a result of such a procedure. That is much the same as the Jehovah's Witness' reaction at the thought of a blood transfusion.

The scriptural texts also make clear that the context of the injunction against "eating blood" is one of rules governing hunting and food preparation. However, Jehovah's Witnesses interpret the rule to apply to taking blood into the body in any form and by any means. Is this a reasonable construction of the scriptural passages cited?

Many Christian groups refrain from acknowledging this and other Old Testament rules by invoking the "new covenant" contained in the New Testament. However, in response to this, Jehovah's Witnesses refer to a New Testament passage that seems to reaffirm that the prohibition against blood applies to Christians as well. The text comes from Acts, in the context of the debate that went on for some time in the early Christian church about how much of Jewish law should be imposed on gentile converts. The elders of the church at Jerusalem met to discuss this question and settled on the following list (conveyed in a letter to the church at Antioch; emphasis is added):

> It is the decision of the Holy Spirit, and our decision, to lay no further burden upon you beyond these essentials: you are to abstain from meat that has been offered to idols, *from blood,* from anything that has been strangled, and from fornication. If you keep yourselves free from these things, you will be doing right. (Acts 15:28–29)

Recently, the group has issued some further clarification of the scope of the prohibition:

> Witnesses view [these scriptures] as ruling out transfusion of whole blood, packed RBCs, and plasma, as well as WBCs and platelet administration. However, Witnesses' religious understanding does not absolutely prohibit the use of components such as albumin, immune globulins, and hemophiliac preparations; each Witness must decide individually if he can accept these. (Dixon and Smalley 1981, 2471)

It should be noted that Jehovah's Witnesses are generally willing to accept responsibility for the risks they choose to run. They usually announce their religious affiliation to the physician at their first contact and are understanding if the physician indicates an unwillingness to treat them. They have tried to persuade surgeons to attempt a variety of surgical procedures (including open heart surgery) without blood transfusions. Furthermore, church leaders have worked with the legal counsel of the AMA to develop a document (Form P-47) in which the patient absolves the physician and hospital of all legal responsibility for harm resulting from their foregoing blood transfusions (Office of the General Counsel 1979, 85), and individual Witnesses are willing to fill out this document. (Indeed, often they bring copies when they enter the hospital.) Most of the problem cases arise in crisis situations, when the need for blood was not anticipated and thus was not discussed in advance.

These cases have frequently been taken to court. The courts have often authorized intervention against the wishes of patient and/or family when the patient is a minor, but they have almost always honored refusals by competent, adult Jehovah's Witnesses who are not ambivalent in their expression of refusal.

2.2.3 Lynn Languish (the Final Chapter)   To give a concrete focus to the discussion of the patient's role in treatment decisions, consider the specific clinical situation of Lynn Languish, first introduced in Chapter 1, Section 1.2.1.B and further developed in Chapter 2, Section 2.3. Now you will hear another chapter of her story.

> Ms. Languish's lymphadenopathy did turn out to be associated with cancer of the breast. Over the 20 months since diagnosis was made, she has gone through numerous and varied treatment modalities.
>
> She refused to submit to a mastectomy (although this was your initial recommendation—she disagreed that it was "a time to rend, and a time to sew"), so you referred her to an oncology team you knew would be open to a lumpectomy procedure. This was followed by a combination of radiotheraphy and chemotherapy.
>
> For some months, things went quite well. Side effects from the treatments were well tolerated. Her emotional adjustment was bolstered by regular visits with you and also by her active involvement in a counseling group associated with the oncology service.
>
> Six months ago, however, she presented with bone pain. Tests confirmed widespread bone metastases. These have since spread to the lumbar spine, despite intensive therapeutic efforts that included hormone therapy.
>
> She has become more and more discouraged as this progression has continued. (This reaction is, of course, understandable; you and the oncology team have felt pretty much the same way.) Nevertheless, her will to live is strong, and although she has hesitated and pondered, she has eventually accepted every new treatment modality offered to her.
>
> For the past ten days, she has been confined to a bed in the Oncology Unit. She is never free from pain. At times the pain is so intense that she is incoherent and disconnected in her attempts at communication. Generally, though, she remains lucid. She is barely able to move. You judge that the end will not be long in coming.
>
> However, the oncologist with whom you and she have been working has not given up hope. Today he has come to discuss with you a new protocol he would like to propose to Ms. Languish. He asks you to accompany him to talk with her about it.

How should you respond to him? Consider the following choices:

1. Agree to help *persuade* Lynn to accept the treatment.

2. Agree to accompany the oncologist to see Lynn, primarily to be sure that the information about risks and benefits is presented to her fully.

3. Agree only to *ask* Lynn if she would like to see the oncologist and hear about his proposal for treatment.

4. Veto in advance any idea of such a presentation.

5. Agree to accompany the oncologist, but plan to see Lynn alone first to let her know in no uncertain terms your professional recommendation that she *not* accept the proposed treatment.

6. Other (specify): _____

2.2.4 Physician Responsibilities Concerning patient-set limits to treatment, the physician has the following responsibilities:

1. *To maintain a presumption on the side of sustaining life, but also actively to attempt to discern the appropriate limits to this policy.*[8]

The AMA Judicial Council endorses a parallel principle and also indicates its limits (see the "Quality of Life" opinion quoted in Section 2.1). When there is reasonable doubt that the "time to die" has arrived, efforts to sustain life should be continued with vigor. However, at the same time, physicians must face the difficult task of prognosis. To *suppress* doubts about the appropriateness of continued life-sustaining measures in a given situation, or to avoid gaining information that could create such doubts, is to shirk one dimension of medical responsibility at this stage of the clinical course. When such doubts arise, they must be investigated as fully and energetically as therapeutic possibilities so that sufficient information is gained to enable all parties to make a sound, well-grounded decision.

When the "time to die" has arrived, it is a *misuse* of medical knowledge and skill to prolong the agony of all concerned. Instead, the goal should become to help patient, family, and caregivers recognize this fact and accept it gracefully.

Thus, in the case of Lynn Languish, hope for this new protocol must be tinctured with a strong dose of realism in assessing her present condition. In general, any form of patient resistance to a treatment recommendation (whether expressed openly or nonverbally through noncompliant behavior) should prompt a reassessment of the clinical decision by the physician. Be sure the recommendation is sufficiently justified to warrant "making a case out of it."

---

8. See recommendation 2 in the President's Commission report *Deciding to Forego Life-Sustaining Treatment*, listed in Appendix II, Section 2.

2. *To provide information, emotional support, and recommendations to patients.*

This is a natural extension of the duty of informed consent, both in its theoretical justification and in its practical execution. This responsibility is most readily carried out within the framework of continuity of care. The steady but gradual process of informed consent described in Chapter 1, Sections 2 and 3, leads naturally, when the irreversibility of the disease process becomes more and more obvious, to sharing *this* information with the patient, assisting her in dealing with it emotionally, and guiding her on this basis toward decisions about the appropriate limits to treatment.

The President's Commission endorses this principle in several places. Its report on informed consent states:

> 7. Patients should have access to the information they need to help them understand their conditions and make treatment decisions. (President's Commission 1982, 4; see Appendix II, Section 1)

In its report on limits to treatment, the Commission offers a recommendation specifically for dealing with decisions concerning seriously ill newborns that could, with only slight modification, be applied to all patients:

> 16. Decisionmakers should have access to the most accurate and up-to-date information as they consider individual cases.
>
> —Physicians should obtain appropriate consultations and referrals.
>
> —The significance of the diagnoses and the prognoses under each treatment option must be conveyed to the [patient,] parents (or other surrogates). (President's Commission 1983, 7; see Appendix II, Section 2)

Along similar lines, the AMA Judicial Council holds that the patient and family should be given information about the options, benefits, and risks, and about how the patient's condition affects the potential for human relationships; in addition, any questions they have should be answered (see "Quality of Life" opinion quoted in Section 2.1).

If this responsibility has been carried out, Lynn should have by now a realistic understanding of her prospects and you, as her physician, should have in turn a thorough understanding of her fundamental values. Unless she has already indicated she will accept no further treatment, the new protocol should be offered to her, but care must be taken to avoid overstating its promise.

If the primary reason for attempting this treatment is to gain knowledge that could be of therapeutic benefit to future patients at earlier stages of disease progression, then it should be proposed only if it has been ascertained previously that research values are important to her. And in that case, the primary purpose ought to be made clear to her. (It should not be thought that this would make her acceptance of the protocol unlikely. Research values are quite important to many patients at this stage. They take great comfort in the hope that they may spare someone in the future from the suffering they are currently going through. These patients are to be admired for such a demonstration of benevolence under difficult circumstances, but care must be taken to ensure that their choice is fully voluntary and not unduly influenced by professional eagerness for knowledge.)

3. *To guide patients to formulate preferences on the basis of their own fundamental values.*

This is an aspect of the comforting and supporting role of the physician. This may be one of the most difficult tasks the physician confronts: to enable the patient to face the disturbing prospect that medical technology will be unable to rescue her and to help her choose between the tragic alternatives that remain.

It is tempting to shield the patient from these decisions and take them upon your own shoulders. However, the same considerations that support giving the patient a voice in less momentous and tragic decisions apply with equal force in this context. Patients have individual values that make a difference in these choices, and they ought to have the opportunity to shape the ending of their lives in terms of these values. Lynn's will to live may reflect a fundamental value of hers, but only she herself can determine whether it is still important enough to justify the treatment now being proposed. Another patient may be ready to give up the fight at an earlier stage. This, too, should be accepted graciously once it is determined that the decision is based on a realistic understanding of the situation and expresses the patient's fundamental values.

If the basis of the patient's refusal is irrational, the physician has an obligation to guide the patient to think the matter through again. (Meanwhile, until this process has been completed, the response to any life-threatening crisis that arises should be dictated by 1) the presumption in favor of sustaining life, and 2) the option that would offer an opportunity for renegotiating the DPA covering this situation.)

4. *To negotiate with the patient a course of action that is mutually acceptable to all parties centrally involved.*

This is an extension of the process of DPA discussed at length in Chapter 1. The physician also may have fundamental values that influence his role in this relationship. The final decision should result from a process of shared decision making involving patient, physician, and others who are significantly affected.

One chief danger is that caregivers will allow their own core values and beliefs to dominate the negotiations. For example, with the goal of supporting the patient's "having hope," caregivers may propose a level of treatment far in excess of what would be needed to achieve this. Rather it is what is required for the maintenance of hope *in themselves*. At this stage of illness, "hope" may mean to the patient no more than an assurance of company and comfort to the end, not a promise of cure or even prolongation of life.

If no mutually acceptable decision can be reached, and the physician cannot in good conscience cooperate with the patient's wishes, then the only recourse may be to sever this doctor-patient relationship and help the patient find another physician who could reach an agreement with her. This tragic outcome should be an absolute last resort. The depth of the relationship may be an important source of support for the patient in this difficult time, and it may not be possible to establish a new relationship of equal depth in the brief span of life that remains. Thus you should search your conscience thoroughly before taking this step, to be quite sure whether, and to what extent, the motive for stepping away from this patient at this time includes considerations such as

1. a "vanity trip"
2. a personal difficulty in dealing with death
3. an emotional reaction to this patient's death
4. an interest in sustaining the institution's image.

To sever a relationship at this stage of care would appear to be justified only on the basis of a clearly defensible moral position or a deep disagreement about fundamental life values.

This is one of many reasons why it is best for physicians and patients to talk about these issues relatively early in the physician-patient relationship, so the general outlines of a DPA covering terminal situations can be developed in advance. It would have to be filled in later with the details of the actual situation, to be sure, but general boundaries can be agreed upon in advance—for example, whether a plan of aggressive life-sustaining treatment is to be continued at all costs, or whether it is regarded as more appropriate to suspend intensive efforts when a realistic prognosis indicates the end is near.

5. *To assist patients in carrying out these mutually agreed-upon goals.*

The physician will play an especially important role in communicating these decisions to the other caregivers, and in relating them to institutional and social policy. If, for example, Lynn Languish decides *not* to accept the protocol, it may fall to you as her primary physician to persuade the aggressive oncologist to accept this decision. On the other hand, if she accepts it (against your better judgment), then the oncologist may have to remind you of the case in its favor. This may be a "time to cast away" treasured judgments (or at least to rethink them thoroughly) so that it can be "a time to keep" your trust with this patient.

When goals of cure have been abandoned, a goal of providing for the patient's comfort and dignity should be substituted. This may require actions that will have the effect of hastening death. (Some of the internal complexities of this stage are discussed in Section 2.4.)

6. *To assist patients in communicating these decisions to family and friends, and to support these people in their process of coping with the decisions.*

At this stage of events, the physician-patient relationship expands to include responsibilities toward the survivors, even if they are not your primary patients. Consideration of the impact of decisions on the survivors ought to be an element in the process of deliberation and negotiation, and care and concern should be shown in guiding them to accept the inevitable outcome and the choices that have been negotiated with the patient.

The family may have reached a state of acceptance in advance of the patient, and thus may be prepared for death to come; indeed, in some cases, the family may be almost eager to "get the ordeal over with." However, if the patient still desires to continue aggressive measures, the family should be guided to see the basis of the patient's position. The same process happens in reverse when the patient is prepared for the inevitable and the family is not.

2.3 Dealing with Families' Decisions

The family and close friends of the patient have a significant influence on the patient's thinking and decisions at every stage of illness, but their role becomes especially important in terminal illness. The death of the patient may be a monumental event in their lives. They are the people whose on-going association with the patient can be a source of deep comfort and support, or in bad circumstances, a considerable hindrance to the accommodation of the patient to his or her terminal state.

Western society pays lip service to the social importance of the family unit. In the situation of terminal illness, the physician must acknowledge this importance in her actions.

2.3.1 Family and the Competent Patient   In the case of the competent patient, the physician may often become a "go-between." Both the patient and members of the family may ask the physician for information about the seriousness of the condition, and they may express thoughts about decisions that have to be made. But often it becomes obvious that they are not talking *to each other* about these things. Indeed, it is not uncommon for several clusters to form within the patient's family and social circle, with none of them communicating fully with the others and the physician unable to determine which of them is preeminent in serving the patient's interests. One useful service the physician can render here is to prompt these parties to communicate openly with one another and to facilitate this communication (which is understandably difficult for all involved) when it does begin to occur.

A. Primacy of Patient Preference   Self-determination is a personal right of the competent, adult patient; thus, when the patient and family are on different wavelengths, the patient's preferences must be honored. However, with proper attention to communication, a confrontation on these issues can be avoided in many cases.

For example, if a patient expresses to you, his physician, definite wishes to withdraw from treatment or not to be resuscitated, you should ask whether he has talked these decisions over with the family. If he has not, offering to assist him in discussing his wishes with the family (or perhaps even to convey his wishes to the family on his behalf) could help avoid future misunderstandings on all sides. If the family finds it difficult to discuss these matters or to accept the patient's decision, you can work with them further—in a gradual and supportive way—to explain the facts of the patient's situation, the basis of the patient's choices, and the importance for the emotional well-being of the patient (and indeed, of the family as a unit) of their understanding and support.

If you are unwilling or unable to dedicate time and effort to sorting out complex family situations, you may want to enlist the assistance of other members of the health-care team to work with the family in depth. In a setting with a coordinated health-care team, it is not necessary for every team member to go over each item of information with the patient and family. A clinical "division of labor" may prevail here. It is imperative, of course, that all relevant information be communicated by someone or other. Responsibility for coordination of information exchange is most naturally assigned to the primary physician. (Similarly, it ought not be necessary to go over all the information with each family member individually. Family members have a duty to share information they have been given among themselves (with a proviso to follow). Family members sometimes invoke a principle of confidentiality to justify keeping to themselves what the physician has told them, but there is no valid principle of confidentiality between family member and physician that would apply in this case.)

This interaction with the family should not be considered a diversion from patient care. If you can generate support and understanding from the family, the effects on the patient may be more significant than large doses of pain control medications or lengthy counseling sessions on your part.

B. Confidentiality and Family Involvement   Discussions with the family may test the principle of confidentiality. Strictly speaking, confidentiality is a right of the individual patient, and one steps beyond the bounds of confidentiality by disclosing *any* information to *anyone* outside the health-care team without express permission from the patient. The ACP Ethics Manual stresses this point:

> The problem should not be discussed with his family unless the patient authorizes such a discussion. . . . Physicians should not breach the confidential nature of the physician/patient relationship by discussing the patient's care with

persons who are not authorized by the patient to be made aware of the patient's diagnosis, prognosis, or treatment. . . . Physicians should understand that mere blood relationship does not by itself allow a family member to know about or authorize the medical treatment of a patient. [ACP 1984a *(Manual)*, 28–29; 1984b *(Annals)*, 265]

However, as the author of Ecclesiastes points out, there is "a time to keep silence, and a time to speak." To insist on the letter of the law here may have a "chilling" effect on important relationships. When a concerned family member encounters you in the hallway of the hospital and asks how the patient is doing, refusing to disclose any information, explaining that you must first get express permission from the patient, may cause a strain in your relationship with an ally with whom you may need to work closely to provide support to and make decisions about the patient in the final stages of his life. This situation can sometimes be avoided by explaining to the patient in advance that you will discuss his case with the family; however, if the patient is having difficulty facing the situation himself and is perhaps finding it awkward to disclose essential information to you, bringing up the possibility of your passing information on to family members may further inhibit him. If the patient expresses a wish that certain matters not be discussed with the family, your response may be to encourage the patient to change his mind and allow open communication, rather than simply accepting his wishes as the last word on the matter. However, disclosure should not proceed unless and until the patient has been persuaded to authorize it.

If you encounter family members with questions, one useful approach is to begin by sounding them out about how much information the patient himself has provided. If the patient has been completely open with them, it does not appear to violate the spirit of the principle of confidentiality for you to correct and interpret the information they already have. However, if it becomes obvious that the patient has been guarded, you would be wise to provide only the most general information until you discuss with the patient the reasons in favor of open communication (or learn from him the reasons why it is inadvisable to provide information to particular persons).

2.3.2 Patients of Questionable Competence   If the competence of the patient is in doubt, family members may be enlisted to assist in *assessing* the degree of impairment. Since they are most familiar with the patient's normal functioning, they are in a good position to provide information relevant to a determination of competence.

The family also may assist in ascertaining the patient's core values. This can be an aspect of determining competence, and it can also form a basis for decision making when the patient is incapable of participating fully in the process.

It is advisable, from both legal and ethical viewpoints, to include the family in decision making. Although it is true that "family members and next of kin have *no legal authority* to make crucial decisions on behalf of *adult* patients unable to make decisions on their own behalf, unless that authority is specifically given by the act of a judge granting guardianship powers (or in several states, by a statute)" (Jonsen et al. 1982, 146–147), it is going too far to say that family members "have no legal, ethical, or moral standing to enforce their desires unless a court declares the patient to be legally incompetent and appoints a guardian to make treatment decisions for the patient" [ACP 1984a *(Manual)*, 28; 1984b *(Annals)*, 265]. The legal status of family involvement in decision making without recourse to the courts has never been addressed explicitly by courts, which is understandable since the cases brought before them can hardly have the feature of not being brought before a court (See President's Commission 1983, 131–132).

However, the moral warrant for including the family in decision making is strong, stemming from principles of respect for the family as a key social unit. [For a sensitive discussion of this point, see *Deciding to Forego* (President's Commission 1983, 127–129).] Even in legal terms, it is still important to consult family members. After all, they will be around after the patient has died, and they may be left with ill feelings toward the action. In other words, they may feel that it is a "time to cast . . . stones" (i.e., through legal action) if they believe the decision was arbitrary (i.e., if they were not included in making it). Furthermore, it can be of benefit both to patient and family in facing the outcome to make them feel "ownership" of the plan of action (or inaction).

The President's Commission wisely counsels involvement of the family in informal ways and avoidance of formal court actions in most situations. (See Appendix II, Section 2, recommendation 9, fifth entry.)

2.3.3 Family and Incompetent Patients   Both the President's Commission and the AMA Judicial Council acknowledge that the patient's family provides the prime candidates for surrogate decisionmakers for incompetent patients. The ACP departs from this view only to endorse seeking official legal guardianship or conservatorship in more cases than the other two groups recommend.

The President's Commission stresses that the standard for decision making ought to be what the patient would have wanted in terms of his or her own deepest personal values. If this cannot be determined (e.g., a patient who was *never* competent to formulate personal values or who never communicated them to others), then the *patient's* best interests ought to be the guideline for decisions.

The physician's responsibilities here include 1) supplying information to family or guardian, on the basis of which the most enlightened decision possible can be made, and 2) providing emotional support to aid in making best use of this information. However, the physician's role does not end here. He must continue to serve as an advocate for the patient, evaluating the family's decision in the light of his own understanding of the patient's values and best interests. If there is reason to believe the family is making an inappropriate decision, the physician should 1) prompt the family to think the matter through again, 2) bring other members of the health-care team into the discussion and/or perhaps consult an institutional review committee, and 3) perhaps initiate court review of the matter if an inappropriate decision still is proposed.

2.3.4 Alternatives to Family Decision   The family is not automatically vested with authority to make decisions for incompetent patients. In some cases, it may be more appropriate for friends of the patient to occupy this role than for any family member, e.g., when the family has not maintained close contact through the years and the friend is in a much better position to know the patient's fundamental personal values.

In the past the patient may have indicated a preference about the person who should make decisions; if so, every attempt should be made to honor this. There are a variety of ways in which the patient might state her preference: 1) through personal communication with you as her physician, or with her minister or some other trustworthy professional; 2) through an annotation on an advance directive ("Living Will") document; and/or 3) through the formal legal mechanism of a durable power of attorney. The last of these has the most solid legal standing (see President's Commission 1983, Appendix E, 390–437). The others may require confirmation through court action. The physician in his role as patient advocate may have the responsibility to initiate the requisite court action and he may also play an important role in the proceedings that result. You should seek the advice of legal counsel about the appropriate procedures in your locality for such situations. You also have an ethical responsibility to assure that the steps taken are indeed in the best interests of your patient and not (for example) primarily undertaken to serve the interests of other parties.

Finally, more and more patients are communicating their preferences about limits to treatment by means of advance directive documents. A growing number of states have statutes that enable and regulate this process; in the states that have not taken such action, a properly executed "Living Will" can carry significant weight in court as evidence of the patient's wishes. Many of these documents are vague and general, however, so it is best for you to explore further the personal values of a patient who presents such a document to you (perhaps encouraging him to add to the document more specific guidelines on which you agree).

2.4 Other Dimensions of Limits to Treatment

In the previous sections, some key elements of decisions to limit treatment have been described. However, numerous other morally relevant dimensions may be present in actual situations in which you face these choices. Table 4-1 contains a list of many considerations commonly cited in connection with such decisions.

The boundaries between some of these items are not sharp and well defined (e.g., items 15 and 16), and others are subject to differences of interpretation (e.g., item 43). Furthermore, actual cases almost always contain complexes of these elements intermingled. The first step in analyzing a case, then, is to identify the elements within it. Then the valence and weight of each element can be determined, and each can be weighed against the others to reach a final judgment.

Three valences are possible. A certain consideration may suggest a given treatment is either:

a. obligatory or morally required
b. optional or morally permissible (i.e., either the choice to treat or the choice not to treat would be justified)
c. prohibited or morally wrong.

For example, that the patient explicitly requests a certain treatment (Table 4-1, item 1)[9] creates a *prima facie obligation (a)* to provide it. That the procedure is without significant risk (cf. item 8) counts toward classifying it as *morally optional (b)*. That the procedure itself involves doing harm (cf. item 39) makes it *prima facie morally wrong (c)*.

If (as often happens) the same proposed treatment has all these features, conflicting factors must be weighed against each other to determine on which side the resultant moral force is found. Consider the following two situations, both of which have the valences described:

Patient A asks the doctor to lance a painful boil, even though it has been explained that the procedure itself will cause some discomfort. Here the harm done (discomfort) seems justified by the patient's acceptance of it and by the fact that it may prevent greater discomfort in the future. Thus, considered on the whole, the act is morally permissible. We can see that it is not morally obligatory because it would be permissible to forego this treatment if the patient has a change of mind at the last minute and decides she prefers some other treatment approach.

Patient B asks the doctor to cut a hole in the side of his nose through which he can hang jewelry in the "punk rock" style. He says he is aware that the procedure will cause some discomfort, and that it will leave a permanent scar. Here the harm done (discomfort, scar) does not seem justified, even though the patient accepts it, since no therapeutic benefit results. Thus, on the whole, it is morally wrong for a physician to perform this procedure.

Let us consider how this sort of analysis works in a concrete case situation.

---

9. Throughout Sections 2 and 3 of this chapter, any citation of "item" with a number refers to the list on Table 4-1.

Table 4-1 Terminating Treatment: Grounds For and Against

A. Consent Elements

1. Patient's informed consent/refusal of treatment/demand for treatment/demand to die
2. Substituted judgment: decision made by another, but based upon an attempt to determine what the patient himself/ herself would choose if competent.
3. Proxy consent/refusal/demand: decision made on behalf of the patient by a designated agent, ideally based upon the agent's judgment as to what is in the *patient's* best interests.
4. Family's or friends' wishes in the matter: decision based upon the best interests, values, etc. of the *family and/or friends themselves.*
5. Consensus judgment: of any or all of the following: patient, family, friends, health-care professionals, hospital ethics committee.

B. Quality of Life Judgments

6. Patient's quality of life: determined wholly from the perspective of the patient himself/herself.
7. Evaluation of the patient's quality of life from the perspective of an observer: e.g., "I don't know what that state of life feels like from the inside, but I consider it unacceptable."
8. Disvalues of treatment: Pain, risks, indignities, uncertainties, displacement, disruption of relationships.
9. To prevent the patient from "losing hope"
10. Family's quality of life: cf. Section D, especially item 24.

C. Medical Judgments

11. Determination that death has already occurred
12. Efficacy of treatment: "Treatment wouldn't do any good anyway."
13. Reversibility of illness
14. Imminence of death: "She doesn't have long to live no matter how much we do."
15. Standard-medical-care policy: assumes that a given procedure is obligatory if its use is "standard medical care" in cases of this clinical type.

16. Medical-indications policy (Ramsey 1978): assumes that a given procedure is obligatory as long as there exist "medical indications" or "biological indices" for its use.
17. Implications of the patient/professional relationship: "Patients expect their physicians to . . . "
18. Principles of professional ethics
19. Goals of medicine: e.g., to extend life, to relieve suffering, to restore health, etc.
20. Educational values: "To attempt to extend this patient's life for a short period could teach me how to save lives of future patients."
21. Research values: "Medical science could learn something from this patient which would save lives of future patients."

D. Other—Regarding Judgments

22. Patient's obligations to others: "The patient owes it to his children to allow them some time to adjust to the prospect of his death," or "The patient owes it to his family to spare them the agony of a prolonged death watch."
23. Family's obligations to patient: "The family owes it to the patient to spare her this suffering," or "The family owes it to the patient to see that everything is done that can possibly be done."
24. Family's obligations to its members and others: "The family members owe it to themselves not to prolong their agony in a protracted death-watch," or "They owe it to his friends to allow them time to adjust to the prospect of his death."
25. Societal obligations to patient: e.g., to provide treatment resources, to spare the patient from pain and indignity.
26. Societal needs: e.g., for the resources required to sustain this patient, for the moral example the patient could provide.
27. Public health issues
28. Allocation of resources issues: e.g., effects of denying resources to others, issues of equity, social worth of patient, expenses of treatment.
29. Effects on health services personnel who must work with the patient

E. Conceptual Elements

30. Ordinary/extraordinary measures distinction
31. Natural/artificial support distinction
32. Killing/allowing-to-die distinction
33. Active/passive measures distinction
34. An "act of mercy"
35. Providing "a good death"
36. To avoid "playing God"
37. To avoid acting "contrary to Nature"
38. To avoid "prolonging dying"
39. To satisfy the precept "do no harm"
40. Deontological religious standards: accordance with God's will, the Ten Commandments, other biblical dictates, etc.
41. To satisfy requirements of law

F. Moral Principles

42. The Golden Rule: "because this is what I would want done if I were in the patient's shoes (or bed)."

43. Principle of sanctity of life
44. Principle of right to life
45. Principle of value of life
46. Slippery slope objections: even though this act may not be wrong in itself, undertaking it may incline us in the future to perform acts that *are* clearly objectionable.
47. Appeal to the "symbolic meaning" of treatment (or nontreatment)
48. Appeal to the long-term consequences of this decision: e.g., disabilities become intolerable; the infirm may feel social pressure to refuse treatment.

G. Factual Appeals

49. "A miracle cure might come along."
50. Appeal to uncertainty of diagnosis, prognosis: "We cannot know for certain that death is near."

2.4.1 Case: A Physician in an Overseas Hospital: Part I The following case has been adapted from Symmers (1968, 442).

A physician, aged 68 years, was admitted to an overseas hospital after a barium meal had shown a large carcinoma of the stomach. He had retired from practice five years earlier, after a severe myocardial infarction had left his exercise tolerance considerably reduced.

The early symptoms of the carcinoma were mistakenly attributed to myocardial ischemia. By the time the possibility of carcinoma was first considered, the disease was already far advanced. Laparotomy showed extensive metastatic involvement of the abdominal lymph nodes and liver.

Palliative gastrectomy was performed with the object of preventing perforation of the primary tumor into the peritoneal cavity, which appeared to the surgeon to be imminent. Histological examination showed the growth to be an anaplastic primary adenocarcinoma. There was clinical and radiological evidence of secondary deposits in the lower thoracic and lumbar vertebrae.

The patient was told of the findings and fully understood their import. He was not asked for, nor did he offer, any expressions of his wishes with regard to resuscitation or aggressive life support measures. His primary physician had indicated nothing about such decisions in the medical record.

In spite of increasingly large doses of pethidine, and of morphine at night, the patient suffered constantly with severe abdominal pain and pain resulting from compression of spinal nerves by tumor deposits.

On the tenth day after the gastrectomy, the patient collapsed with classic manifestations of massive pulmonary embolism and suffered cardiac arrest. A staff physician happened to be on the unit when the arrest occurred. His first impulse was to order full resuscitation measures and to undertake an emergency pulmonary embolectomy. But he hesitated a moment, wondering whether this was the right thing to do with this particular patient.

Consider the following questions:

1. If you faced this decision, what would *you* do? Why?

2. Do you see this decision as a *dilemma* (i.e., an option with strong moral considerations weighing both for and against each alternative)? List the moral considerations involved in the choice.

3. What measures (if any) could have been taken in advance to prevent this choice becoming a dilemma for the staff physician?

The chief difficulty in making a decision in this situation is the absence of information about *consent elements* (items 1–5). One can question why this information was not obtained from the patient earlier, but the fact remains that at this point it is too late to gather any information about the patient's wishes, nor is there time to discuss the matter with the staff of the unit to reach a consensus judgment.

Judgments about the patient's *quality of life* are obviously an important factor in the decision. But notice that, absent a discussion with the patient, quality of life must be judged from the standpoint of an observer (item 7) rather than from the patient's own assessment (item 6). A reliable judgment on this basis would require a much closer relationship with the patient than the staff of this unit had experienced in the brief time they had cared for him. Furthermore, the state of life of this patient immediately prior to the arrest was not obviously below the threshold of a worthwhile quality of life. He was conscious, alert, and capable of communicating with those around him. He appeared to have been reasonably mobile. Although his pain was considerable, it was not so severe as to cloud his consciousness or to prevent meaningful mental activity.

Determinations of the *efficacy of treatment* (item 12) and the *reversibility of illness* (item 13) will vary depending upon the basis on which the judgment is made. Resuscitation and embolectomy offer a fairly good prospect of reversing the cardiac arrest. However, even if they are successful in achieving this limited objective, the patient's underlying cancer and heart disease will not be reversed. Thus, from a perspective of the overall condition of the patient, the proposed treatments must be ruled ineffective and the conditions irreversible.

A *standard-medical-care policy* (item 15) or a *medical-indications policy* (item 16) faces similar difficulties. Determinations of "standard" care or medical "indications" are often made from the limited perspective of efficacy regarding the immediate medical crisis, with little attention to the overall life prospects of the patient. Overcoming the immediate problem benefits the patient little if the life situation to which he is restored is painful, hopeless, and/or unwelcome.

In this situation little is known of the patient's family or other social relationships, so the *other-regarding elements* (items 22–24) cannot be ascertained sufficiently to make them a major factor in the decision.

None of the *conceptual elements* (items 30–40) appears to offer a decisive basis for choice in this situation either. One might argue that refraining from resuscitating this patient would be an "act of mercy" (item 34) that would provide a "good death" (item 35) and avoid prolonging the dying process (item 38). However, without any indication from the patient that he finds his condition intolerable, to make such a judgment would be an extremely presumptuous exercise of paternalism.

The application of the distinctions in items 30–33 does not entail one conclusion rather than the other. Resuscitation might be classified as an *ordinary* measure (and thus perhaps as morally obligatory), but a case might be made for considering the emergency embolectomy as an *extraordinary* measure. If resuscitation is foregone, the patient would have been *allowed to die* rather than killed (item 32), and his death would have resulted from *passive* rather than active death-dealing measures (item 33). These factors might indicate that foregoing resuscitation would be morally permissible, but they do not provide a decisive reason for or against this choice.

Most of the *moral principles* listed (with the possible exception, in this case, of item 42) dictate sustaining life, but they would be challenged by many people in precisely this sort of situation. The *factual appeals* (items 49–50) seem clearly misguided if applied to this situation: the diagnosis has been thoroughly confirmed, and the patient's medical problems are so overwhelming that the possibility of a cure is virtually nonexistent.

The *law* (item 41) leaves decisions in such situations to the discretion of the physician present (wisely, in our judgment), but this means that it cannot be looked to as a basis for decision.

On what basis, then, is a decision to be made in this situation? Without decisive indications of the patient's wishes or other consent elements and decisive negative quality of life judgments, the most reasonable basis for choice is to invoke what the President's Commission describes as a "presumption in favor of sustaining life" [see Appendix II, Section 2, recommendation 2] This presumption, in turn, is rooted in the principle of the value of life (item 45).

Thus, we conclude that resuscitation is morally obligatory in this situation. And that, indeed, is the decision that was made in the actual case, as you shall now see.

2.4.2 Case: Part II

The staff physician decided to proceed with resuscitation and emergency pulmonary embolectomy. The patient was successfully resuscitated and stabilized.

When the patient had recovered sufficiently, he expressed his appreciation of the good intentions and skill of his young colleague. At the same time, he asked that if he had a further cardiovascular collapse no steps should be taken to prolong his life, for the pain of the cancer was now more than he would needlessly continue to endure. He himself wrote a note to this effect in his case records, and the staff of the hospital were made aware of his feelings.

Two weeks after the embolectomy, the patient collapsed again—this time with acute myocardial infarction and cardiac arrest. (adapted from Symmers 1968, 442)

Consider the following questions:

1. Should the patient be resuscitated this time? Why or why not?

2. Do you see this decision as a *dilemma?* List the moral considerations involved in the choice.

3. What further measures (if any) could have been taken in advance to prevent this choice becoming a dilemma for the staff?

What elements are relevant to the choice in this new situation? Clearly it is of great importance that the patient has emphatically expressed his own wishes in the matter. At this point the staff is provided with the strongest sort of consent element: an informed judgment to refuse treatment made by the patient himself (item 1). This consideration heavily favors the judgment that further resuscitation would be *morally wrong.* In legal terms resuscitation would constitute a battery, and the moral assessment here would concur with the law.

Furthermore, the patient has supplied a clear and emphatic personal assessment of his quality of life (item 6). An observer might not agree with this assessment (item 7), but there is little (if any) basis for preferring an external assessment to the patient's own in this case. A quality-of-life judgment is made up of at least two elements: 1) a prediction about what future life events are in prospect for the patient, and 2) an evaluation of these life events based on the patient's fundamental values. In some cases an observer might be in a better position than the patient himself to make judgments of the first type—e.g., a physician making a technical prognosis based on her past professional experience with similar cases. There might even be some situations in which an observer can ascertain the patient's fundamental values better than the person himself—e.g., a friend who knows that the person is likely to get over his broken heart and find a new romantic interest in time, whereas the lovestruck one insists, "There will never be anyone else for me." However, neither of these sorts of situations apply in the present case. This patient is likely to know his central values, and he understands the prospects for satisfaction of those values. Thus his own quality-of-life judgment must prevail.

What (if anything) would favor a decision to resuscitate under these conditions? There is the consideration that the immediate condition is probably reversible (item 13), although the fact remains that the underlying conditions are not. A strong sanctity-of-life principle (item 43) would emphatically favor resuscitation. There is enough ambiguity in the law on these matters (item 41) to make one nervous about any decision reached, but one is more likely to encounter civil suits and/or criminal prosecution as a result of nontreatment than from an error in the opposite direction.

However, disturbing as this legal situation might be, protecting oneself from suit is not as weighty a factor in moral terms as the consent and quality-of-life elements. Thus, the weight of moral considerations in these circumstances would make nonresuscitation not only *morally permissible,* but even *morally obligatory.*

The "time to heal" is past, Instead, it is now "a time to embrace," "a time to love," and otherwise a time to comfort and sustain this patient as he faces the inevitable "time to die." It is now time to acknowledge the statement of the ACP Ethics Manual that "the physician has a responsibility to ensure that his hopelessly ill patient dies with dignity and with as little of suffering as possible" [ACP 1984a *(Manual),* 26; 1984b *(Annals),* 265].

Read on to see what was actually done in this case.

2.4.3 Case: Part III

His wish notwithstanding, the patient was again revived by the hospital's emergency resuscitation team. His heart stopped on four further occasions during that night, and each time was restarted artificially.

The body then recovered sufficiently to linger for three more weeks, but in a decerebrate state, punctuated by episodes of projectile vomiting accompanied by generalized convulsions.

Intravenous nourishment was carefully combined with blood transfusions and measures necessary to maintain electrolyte and fluid balance. In addition, antibacterial and antifungal antibiotics were given as prophylaxis against infection, particularly pneumonia complicating the tracheotomy that had been performed to ensure a clear airway.

On the last day of his illness, preparations were being made for the work of the failing respiratory center to be given over to an artificial ventilator, but the heart finally stopped before this endeavor could be realized. (adapted from Symmers 1968, 442)

Consider the following questions:

1. Analyze the considerations for and against each of the measures that were taken in this case:

   a. the initial resuscitation

   b. the four additional resuscitations required that same night

   c. intravenous nourishment

   d. blood transfusions

e. measures necessary to maintain electrolyte and fluid balance

f. tracheotomy

g. mechanical ventilator

2. Do you see these choices as *dilemmas?*

3. What measures (if any) could have been taken in advance to prevent these choices becoming a dilemma for the staff?

These actions go beyond any reasonable presumption in favor of life. Instead, they appear to involve a blind *inertia* to "keep trying" or perhaps an unthinking sanctity-of-life principle. As indicated earlier, we contend that the patient's explicit request and his own quality-of-life assessment were sufficient to show that the first resuscitation attempt in this series was morally prohibited. However, even if this had not been so, surely once that effort was completed and the patient's resulting mental status was assessed, it should have been obvious that the patient's quality of life was so low as to make further life-sustaining efforts morally optional at best or even morally wrong.

Each step taken moved further in the direction of heroic or extraordinary measures (item 30). The introduction of intravenous nourishment and substances to maintain electrolyte balance was clearly an artificial means of sustaining this life (item 31) and, as such, morally optional or questionable in this context. Even if these were introduced before the patient's mental status could be determined, to withdraw them once the patient's quality of life became clear would not be an act of killing (item 32). The quality of life is so low here as to be below the threshold that creates an obligation to sustain life.

All in all, the reaction at this stage seems to be undeniably a case of *misuse* of medical techniques and technology, serving no valid purpose. Lest you take comfort from supposing that this could only happen in an "overseas" hospital and not in our society, you should notice that this case is taken from a British medical journal. The "overseas" hospital may have been in the United States.

2.4.4 Conclusions[10]

1. *No one of these considerations is decisive by itself.*

The strongest individual factor is the personal consent element (item 1). However, even this does not establish conclusively an obligation on its own. If a patient with a critical but fully reversible illness such as bacterial meningitis emphatically refuses treatment, many physicians would find it unconscionable to honor this request. [For extended discussion of such a case, see Jonsen et al. (1982, 78–80).]

---

10. The conceptual elements in Table 4-1 (items 30–33) are addressed in many of the works listed in the "Further Reading" section, so they will not be treated in detail here. For an especially thorough and balanced discussion, see *Deciding to Forego Life-Sustaining Treatment* (President's Commission 1983, 60–90; see also recommendation 5 in Appendix II, Section 2).

Absent a quality-of-life judgment, a judgment about the irreversibility of the condition, or a prognosis of the imminence of death that makes sense of this refusal, it does not carry sufficient weight to make honoring it obligatory. At the very least, a physician would be justified in refusing to carry out the patient's request on grounds of conscience. (However, there would be questions about the conscience of any other professional who allowed the patient to carry out this request.)

The Golden Rule (item 42) is often cited as a sufficient standard by itself. Upon analysis, however, the Golden Rule has a limited usefulness. It can point out certain fairly obvious moral wrongs in a context of shared values. ("Stop biting people. How would you like it if people bit *you?*" This is, of course, even more effective if accompanied by a demonstration.) But this principle by no means provides the basis for the whole of morality.

The Golden Rule is especially troublesome in circumstances in which value pluralism reigns, because it invites us to impose our own personal values on other people. If my personal distaste for eating snails is so strong that I would not want anyone even to *offer* me snails, for example, the Golden Rule might lead me to propose outlawing the eating of snails altogether.

More to the point here, one might have personal values at present that strongly oppose any measure to limit treatment—for example, a desire to exhibit courage and endurance in the face of suffering, which might lead her to judge that requests by others to avoid prolonging suffering ought to be ignored. At the extreme, she might even decide now not to have granted a future request of her own to cease treatment, since she can only assume that she would have lapsed into irrationality before making such a request. There might be justification for her adopting such a policy in her own case (through specification on an advance directive document). The objectionable move is for her to employ the Golden Rule argument to impose the same policy on others.

Similarly, a unilateral quality-of-life judgment (items 6 and 7) is not generally a reliable guide to decision. Since quality-of-life judgments are composed of both a "subjective" or personal element as well as an "objective" or predictive element, it is ethically problematic for any person to make such assessments alone. The physician may be able to predict with precision the level of comfort and functioning in store for the patient, but only the patient can decide whether this state is worthwhile. A long-term knowledge of the patient can give strong clues here, but even this cannot provide a solid base for judgment, since the patient's assessment may change when conditions of illness are actually encountered. In the last analysis, then, it is hazardous for anyone other than the patient him- or herself to make these judgments. And the patient may not be able to understand fully the predictive element in such judgments. (For a useful catalog of subjective factors that might affect unilateral quality-of-life judgments, see Appendix III for the excerpt from the ACP Ethics Manual entitled "Quality of Life.")

Quality-of-life judgments, then, are inherently problematic. They may have a role in treatment/nontreatment decisions, but they must be employed with extreme caution.

Judgments of medical indications (item 16) are problematic in the same way. The probability that the *immediate* medical crisis can be reversed might be quite high. However, if this leaves an irreversible underlying condition, then the value of successfully achieving this limited objective can be assessed only by determining its contribution to the patient's quality of life.

2. *No* one *of these considerations is irrelevant to a decision.*

Some of them may turn out to carry very little weight in the final assessment of an action, but none can be discounted entirely. And in certain circumstances the relatively small weight of one factor may "tip the scales" in one direction.

Many commentators eschew reference to financial considerations in connection with these decisions. It is tragic, for example, when a patient feels it necessary to reject further treatment on the grounds that its cost would ruin his family financially (item 22). However, this sense of tragedy may be due largely to a belief that society owes it to the patient and family (item 25) not to allow them to be driven to a choice such as this; this belief overlooks the harsh fact that parallel choices must be made at a societal level (items 26 and 28). Although these are usually addressed in abstract rather than personalized terms, a specific case could arise in which the costs of life-sustaining measures were so exorbitant that we could not permit allocation of this proportion of societal resources to this one patient. Thus, the question is *how much* weight to give this factor, not whether to weigh it in at all.

Similarly, educational values (item 20) and research values (item 21), although they should not be elevated in importance above the best interests of the patient, may be factored into the decision. Occasionally they may be decisive in the choice between two treatments that are closely balanced in the extent to which they serve the patient's best interests.

3. *A priorities list for urgent situations can be constructed.*

When a decision about a life-sustaining treatment must be made immediately, the following order of considerations is appropriate:

1. Consent elements, especially item 1
   a. If a clear directive has been offered by the patient (as it should have been in most cases if the advance work of the DPA has been carried out), it should be honored.
   b. If there is no clear directive that covers the case at hand, proceed to the next item.

2. Imminence of death *without* treatment
   a. If death is imminent and the need for action is urgent, the presumption in favor of sustaining life may dictate initiating action immediately, without further consideration.
   b. If time allows further reflection, then proceed to the next item.
3. Efficacy of treatment from a limited perspective
   a. If the odds are high that the treatment will be ineffective in overcoming the immediate crisis, there is little point in initiating it.
   b. If there is a reasonable chance that the immediate crisis can be combated successfully, proceed to the next item.
4. Disvalues of treatment
   a. If the disvalues of treatment are so great that they vastly outweigh the benefit of overcoming the immediate threat, it would be a net harm to the patient to initiate it.
   b. If the disvalues are within reasonable limits, proceed to the next item.
5. Imminence of death *with* treatment
   a. If reversing this condition restores the patient to an overall life situation with little prospect of long-term survival, it seems pointless to undertake it.
   b. If the patient's overall life prospects are more hopeful, proceed to the next item.
6. Quality of life
   a. If your evaluation of the patient's net quality of life is overwhelmingly negative and well grounded, there seems no moral justification to act to sustain this life.
   b. If your evaluation is affirmative, proceed to the next item.
7. Financial burden
   a. If the treatment imposes no financial burden, there is every reason to undertake it.
   b. If the treatment imposes a severe financial burden, weigh this negative factor against the benefits to be derived from treatment.

3 Seriously Ill Newborns

3.1 Issues

Decisions about treatment for seriously ill newborns are parallel in many (but not all) crucial respects to decisions for an incompetent adult patient. Among the chief *differences* are:

1. The infant has had no opportunity to develop personal values and plans of her own to form a basis for a substituted judgment (item 2); thus the best interests

standard (item 3) is the only patient-oriented basis for judgments. (This trait is shared by some adult patients, i.e., those who have been significantly mentally retarded from birth. See, for example, the court case of Joseph Saikewicz in "Further Readings.")

2. A prognosis of irreversibility is even more uncertain here than with adult patients, due to both the remarkable healing potential of the infant metabolism and the dramatic and rapid developments in neonatology. (There may be near-parallels to this in certain volatile adult conditions.)

3. The role of parents is unusually forceful with regard to infants and children. This stems largely from the child-rearing responsibility that society has entrusted to the parents.

The key question is how far the authority of parents extends. In general, parents are given wide latitude in carrying out their responsibilities, bounded by certain social policies. Parents are free to choose among a variety of forms of schooling for their children, but they are not free to avoid education for them altogether. Child abuse and neglect are prohibited by the state acting in its role as parent of last resort (i.e., *parens patriae*). However, many of these limits to parental responsibility have been recognized only relatively recently, and in some jurisdictions some restrictions are still only weakly enforced. (See Marsh 1981, especially Chapter 2: "The Historical Perspective of Children's Rights.")

The Judicial Council of the AMA endorses giving parents a dominant role in these decisions (see the second paragraph from the opinion on "Quality of Life," quoted in Section 2.1).

In contrast, the Federal Government has in recent years proposed a series of regulations dealing with these decisions that does not acknowledge any discretionary authority on the part of the parents. These rules, which have come to be called "Baby Doe regulations," if enacted would employ the mechanisms of civil rights enforcement to police decisions regarding limits to treatment for seriously ill newborns. Several versions of such regulations have been struck down by the courts (wisely, in our judgment). The latest version, passed by the US Congress in October 1984 after lengthy negotiations between several interested parties, moves away from this civil-rights model. Instead, it requires state child protective services agencies to establish definitions of and responses to forms of child neglect and abuse involving medical treatment. This brings these decisions more into line with the bounded domain of authority characteristic of parental responsibilities.

The legislation defines "withholding medically indicated treatment" as

> the failure to respond to the infant's life-threatening conditions by providing treatment (including appropriate nutrition, hydration, and medication) which, in the treating physician's or physicians' reasonable medical judgment will be most likely to be effective in ameliorating or correcting all such conditions.

Failure to treat does *not* apply when, "in the treating physician's or physicians' reasonable medical judgment,
(A) the infant is chronically and irreversibly comatose;
(B) the provision of such treatment would
  1) merely prolong dying
  2) not be effective in ameliorating all of the infant's life-threatening conditions, or
  3) otherwise be futile in terms of the survival of the infant; or
(C) the provision of such treatment would be virtually futile in terms of the survival of the infant and the treatment itself under such circumstances would be inhumane." (Public Law 98-457)

3.2 Conclusions

Parents, as surrogates for the infant, should fully share in decision making at every stage. In the same ways in which adult patients are informed, sustained, and consulted about decisions in their own cases, parents should participate in making decisions about infants.

The basic principles governing decisions for newborns should be the same as those for adult patients; i.e., if there is a realistic possibility that the infant could benefit significantly from treatment, it ought to be initiated. This judgment of benefit is arrived at (as in adult cases) by weighing and balancing the full complex of elements listed in Table 4-1, especially

1. the imminence of death without treatment (item 14)
2. the imminence of death with treatment
3. the efficacy of treatment (item 12) and the irreversibility of the illness (item 13), from a broad life perspective
4. a realistic assessment of the prospects for the child receiving the intensive and enthusiastic level of post-hospital care that will be required to realize his full potential—whether this will be from the family (items 10, 23, and 24) or from social institutions
5. the present and prospective quality of life (item 7).
6. the financial burden to the family and to society (Items 10, 26, and 28).

In many cases of seriously ill newborns, residual disabilities make the fourth item especially important. One may argue that the family and/or society have a strong obligation to provide resources to allow the child to develop to her full potential. The President's Commission (1983, 205–207) states the case for this ably. However, if it appears unlikely that this obligation will be met, it is unrealistic to make a decision based on the assumption that it will be. Any attempt to force unwilling parents to live up to what *we* perceive to be their duty is unlikely to succeed. Prospects for success in persuading society to live up to its duty here may be somewhat greater, if we are willing to work at it, but success is unlikely to come swiftly enough to be of much help to *this* baby.

If the parents express definite wishes regarding treatment of their newborns (and they should be guided to do so), their judgment should be determinative in situations in which the options are relatively evenly balanced. They may be overruled in some situations, but only when the benefits of the treatment they wish to forego (or the harms of the treatment they are insisting on instituting) are so clear that to carry out their wishes would amount to a form of child abuse.

The authority of parents to volunteer their infants and children for procedures whose orientation is more experimental than therapeutic is sufficiently in doubt that such decisions should routinely be ratified by some carefully chosen third party or parties.

4 Abortion

The issue of abortion extends the questions of the previous section yet a step further. The moral standing of any infant is called into question because of a paucity of any previous moral relationships, but the standing of the fetus is even more questionable in this regard—although recent developments in *in utero* surgery and diagnostic tests add to the inventory by establishing a physician-patient relationship with the fetus. Current policy with regard to seriously ill newborn infants implies that an independent right to life is subordinated in practice to the moral authority of parents to determine whether this right is exercised or waived; thus any such claim of a right to life for a zygote or fetus will be even more controversial. Whatever limits are placed on the authority of parents to make life-and-death decisions for newborn infants, these are generally regarded as exceeded by the authority of a pregnant woman to end her pregnancy during the first trimester.

Clearly a central question in this debate is whether or not the fetus is to be regarded as an independent member of the moral community, i.e., as a "person" or a "human being" in his/her/its own right. Like the question of demarcating the threshold of death (discussed in Section 1), this is fundamentally a philosophical question: What traits and/or relationships must a being have in order to be considered "one of us," a member of the moral community of persons? This question has been debated at length in philosophical and theological circles for centuries, and it is unlikely that one of the several competing answers will be declared the winner of the debate in the immediate future. Some of the many definitions of the beginning of moral personhood that have been proposed are shown in Table 4-2. However, although the question of the moral personhood of the fetus is certainly a central issue in connection with abortion, it is important to recognize that it does not, by itself, competely resolve the question of the moral justification of abortion.

Table 4-2 Beginning of Moral Personhood

Transition Point	Underlying Philosophical Rationale
Pre-conception	Transmigration of souls, reincarnation—the personal identity (soul) exists before and independent of embodiment.
Conception	Identification of personal identity and/or potentiality with genetic integrity.
Conception + 14 days	Past twinning limit, assumes that individuation of soul, identity, or life is established once genetic integrity is firm.
Implantation	Acknowledging the high frequency of spontaneous abortions before this stage; thus individual identity or potentiality is tied with the *probability* of live birth.
Organ function	The beginning of "life" is sometimes dated from the initiation of the functioning of certain key organs, such as the heart or the brain. This is an attempt to make the criterion of the beginning of life parallel to the operational criterion of death.
Quickening	Reflects ancient view that the fetus was inert matter until a certain point and then it "came alive." The change was usually ascribed to ensoulment. (See next item.)
Ensoulment	Infusion into the fetus of a soul.
Viability	Emphasizes possibility of independence as the identifying feature of a person.
Birth	Emphasizes actual independence, direct relationship as the crucial feature of membership in the moral community.
"Personhood"	Usually correlated with certain landmarks in mental and social development—such as, a concept of self. Usually based on an analysis of rights.

Even if it were agreed that the fetus is a person with all the "rights, privileges, and responsibilities thereunto appertaining," it would not follow that abortion is *never* morally justified. The fetus' physiological ties to the mother may create conditions that pose a threat to the life or health of the mother; thus a plausible case, in terms of a sort of self-defense, might be made to justify abortion.

On the other hand, even if it were agreed that the fetus is *not* a person but only a mass of tissue, moral arguments *against* abortion might still be plausible in many circumstances. One of the strongest such arguments would stem from the father's rights and/or tacit or explicit promises the mother might have made to him. If a couple had agreed to have a child and had taken action to initiate pregnancy based on that agreement, then certain legitimate expectations are created in the mind of the father; thus the mother does not have a right to make a unilateral decision to end the pregnancy.

Another limiting argument rests on the question of whether a person has a right to maim himself without some morally significant justification. Few people feel qualms about piercing ears for aesthetic reasons, but many in our society would think it unjustified to pierce one's nose or cheek in order to hang jewelry. And if someone proposed to cut off two fingers to achieve the aesthetic result of having four fingers on each hand, or if a woman golfer proposed to remove a breast to improve her golf swing, or if a man proposed to submit to castration to affect his singing voice, the revulsion with which we would react invokes a moral principle.[11] Similarly, even if the fetus is regarded as nothing more than a mass of cells, it is doubtful that there would be moral justification to remove them merely because their presence is an *inconvenience* to the mother. Some more serious reason than this would at least be required.

Another important issue that arises in connection with abortion has to do with personal conscience. The law and institutional policies have generally attempted to honor personal conscience even while legalizing abortion by providing that anyone who has moral objections may decline to participate in the practice. However, generally the proviso is added that some arrangement must be made to refer the patient to a provider or institution that will grant her request for an abortion, and many who object to abortion think that even this much personal cooperation is morally wrong. Here is a classic example of a conflict of conscience. Meeting one's responsibilities to patients may go against personal conscience on this issue. Honoring conscience may compromise duties to patients. This dilemma is even more acute in a community in which some institutions or practitioners to which patients might turn without guidance provide services you would regard as less than fully satisfactory in terms of safety and medical science. In this situation, you must carefully and thoughtfully balance qualms of conscience about cooperating in abortion against duties to protect the interests of patients. Given that the role in abortion in this situation is so indirect and remote, it is hard to avoid the conclusion that the high stakes in terms of patient safety outweigh qualms of conscience regarding abortion.

5 Reproductive Technologies

Current and developing reproductive technologies bring up additional questions of responsibilities toward potential life. If a sanctity-of-life principle were carried to its logical extreme, it would dictate that every ovum of every fertile woman be fertilized and developed to term, for each has the potential to become a person. Only slightly less extreme would be the requirement that technology be developed to enable every ovum that becomes fertilized in the natural course of events to be developed. If life is truly sacred and valuable beyond price, then it follows that every instance of it ought to be promoted—no matter what the cost. And the cost of either of these proposals would be enormous, not only because of the expense of the technology that would have to be developed and used to carry out this task, but also from consequences of the resulting overpopulation of the planet.

---

11. Roman Catholic moral theology makes the principle explicit. Called the "Principle of Totality," it specifies that inflicting a harm on oneself is justified *only when* a more serious harm to the organism as a whole is thereby avoided, such as when one submits to surgery to repair a life-threatening condition.

The other pole of reaction to reproductive technologies is to condemn them all because they make "artificial" what is proper only through "natural" means. However, the distinction between the natural and the artificial is exceedingly difficult to draw with precision; when it is clarified, it is not obvious that it can bear the moral weight placed on it. For example, the life of a diabetic is maintained by the artificial procedure of injecting insulin to replace the missing natural production within the body. How is this different, in a morally relevant way, from the artificial juxtaposition of sperm and ovum in a culture medium when the blockage of the fallopian tubes impedes the natural process? To move to a more controversial example, how is the harvesting and fertilization of multiple ova, followed by removing all but one from the culture dish at the blastocyte stage, different in moral terms from the quite common natural process of fertilization of multiple ova and sloughing off most of them in the uterus? Here the natural process is mimicked to preserve the wisdom of nature in avoiding the dangers of ova separation before fertilization and in providing the "fail-safe" and "quality control" advantages of multiple fertilizations.

Of course, the potential for introducing harm to the resulting child by not mimicking nature *fully enough* needs to be taken quite seriously. Experimentation on human genetic materials is unjustified before these dangers have been reduced to a reasonable level through laboratory studies. Overzealous pursuit of new knowledge (much less of new publications in one's name) is to be guarded against with extreme caution in an area such as this, where the risks to the resulting child and his or her parents are grave.

Another fundamental issue that arouses moral concern is the allocation of resources. Is there a fundamental "right to reproduce"? Even if there is, what priority should it be assigned relative to other medical needs? These are questions that ought to be worked through to answers before vast sums of money are allocated to this area of research and treatment.

These technologies may bring great benefits to mankind. For one thing, they may help to resolve some of the dilemmas concerning abortion by making it possible to end a pregnancy without necessarily ending the process of development of the fetus. Further exploration into the process of human development may discover ways to prevent genetic diseases that now cause great suffering. However, here as in other areas of experimentation, we must proceed with moral as well as scientific caution.

References

ACP: *See* American College of Physicians

Alexander M: "The Rigid Embrace of the Narrow House": Premature burial and the signs of death. *Hastings Cent. Rep.* 10:25–31, 1980.

American College of Physicians: *Ethics Manual.* American College of Physicians, Philadelphia, 1984a.

———: American College of Physicians Ethics Manual. *Ann. Intern. Med.* 101:129–137, 263–274, 1984b.

Dixon JL, Smalley MG: Jehovah's Witnesses: The surgical/ethical challenge. *JAMA* 246:2471–2472, 1981.

Jonsen AR, Siegler M, Winslade WJ: *Clinical Ethics: A Practical Approach to Ethical Dimensions in Medicine.* Macmillan, New York, 1982.

Judicial Council of the American Medical Association: *Current Opinions of the Judicial Council of the American Medical Association–1984.* American Medical Association, Chicago, 1984.

Marsh FH: *The Emerging Rights of Children in Treatment for Mental and Catastrophic Illnesses.* University Press of America, Washington DC, 1981.

Office of the General Counsel/American Medical Association: *Medicolegal Forms with Legal Analysis.* American Medical Association, Chicago, 1979.

Peschel RE, Peschel ER: Ritual and the death certificate: Case histories, literary histories. *The Pharos,* 11–16, Spring 1983.

President's Commission for the Study of Ethical Problems in Medicine and Biomedical and Behavioral Research: *Defining Death: Medical, Legal and Ethical Issues in the Determination of Death.* US Government Printing Office, Washington DC, 1981.

———. *Making Health Care Decisions: The Ethical and Legal Implications of Informed Consent in the Patient-Practitioner Relationship. Vol. 1: Report.* US Government Printing Office, Washington DC, 1982.

———. *Deciding to Forego Life-Sustaining Treatment: Ethical, Medical and Legal Issues in Treatment Decisions.* US Government Printing Office, Washington DC, 1983.

Ramsey P: *The Patient as Person.* Yale University Press, New Haven CT, 59–112, 1971.

———. *Ethics at the Edges of Life.* Yale University Press, New Haven CT 1978.

Shem S.: *The House of God.* Dell, New York, 1978.

Symmers W StC Sr: Not allowed to die. *Br. Med. J.* 1:442, 1968.

Veatch RM: *A Theory of Medical Ethics.* Basic Books, New York, 1981.

Further Reading

Determination of Death

A definition of irreversible coma: Report of the Ad Hoc Committee of the Harvard Medical School to Examine the Definition of Brain Death. *JAMA* 205:337–340, 1968.

Abrams N, Buckner MD (eds.): *Medical Ethics: A Clinical Textbook and Reference for the Health Care Professions.* The MIT Press, Cambridge MA, Section I.D (28–37), 1983.

Bernat JL, Culver CM, Gert B: On the definition and criterion of death. *Ann. Intern. Med.* 94:389–394, 1981.

———: Defining death in theory and practice. *Hastings Cent. Rep.* 12:5–9, 1982.

Black P McL: Brain death. *N. Engl. J. Med.* 299:338–344, 393–401, 1978.

Brain death (editorial). *Lancet* 1:363–365, 1981.

Byrne PA, O'Reilly S, Quay PM: Brain death—An opposing viewpoint. *JAMA* 242:1985–1990, 1979.

Capron AM: Determining death: Do we need a statute? *Hastings Cent. Rep.* 3:6–7, February 1973.

————: The purpose of death: A reply to Professor Dworkin. *Indiana Law Journal* 48:640–645, 1973.

Capron AM, Kass LR: A statutory definition of the standards for determining human death: An appraisal and a proposal. *University of Pennsylvania Law Review* 121:87–118, 1972.

Conference of Royal Colleges and Faculties of the United Kingdom: Diagnosis of brain death. *Lancet* 2:1069–1070, 1976.

Dillon WP, Lee RV, Troudone MJ, et al: Life support and maternal brain death during pregnancy. *JAMA* 248:1089–1091, 1982. Cf. Editorials, 248:1101–1103.

Dworkin RB: Death in context. *Indiana Law Journal* 48:623–639, 1973.

Englehardt HT Jr: Defining death: A philosophical problem for medicine and law. *Am. Rev. Respir. Dis.* 112:587–590, 1975.

Fletcher JF: Indicators of humanhood: A tentative profile of man. *Hastings Cent. Rep.* 2:1–4, November 1972.

Green MB, Wikler D: Brain death and personal identity. *Philosophy and Public Affairs* 9:105–133, 1980.

Guidelines for the Determination of Death: Report of the Medical Consultants on the Diagnosis of Death to the President's Commission for the Study of Ethical Problems in Medicine and Biomedical and Behavioral Research. *JAMA* 246:2184–2186, 1981.

High DM: Death: Its conceptual elusiveness. *Soundings* 55:438–458, 1972.

Jonas H: *Philosophical Essays: From Ancient Creed to Technological Man.* Prentice-Hall, Englewood Cliffs NJ, 132–140, 1974.

Kass LR: Death as an event: A commentary on Robert Morison. *Science* 173:698–702, 1971.

Korein J (ed.): Brain death: Interrelated medical and social issues. *Ann. NY Acad. Sci.* 315:1–454, 1978.

Morison RS: Death: Process or event? *Science* 173:694–698, 1971.

Parisi JE, Kim RC, Collins GF, et al: Brain death with prolonged somatic survival. *N. Engl. J. Med.* 306:14–16, 1982. Cf. Correspondence, 306:1361–1363.

Reich WT (ed-in-chief): *Encyclopedia of Bioethics.* Macmillan and the Free Press, New York, 1978.
Death, Definition and Determination of
I. Criteria for Death (Molinari GF)
II. Legal Aspects of Pronouncing Death (Capron AM)
III. Philosophical and Theological Foundations (High DM)

Steinfels P, Veatch RM (eds): *Death inside out.* Harper & Row, New York, 1975.

Task Force on Death and Dying of the Institute on Society, Ethics and the Life Sciences: Refinements in criteria for the determination of death: An appraisal. *JAMA* 221:48–53, 1972.

Veatch RM: The whole-brain-oriented concept of death: An outmoded formulation. *Journal of Thanatology* 3:13–30, 1975.
————. *Death, Dying and the Biological Revolution.* Yale University Press, New Haven CT, 21–76, 1976.

Veith FJ, Fein JM, Tendler MD, et al: Brain death: I. A status report of medical and ethical considerations. *JAMA* 238:1651–1655, 1977.
————: Brain death: II. A status report of legal considerations. *JAMA* 238:1744–1748, 1977.

Walton DN: *On Defining Death.* McGill-Queen's University Press, Montreal, 1978.
————: *Brain Death: Ethical Considerations.* Purdue University, West Lafayette IN, 1980.

Youngner SJ, Bartlett ET: Human death and high technology: The failure of the whole-brain formulations. *Ann. Intern. Med.* 99:252–258, 1983.

Other Limits to Treatment

Abrams, Buckner: *Medical Ethics,* Sections I.E (38–45) and III.B (312–389), 1983.

Angell M: Respecting the autonomy of competent patients (editorial). *N. Engl. J. Med.* 310:1115–1116, 1984.

Annas GJ: *The Rights of Hospital Patients: The Basic ACLU Guide to a Hospital Patient's Rights.* Avon Books, New York, 1975.

Annas GJ, Glantz LH, Katz BF: *The Rights of Doctors, Nurses, and Allied Health Professionals: A Health Law Primer.* Ballinger Publishing, Cambridge MA, 1981. See especially Chapter IV: "Informed Consent and Refusing Treatment" and Chapter XI: "Care of the Dying."

Battin MP: *Ethical Issues in Suicide.* Prentice-Hall, Englewood Cliffs NJ, 1982.

Battin MP, Mayo DJ: *Suicide: The Philosophical Issues*. St. Martin's Press, New York, 1980.

Bayer R, Callahan D, Fletcher J, et al: The care of the terminally ill: Morality and economics. *N. Engl. J. Med.* 309:1490–1494, 1983.

Bedell SE, Delbanco TL: Choices about cardiopulmonary resuscitation in the hospital. *N. Engl. J. Med.* 310:1089–1093, 1984.

Behnke JA, Bok S (eds): *The Dilemmas of Euthanasia*. Doubleday Anchor, New York, 1975.

Bok S: Personal directions for care at the end of life. *N. Engl. J. Med.* 295:367–369, 1976.

Fried C: Terminating life support: Out of the closet. *N. Engl. J. Med.* 295:390–391, 1976.

Imbus SR, Zawacki BE: Autonomy for burned patients when survival is unprecedented. *N. Engl. J. Med.* 297:308–311, 1977. See accompanying editorial "Autonomy and Ethics in Action" (Cassell EJ), 297:333–334.

Jackson DL, Youngner S: Patient autonomy and "death with dignity": Some clinical caveats. *N. Engl. J. Med.* 301:404–408, 1979. Cf. Correspondence, 302:125–126, 1980.

Jonsen AR: A concord in medical ethics. *Ann. Intern. Med.* 99:263, 1983.

Judicial Council of the American Medical Association: *Current Opinions of the Judicial Council of the American Medical Association–1984*. American Medical Association, Chicago, 1984. 2.13 Organ Transplantation Guidelines

Kohl M (ed): *Beneficent Euthanasia*. Prometheus Books, Buffalo, 1975.

Ladd J (ed): *Ethical Issues Relating to Life and Death*. Oxford University Press, New York, 1979.

Lo B, Dornbrand L: Guiding the hand that feeds: Caring for the demented elderly. *N. Engl. J. Med.* 311:402–404, 1984.

Optimum care for hopelessly ill patients: A report of the Clinical Care Committee for the Massachusetts General Hospital. *N. Engl. J. Med.* 295:362–364, 1976.

Rabkin MT, Gillerman G, Rice N: Orders not to resuscitate. *N. Engl. J. Med.* 295:364–366, 1976.

Reich: *Encyclopeida of Bioethics*, 1978. Blood Transfusion (Garland MJ) Death and Dying: Euthanasia and Sustaining Life
  I. Historical Perspectives (Gruman GJ)
  II. Ethical Views (Bok S)
  III. Professional and Public Policy (Veatch RM)
Death, Attitudes Toward (Kalish RA) Life,
  I. Value of Life (Singer P)
  II. Quality of Life (Reich WT)
Life-Support Systems (Jonsen AR, Lister G)
Religious Directives in Medical Ethics
  I. Jewish Codes and Guidelines (Trainin IN, Rosner F)
  II. Roman Catholic Directives (Haring B)
  III. Protestant Statements (Derr TS)
Right to Refuse Medical Care (Capron AM) Suicide (Smith DH, Perlin S)

Robertson JA: *The Rights of the Critically Ill*. Bantam Books, New York, 1983. See especially Chapter III: "The Right to Commit Suicide" and Chapter IV: "The Right to Refuse Treatment."

Simpson MA: Planning for terminal care. *Lancet* 2:192–193, 1976.

Steinbock B (ed): *Killing and Letting Die*. Prentice-Hall, Englewood Cliffs NJ, 1980.

Veatch: *Death, Dying, and the Biological Revolution*, 1976.

Wagner A: Cardiopulmonary resuscitation in the aged: A prospective survey. *N. Engl. J. Med.* 310:1129–1130, 1984.

Wallace SE: *After Suicide*. Wiley-Interscience, New York, 1973. Interviews with the families of several suicides to study the impact of suicide on them.

Wallace SE, Eser A: *Suicide and Euthanasia: The Rights of Personhood*. University of Tennessee Press, Knoxville, 1981.

Wanzer SH, Adelstein SJ, Cranford RE, et al: The physician's responsibility toward hopelessly ill patients. *N. Engl. J. Med.* 310:955–959, 1984. Cf. Correspondence, 311:334–336, 1984.

Key Court Cases

Quinlan (1976)—A father withdraws the respirator from his permanently comatose daughter. [*In re Quinlan,* Supreme Court of New Jersey, 1976. 70 N.J. 10, 355 A.2d 647.]

Saikewicz (1977)—Nontreatment of acute myeloblastic monocytic leukemia in a 67-year-old man who had been profoundly retarded since birth. [*Superintendent of Belchertown State School v. Saikewicz,* 373 Mass. 728, 370 N.E.2d 417 (1977).]

Candura (1978); Northern (1978)—Refusal of treatment by patients of questionable competence. [*Lane v. Candura,* Mass. Adv. Sh. 588 N.E.2d 1232 (1978); *Department of Human Services v. Northern,* 563 S.W.2d 197 (Tenn. Ct. of Appeals, 1978).]

Dinnerstein (1978)—Do-not-resuscitate order for patient in terminal stages, agreed to by family. [*In the Matter of Dinnerstein,* Mass. App, 380 N.E.2d 134 (1978).]

Chad Green (1978)—Three-year-old boy with acute lymphocytic leukemia whose parents refuse chemotherapy in favor of an approach combining megavitamins, diet, and laetrile. [*Custody of a Minor,* 379 N.E.2d 1053 (Mass 1978), reviewed & aff'd, Mass Adv. Sht. 2124 (1979).]

Phillip Becker (1979)—Eleven-year-old boy with Down's syndrome and ventral septal defect whose parents refuse cardiac surgery. [*In re Phillip B.,* 92 Cal.App.3d 796, 156 Cal.Rptr. 48 (1979). Cf. *Guardianship of Phillip Becker,* Superior Court, Santa Clara County, Cal., No. 10198 (Aug. 7, 1981).]

Eichner v. Dillon (1980)—Withdrawal of ventilator from an 83-year-old monk with massive brain damage following routine surgery. The religious leader of the order made the decision, acting on prior remarks by the patient about cases of this sort. [*Eichner v. Dillon,* 73 A.D.2d 431, 426 N.Y.S.2d 517 (1980), reviewed & aff'd, N.Y. Ct. of Appeals—420 N.E.2d 64 (1981).]

Earle Spring (1980)—Discontinuation of dialysis for a 78-year-old, senile man at the request of his wife and adult son. [*In re Spring,* 405 N.E.2d 115 (Mass 1980).]

John Storar (1981)—Fifty-two-year-old profoundly retarded man with cancer of the bladder whose mother requested discontinuation of life-sustaining blood transfusions. [*In the Matter of John Storar,* 52 N.Y.2d 363, 420 N.E.2d 64, 438 N.Y.S.2d 266 (1981).]

Barber & Nedjl v. Calif. (1983)—Physicians charged with manslaughter for withdrawing nutrition from a brain-damaged patient.

Conroy (1983)—Eighty-four-year-old woman with organic brain syndrome whose nephew (and guardian) requests removal of a feeding tube.

Stephen Dawson (1983)—Severely retarded child whose parents refused permission for therapy to replace cranial shunt (Canada).

Pamela Hamilton (1983)—Twelve-year-old girl with Ewing's Sarcoma whose father refuses chemotherapy and radiotherapy on religious grounds.

Elizabeth Bouvia (1984)—Twenty-seven-year-old quadraplegic who requests hospital's assistance as she starves to death; contrast with New York case in which force-feeding was *not* authorized.

Seriously Ill Newborns

Abrams, Buckner: *Medical Ethics,* 368–389, 1983.

Ackerman TF: The limits of beneficence: Jehovah's Witnesses and childhood cancer. *Hastings Cent. Rep.* 10:13–18, 1980.

Brandt R: Defective newborns and the morality of termination. *In* Kohl M (ed): *Infanticide and the Value of Life.* Prometheus Books, Buffalo NY, 46–57, 1978.

Engelhardt HT Jr: Ethical issues in aiding the death of young children. *In* Kohl M (ed): *Beneficent Euthanasia.* Prometheus Books, Buffalo NY, 180–192, 1975.

Fost N: Ethical issues in the treatment of critically ill newborns. *Pediatr. Ann.* 10:16–22, 1981.

Gustafson JM: Mongolism, parental desires, and the right to life. *Perspect. Biol. Med.* 16:529–555, 1973.

Jonsen AR, Garland MJ: *Ethics of Newborn Intensive Care*. Institute of Government Studies, Berkeley CA, 1976.

Kipnis K, Williamson GM: Nontreatment decisions for severely compromised newborns. *Ethics* 95:90–111, 1984.

Lorber J: Selective treatment of myelomeningocele: To treat or not to treat? *Pediatrics* 53:307–308, 1974.

Reich: *Encyclopedia of Bioethics*, 1978.
Children and Biomedicine (Fost NC)
Infants
    I. Medical Aspects and Ethical Dilemmas (Hemphill JM, Freeman JM)

II. Ethical Prespectives on the Care of Infants (Reich WT, Ost DE)
III. Public Policy and Procedural Questions (Reich WT, Ost DE)
IV. Infanticide: A Philosophical Perspective (Tooley M)

Robertson JA: Involuntary euthanasia of defective newborns: A legal analysis. *Stanford Law Review* 27:213–269, 1975.

Tooley M: *Abortion and Infanticide*. Oxford University Press, Oxford, 1984.

Abortion

Abrams, Buckner: *Medical Ethics*, Section III.C (428–443), 1983.

Bracken MB, Klerman LV, Bracken M: Abortion, adoption, or motherhood: An empirical study of decision-making during pregnancy. *Am. J. Obstet, Gynecol.* 130:251–265, 1978.

Callahan D: *Abortion: Law, Choice, and Morality*. Macmillan, New York, 1970.

Cates W Jr, Gold J, Selik RM: Regulations of abortion services—For better or worse? *N. Engl. J. Med.* 301:720–723, 1979.

Cohen M, Nagel T, Scanlon T (eds): *The Rights and Wrongs of Abortion*. Princeton University Press, Princeton NJ, 1974.

Engelhardt HT Jr: The ontology of abortion. *Ethics* 84:217–234, 1974.

Feinberg J (ed): *The Problem of Abortion*, ed 2. Wadsworth, Belmont CA, 1984.

Glover J: *Causing Death and Saving Lives*. Penguin Books, New York, Chapters 9–11, 1977.

Institute of Medicine: *Legalized Abortion and the Public Health*. National Academy of Sciences, Washington DC, 1975.

Judicial Council of the American Medical Association: *Current Opinions–1984*, 1984.
2.01 Abortion

Reich: *Encylopedia of Bioethics*, 1978.
Abortion
    I. Medical Aspects (Hellegers AE)
    II. Jewish Perspectives (Feldman DM)
    III. Roman Catholic Perspectives (Connery JR)
    IV. Protestant Perspectives (Nelson JB)
    V. Contemporary Debate in Philosophical and Religious Ethics (Curran CM)
    VI. Legal Aspects (Finnis JM)
Fetal-Maternal Relationship (Mahoney MJ)
Fetal Research (Hellegers AE)
Person (van Melsen AGM)
Prenatal Diagnosis
    I. Clinical Aspects (Milunsky A)
    II. Ethical Issues (Fletcher JC)

Schneider CE, Vinovskis MA (eds): *The Law and Politics of Abortion*. DC Heath, Lexington MA, 1980.

Thomasma DC: *An Apology for the Value of Human Life*. The Catholic Health Association of the United States, St. Louis MO, 1983.

Toward a definition of fetal life: Ethical and legal options and their implications for biologists and physicians. *Clin. Res.* 23:210–237, 1975.

Reproductive Technologies

Abrams, Buckner: *Medical Ethics*, Section III.C (443–486), 1983.

Edwards RG, Steptoe P: *A Matter of Life*. William Morrow, New York, 1978.

Gorovitz S: *Doctor's Dilemmas: Moral Conflict and Medical Care*. Macmillan, New York, 164–178, 1982.

Law and Ethics of A.I.D. and Embryo Transfer. Ciba Foundation Symposium 17, Associated Scientific Publishers, New York, 1973.

Ramsey P: Shall we "reproduce"? *JAMA* 220:1346–1350, 1480–1485, 1972.

Reich: *Encyclopedia of Bioethics*, 1978.
Reproductive Technologies
  I. Sex Selection (Largey G)
  II. Artificial Insemination (Frankel MS)
  III. Sperm and Zygote Banking (Frankel MS)
  IV. In Vitro Fertilization (Mastroianni L Jr)
  V. Asexual Human Reproduction (Sinsheimer RL)
  VI. Ethical Issues (McCormick RA)
  VII. Legal Aspects (Robertson JA)
Sterilization
  I. Medical Aspects (Hellman LM)
  II. Ethical Aspects (Lebacqz K)
  III. Legal Aspects (Friedman JM)

Tiefel HO: Human in vitro fertilization: A conservative view. *JAMA* 247:3235–3242, 1982.

Walters W, Singer P: *Test-Tube Babies: A Guide to Moral Questions, Present Techniques, and Future Possibilities*. Oxford University Press, Melbourne, 1982.

Chapter Five

Who Gets What?

You have not yet prepared that report on injuries of the great toe assigned by your attending on this orthopedics clerkship to present at tomorrow's teaching rounds, and you are eager to get over to the library to begin the inevitable long evening of research. And yet you said to yourself earlier today that you would make one more try at adjusting Brokka Legg's traction to relieve the discomfort it has been causing her. But that can really wait until morning, for unless you get busy looking up every arcane detail about the bones of the foot, Dr. Picayune will ask a question you can't answer and then will make a big deal of the gap in your knowledge in front of all your associates.

Here you face one form of a classic and recurrent dilemma: the problem of allocating scarce resources. In this case (as in many such cases), the resource in question is your time. In other cases the resource may be different, e.g., a drug, a technology, an organ. How is it to be decided who gets what when it is impossible for everyone to get everything? Variations on this question are the chief topic of this chapter.

1 Allocation of Resources

1.1 Life and Death Resources

The most gripping form of this dilemma arises when the resource in short supply means the difference between life and death. The classic instance of this, much discussed in the medical ethics literature, arose in the early days of development of renal dialysis when there were only a few machines available in the country.

The long-term solution in the case of kidney dialysis was to increase the availability of the resource to the point that nowadays no one who could benefit from dialysis need be deprived of it. But this does not resolve the short-term problem: how are recipients to be selected until the supply of the resource is increased? And the problem is a recurrent one. There will always be some developing technology or other resource in short supply—yesterday it was kidney machines, today it is interferon and artificial hearts, tomorrow it may be implantable artificial lungs; and always there will be a limited supply of cadaver organs. Furthermore, as you will see in Section 2, the long-term solution that worked in the case of kidney machines may not be viable as an option for other resources in today's cost-containment era.

1.2 Principles of Allocation

The following are some criteria of selection proposed for situations in which resources are scarce:[1]

1.2.1 Equality A principle of distributive justice that receives high regard in modern Western societies is the principle of equality. Every person is considered to be of equal worth and thus to be equally entitled to the goods and services society has to offer. If such public services as police protection or water mains were made available only to certain citizens and denied to others, people would be justifiably outraged. Similarly, lavishing exotic medical treatments on some might make routine levels of care unavailable to others, and this would be generally regarded as objectionable. However, as important as this principle is, it cannot form the whole basis for allocation decisions in medicine:

"Radical egalitarianism" is a position based *solely* on a principle of equality, requiring allocation of goods and services in precisely equal shares, regardless of need. Thus, if Beulah suffered from bronchial asthma and Barney did not, both would still receive equal doses of theophylline. If there was not enough available to provide a therapeutic dose for everybody, each would still receive the same, subtherapeutic dose.

Surely it makes little sense to consider giving such a resource to those who have no need of it, or when the resource is in short supply, even to consider giving any to those whose need is not *urgent*. But this is to say that a principle of equality is not the only—or even the most important—criterion for allocation of medical resources. A higher priority is assigned to a principle of medical need.

1.2.2. Medical Need This is clearly a background principle of the greatest importance. Virtually every system of allocation that has been proposed or put into practice includes reference to medical need. What is not often recognized is that this amounts to assigning priority to a principle of medical efficiency or "medical indications" above principles of equality (and possibly above other principles as well, as you shall see).

Central judgments here include *judgments of medical appropriateness* and *judgments of medical necessity*.

---

1. For a description of one hospital's approach to these decisions, which shows some of these criteria "in action," see Shana Alexander (1962).

A. Judgments of Medical Appropriateness   If kidney dialysis is the resource being distributed, there is no point in employing it on those who have unimpaired kidney function. To do so would be, at best, useless and perhaps harmful. Thus these people can immediately be ruled out as candidates for the resource.

But what about a terminally ill cancer patient whose kidneys have failed? Dialysis would offer some benefit to this patient (or, at least, to his organic functioning), but is this short-term and limited benefit an appropriate use of this resource? As you saw in Chapter 4, these questions arise even when there is no scarcity of resources. Thus there might be reasons independent of allocation issues for ruling out these patients as candidates for the life-extending treatment. However, this move is controversial; some physicians (as well as some patients) would want to continue aggressive measures like this even if death were imminent.

Furthermore, what about a schizophrenic patient? Some studies suggest that dialysis may be of assistance in counteracting schizophrenia in some patients. Does this possiblity warrant making the resource available to schizophrenics? What if a particular patient or a member of her family explicitly *requests* that this form of treatment be attempted? If dialysis services were available in plentiful supply, one might consider honoring such a request both 1) to respect the wishes of the patient and/or her representative and 2) to gather further evidence to test this possibility. However, this request would generally not carry great weight if dialysis were in scarce supply.

Defining medical need is not a straightforward exercise of technical reasoning. At least two elements are essential to constitute a medical need: 1) the presence of a disease condition and 2) endangerment, i.e., the judgment that the condition is likely to alter the life course of the patient in an undesirable way. And the second of these is as much a value judgment as a technical judgment. Further complications are introduced if, for example, a screening test uncovers a disease condition that is asymptomatic at present and has an uncertain future course [e.g., the HTLV-III screen for acquired immunodeficiency syndrome (AIDS)]. Does this patient have a medical need? Or, if the disease condition obviously has been a long-standing one, the patient-perceived need prompting presentation to a physician may be only tangentially related to it. In addition, the exploration required to uncover and measure the extent of the need may itself be likely to cause harm, and judgments of need are bound to be influenced by considerations of the possibility of alteration through treatment, as well as by assessments of the likely cost (in terms of both effort and expenses) of alteration.

Finally, even if all possible inappropriate candidates were screened out, there might still be more candidates than could be served with the supply of the resource available. Some further basis of selection must be found.

B. Judgments of Medical Necessity A further screening criterion might be developed in terms of judgments about the degree of medical need: whose need for the resource is *urgent*? For example, the patient in end-stage kidney failure will die without access to dialysis, whereas the schizophrenic's life is not at stake. Another variation arises from estimates of the probability of successfully reaching the goal sought. One candidate may have a 90% chance of survival if given the resource, whereas another may have only a 50% chance even if the resource is provided.

However, these judgments cannot fully resolve allocation questions. In the first place, how need is to be taken into account in allocation decisions is unclear. Is priority to be given to the *neediest* person? Then it would go to the patient who has only a 50% chance of survival even with the resource. However, this conflicts with a standard of efficient use of the resource, which would dictate giving it to the patient with a 90% chance, if there is only enough to provide for one of these two patients.

Furthermore, it appears that judgments of necessity are themselves influenced by considerations of availability of resources. For example, the availability of intensive care unit (ICU) beds may influence the threshold of risk that a physician is willing to tolerate. If only one or two beds are available in the unit, she might be willing to "take a chance" by putting a patient on a regular ward, whereas if a half dozen beds in the ICU are vacant, she would prefer to have the patient monitored "just in case."[2] This suggests that judgments of medical necessity are probabilistic and variable. One physician's threshold may be markedly higher or lower than another's, and the same physician's threshold may vary in different circumstances.

Even though they cannot serve as the whole basis of decision making, judgments of medical need of both these types can be employed in an initial medical screening to identify the group whose need is compelling and to screen out others whose need could be met in alternative ways. Then, if a surplus of candidates remains, perhaps some principle of distributive justice can be employed to make the final selection.

1.2.3. Lottery The principle of equality might be applied via *randomness*. Thus, one method often proposed to preserve equality in the face of shortage is a lottery of some sort; each person has an equal *chance* of receiving the benefit.

1.2.4. "First Come, First Served" Some theorists regard a procedure of "first come, first served" as equivalent to a lottery (Ramsey 1970, 252–259; Childress 1970). However, this overlooks the serious problems of differential access that may affect one's position at any point at which scarce benefits are to be allocated.

---

2. For a careful discussion of decision making with regard to the ICU see Albert G. Muley, "The Allocation of Resources for Medical Intensive Care" (President's Commission 1983c, 285–311).

1.2.5. Merit/Past Contribution   With this criterion, one person would be favored over another if he or she had made a more significant contribution to society in the past or had acquired moral merit according to some standard. Thus the upstanding citizen would be favored over the person with a criminal record; the Pulitzer-Prize-winning poet would be favored over the ne'er-do-well. This, for example, is the basis for the program of veteran's benefits.

1.2.6. Social Worth/Future Contribution   This criterion would allocate resources to persons on the basis of their future promise rather than their past achievements. It can be viewed as society pursuing maximum return on its investment in the resource; thus the young would be favored over the old (assuming, of course, that they show promise).

1.2.7. Social Responsibilities   In allocation exercises, people are often favored if they are married, and especially if they have dependent children. This can be viewed (cynically) as society aiming to minimize its future burdens by keeping alive those who would leave the most dependents for society to care for. Less cynically, it can be viewed as a way of supporting those who have accepted social responsibilities.

1.2.8. Entitlement Theory   This theory designates a process of acquisition as the foundation of just possession rather than some end goal such as equality or allocation according to merit. One is entitled to have and to keep whatever one acquires by a fair, nonexploitive process, e.g., by initiative or ingenuity, or through a contractual agreement. In practice, this view often leads to a system of distribution based on commercial exchange in a free enterprise economic system. Thus one is entitled to the health care that one has earned money enough to *pay for*—no more and no less.

1.3 Case: Who Gets the Protection?

Consider the principles just described in connection with the following case:[3]

> Hepatitis B immune globulin (HBIG) is a drug indicated for prophylaxis to be administered as soon as possible following direct exposure to type B hepatitis. Because it is a very expensive drug, Community Hospital stocks a supply of only about five doses. Cornfield General Hospital, a small hospital in a nearby community, stocks none at all and has customarily relied on the pharmacy at Community Hospital to supply this drug when it is needed.

---

3. Case and questions adapted from *Can I? Should I? Must I? . . . Will I? A Symposium on the Ethical, Moral, and Legal Issues Confronting the Hospital Pharmacist of Today* (The University of Tennessee Memorial Research Center and Hospital, Knoxville, April 23, 1982).

This supply usually meets the needs of the community adequately, but today is the resounding exception. The staff dentist in the Dental Clinic of Community Hospital urgently requests two doses of HBIG for himself and a dental assistant who have just received word from the lab that a patient they treated two days ago has active hepatitis B. Almost immediately after this call, the pharmacist from Cornfield General calls with an urgent request for two doses of HBIG—one for an infant just born there whose mother had documented hepatitis B infection during the last trimester of pregnancy and another for a nurse exposed through a needle stick involving the mother.

To make matters worse, the Emergency Room (ER) physician from Community Hospital appears in person to demand three doses for herself and two nurses who were exposed when a hepatitis B patient (also confirmed, after the fact, by lab reports) was brought in with gunshot wounds and they had to wade in up to their elbows in blood to stop the bleeding. The employee health nurse repeats the request for doses for the dental assistant and the ER nurses, and also asks for an additional dose for a floor nurse who was exposed through a needle stick involving the gunshot wound patient after he had been transferred to the floor.

The hospital pharmacist calls around to hospitals in the area only to find that there is no additional HBIG at all in the vicinity. A call to the drug supplier brings word that the company does not have any in stock and cannot get any in before the end of the week, due to a general airline strike paralyzing transportation.

The Sheriff's office calls explaining that the man they have in custody for shooting your ER patient is claiming that he and the patient have had a homosexual relationship for the last seven months, with their last sexual encounter occurring just before the shooting. The Sheriff demands a dose of HBIG to give to the prisoner.

As chief of staff, you are called on to make the decision as to who should receive the available doses of the drug. You face *nine* requests for *five* doses of the drug. In the order in which the requests were received, they are:

1,2	staff dentist, dental assistant
3,4	infant, floor nurse at Cornfield General
5,6,7	ER—physician, nurse 1, nurse 2
8	floor nurse at Community Hospital
9	prisoner

Consider the folowing questions:

1. The solution most in line with *radical egalitarianism* would be to give each of the nine people $5/9$ of a dose. However, this would not protect *anybody* adequately. A second procedure suggested by this principle would be to put the nine names into a hat and draw five out. Would this be a reasonable way to allocate the supply? (Read the additional considerations cited before accepting this alternative).

2. The following considerations are relevant to measurement of *medical need.* What difference should these factors make to the decision about who is to get the drug?

   a. The efficacy of HBIG for an infant whose mother was infected has not been established.

   b. The probability of infection is lower for exposure during a dental procedure than for exposure through a needle stick or contact with the patient's blood.

   c. The prisoner already may have active hepatitis B; if so, it is too late for a prophylactic agent like HBIG to do any good.

3. Would the principle of *"first come, first served"* be a reasonable basis for decision?

   a. Would it make a difference here if you learned, for example, that the only reason that the Dental Clinic called you before the ER did was that the laboratory technician is a good friend of the dental assistant and therefore called the results to her before calling the ER?

   b. Suppose the priority were a result of a *negative* factor; i.e., suppose you learned that the laboratory technician had deliberately delayed calling the ER because she has a long-standing grudge against one of the ER nurses? How would this influence your view of the principle of "first come, first served"?

   c. What if you learned that the specimen from the ER had been delivered to the laboratory *before* the one from the Dental Clinic?

4. Would considerations of *merit or past contribution* make a difference to the choice?

   a. What if you knew, for example, that one of the nurses had been a faithful employee of the hospital for more than 20 years, whereas all the others had been associated with their respective hospitals for less than five years? Should this make a difference to your choice?

   b. What effect does the prisoner's criminal status have on his eligibility?

   c. What effect does the prisoner's homosexuality have on his eligibility?

   d. Issues of *personal responsibility* for the exposure are also relevant to the principle of merit. What difference (if any) do these factors make in this sort of situation? Consider the following:

      1) Obviously, the prisoner's exposure was the result of a deliberate choice he made—to engage in homosexual acts with the patient. Would it affect your choice if you knew that the prisoner continued homosexual relations with the patient even after learning that the latter had hepatitis and that the disease might be spread through sexual contacts?

    2) The nurses exposed through needle sticks could be accused of careless nursing practice.

    3) Dental Clinic and ER personnel could have taken precautions (e.g., wearing rubber gloves for every patient) that would have prevented or minimized their exposure to hepatitis.

5. Would considerations of *social worth or future contribution* make a difference to the choice?

    a. The infant offers the greatest potential time span over which to make social contributions. Should this influence your choice?

    b. What if you learned that one of the nurses is about to receive certification in a much-needed specialization? Should this influence your choice?

    c. What if you were told that the prisoner is a graduate student who is credited with a scientific breakthrough in his doctoral research? Should this influence your choice?

6. Would considerations of *social responsibilities* make a difference to the choice? Suppose you learned that

    3 of the candidates are unmarried

    2 are married but have no children

    1 has one child

    2 have two children each, and

    1 is the sole financial support of five children.

Should this information make a difference to your choice?

7. A number of factors are relevant to *entitlement theories*. Consider the following:

    a. What difference does it make (if any) that the supply of the drug to be allocated is *owned* by this hospital? That it has been carried in inventory (and thus as an expense) for some time, and that the hospital stocked the drug in anticipation of just such a crisis?

    b. Should Cornfield General's willingness to *pay* for its supply of the drug be a reason in favor of allocating some to it?

    c. One way to allocate the supply is to sell it to the highest bidder. Would this be a *just* system of distribution? Why or why not?

    d. At Community Hospital, all those exposed are employees of the hospital, *except the ER Physician*, who is a member of a medical group that contracts with the hospital to provide ER coverage. Does this difference in affiliation make any difference in the hospital's responsibilities toward this individual?

e. Should your decision be influenced by *the status of the person making the request*? You received requests from (in temporal order):

a dentist

a pharmacist

a physician

an employee health nurse

a sheriff.

What authority do you have to *refuse* the request of the physician? The sheriff? The hospital's employee health nurse? The others?

f. Should your decision be influenced by *the authority and status of the individuals who would* receive *the medication*? If so, how and why? If not, why not?

g. What legal and moral status is created by the past customary practice of supplying the drug to Cornfield General Hospital? In the absence of any sort of formal agreement between the two hospitals, does such customary practice create any basis for a claim on the drug by Cornfield General?

8. It has been said that "possession is nine points of the law." Is this true? What *counts* as "possession" or a commitment already made in these circumstances? Consider the following:

a. Suppose the request from Cornfield General had been received well in advance of the remaining requests, and the drug had been dispatched but had not yet reached its destination at the time the other requests were received. Would it be morally permissible to contact the delivery vehicle by radio and order the drug returned to your hospital, or would a commitment already have been made?

b. Suppose the drug had been dispatched to the Dental Clinic and placed on a shelf there but had not yet been administered by the time the other requests were received. Would it be morally permissible to go to the Dental Clinic and retrieve it, or would a commitment already have been made?

c. When you got to the Dental Clinic to retrieve the drug, suppose it had been drawn into a syringe and the dental assistant was preparing to have it injected into her arm. Would it be morally permissible to postpone this injection until it could be decided whether this was the best use of the drug, or would a commitment already have been made?

9. Suppose your hospital has a functioning Ethics Committee. Would it be appropriate to turn to it for asistance in this case? What role should the committee be expected to play here? To make the decision? To issue an advisory ruling? Merely to talk the issue through?

1.4 Triage

An area in which allocations are regularly made is that group of decisions known as "triage." One common definition of triage is

> the medical screening of patients to determine their priority for treatment; the separation of a large number of casualties, in military or civilian disaster medical care, into three groups: those who cannot be expected to survive even with treatment, those who will recover without treatment, and the priority group of those who need treatment in order to survive. *(Stedman's Medical Dictionary* 1982, 1479)

However, this area does not yield principles likely to be helpful in the whole range of allocation decisions.

1.4.1 Disaster Triage The selection principles indicated in the definition are most fully illustrated in disaster situations, such as battlefield and large-scale community emergencies, in which the shortage of medical personnel and supplies is drastic. These principles cannot be taken over directly as general guidelines for other allocation situations, however, because the goal of selection embodied in them is not justice (i.e., not the candidates' level of need or desert), but rather efficiency in serving the common good, or some all-encompassing principle such as enhancing the military effort.

1.4.2 Emergency Room Triage A typical hospital emergency room uses these triage categories:

1. *Emergent:* Patients whose conditions are life threatening or will cause serious permanent physical impairment if not treated immediately. These patients are taken immediately to the appropriate treatment areas.
2. *Urgent:* Patients whose conditions require care within 30 minutes to 2 hours. Their conditions would not generally cause loss of life or serious permanent impairment if treatment is deferred. They will be placed in the appropriate treatment area after completing the registration process.
3. *Nonurgent:* Patients whose conditions are minor; the time of evaluation is not a critical factor. These patients will be taken to the appropriate treatment area within a reasonable amount of time after completing the initial assessment and registration process.

This is obviously based on a quite different set of principles from disaster triage. The patients who would be passed by in the disaster situation (e.g., those who will die with or without treatment) are given high priority for attention in the less catastrophic emergency room setting. The difference stems largely from the fact that scarcity of resources is not quite so acute in these situations. The result is that full medical goals—as well as decisions based on justice—can be attempted.

1.5 Patient Loyalties and Demands of Justice

To complicate further the case described in Section 1.3, suppose the floor nurse at Community Hospital (i.e., candidate 8) was a private patient of yours. Would this be a reason for you to favor her in allocating the drug? Why or why not?

This complication raises in acute form an issue underlying all these micro-allocation dilemmas: demands of justice may conflict with demands of loyalty to your patient. As discussed in Chapter 3 (Section 2.2), a component of the moral center of medicine is the expectation that the physician will go "all out" for his or her patients. As Charles Fried (1974) puts it:

> The traditional concept of the physician's relation to his patient is one of unqualified fidelity to that patient's health. He may certainly not do anything that would impair the patient's health and he must do everything in his ability to further it. (pp. 50–51)

> . . . According to the model embodying the ideal of personal care this doctor would have the obligation to care for his patient in every way that serves that patient's interest in health. (pp. 117–118)

The American College of Physicians (ACP) Ethics Manual asserts the same principle:

> The guiding principle must be that the physician should concentrate his energy and attention on providing the patient with the best possible medical care within the context of practicing humanistic, scientific, efficient medicine. . . . In the final analysis, no external factors should interfere with the dedication of the physician to provide optimal care for his patient. [ACP 1984a (*Manual*), 31; 1984b (*Annals*), 266]

But, of course, it is impossible to realize this ideal fully in a situation in which resources are too limited to permit it, i.e., in the face of what the Manual describes as "external pressures resulting from limited institutional resources [that] prevent the physician from providing optimal care" [ACP 1984a (*Manual*), 31; 1984b (*Annals*), 266]. The resolution of this dilemma may vary depending on other features of the situation. Consider, for example, the following three variations.

1.5.1. Conflicts Between Two Nonpatients This is the most straightforward choice, since no prior loyalty is owed either party. In the simplest of these cases, decisions can be based entirely on the principles of justice.

In some cases the choice may involve establishing a future physician-patient relationship with one of the parties; if so, then *future* loyalties and the conflicts these might cause must be taken into account in arriving at a judgment. Fried (1974a, 75) describes this situation: "The notion is one of doing unstintingly what it is that one does, though choosing with care the occasions on which one will do it." This sort of situation would arise, for example, if one were choosing not simply who should receive the one-time doses of a vaccine, but rather whom to accept for a long-term therapy program in which only a limited number could be accommodated.

You have no prior obligation to any of these prospective patients (although it would be a tragedy, and perhaps an injustice toward them all, to allow the resource to remain unused when need for it exists). However, once a choice has been made and a physician-patient relationship has been established, loyalty does come into play. It would be unjust, for example, to remove access to a given resource from a patient just because a more medically suitable candidate comes along, although this difference would have been a valid reason for *preferring* the more suitable candidate if they had both presented at the *same time*.

1.5.2. Conflicts Between Your Patient and Another's   One common example of this sort of allocation decision is the case of another physician requesting that you release a patient from the ICU in order to provide a bed for a patient of his. You may acknowledge that his patient's need for the resource is more pressing than yours, but if you judge that the safety of your patient would be jeopardized by removal from the sort of close monitoring possible only in the ICU, is it appropriate for you to accede to his request? To do so would be to subordinate the principle of loyalty to your patient to the principle of justice. Some institutions seek to avoid placing individual physicians in this dilemma by leaving triage decisions of this sort to an ICU director or some other third party, thus converting this into a puzzle of the first type.

1.5.3. Conflicts Between Two of Your Own Patients   This is in some ways the most complicated of all three puzzles. When the needs of two of your own patients conflict and you cannot manage to accommodate them both, you must appeal to a principle of justice to temper *both* principles of loyalty. The result may be that you do less for each patient than you would have done had the conflict not arisen.

1.6 Office Scheduling as an Allocation Problem

These dilemmas are not confined to the rare, life-or-death situation. Parallel questions arise in daily practice—even with regard to so mundane an issue as office scheduling practices.

The procedure best embodying the *principle of equality* would be to stick invariably to a uniform time allocation (say, fifteen minutes) for each and every patient. This would minimize waiting times by keeping everything right on schedule, and in this way it might be agreeable to patients; but, of course, it would not take into account differentials of medical need and thus would fall short of standards of acceptable quality.

At the other extreme, the *principle of patient loyalty* dictates taking as much time as you felt necessary to deal with the problems of each patient, no matter how long other patients had to wait. This is obviously a recipe for frustration and anger on the part of patients in your waiting room. One could avoid this problem by scheduling only one patient every hour, but this remedy may require an unacceptable personal financial sacrifice by either the patient (if fees were set for this period of time at a level that generates a satisfactory income for the physician), or for the physician (if fees were kept at roughly their present levels per visit), or for both (if fees per visit were raised significantly but not enough to sustain present income). For the physician to bear the whole financial brunt of this shift involves a personal financial sacrifice far greater than any duty to patients could demand.

What is required for an acceptable scheduling practice is a process that balances all these needs within practical limits; i.e., one that is sensitive to 1) patients who must take time off from work and other duties to wait to see you, 2) the medical needs of the patients once it is their turn to be seen, and 3) the efficiencies of a medical office as a business enterprise and the realities of medical practice as a source of your livelihood and that of your employees, as well as the means to your own career goals.

2 Allocation on the Social Scale

Usually, the scarcity that necessitates allocation decisions between individual patients is the result of background decisions on a wider scale to limit the resource. These decisions Calabresi and Bobbit (1978, 19) call "first-order determinations." For example, in the case discussed in Section 1.3, a decision by the hospital officials resulted in only five doses of the drug being available. If the officials had stocked ten doses instead, no dilemma of allocation would have arisen on this occasion, although a situation might arise at another time in which eleven demands for the medication would be received. A judgment about how much of a resource to make available determines, as a consequence, how frequently individual allocation decisions will arise and how acute they will be.

Options for the first-order decision in the early days of kidney dialysis included:

1. not developing the resource at all, thus achieving equality by denying it to everybody
2. not using the resource until it was available in sufficient quantity to meet the total need
3. making enough of the resource available to meet only part of the need, and meeting as much of the need as possible while additional quantities of the resource were being developed.

The first option would have led to considerable loss of life, as would the second, since it would have meant that a number of patients who could have benefited would have been denied this life-saving resource during the period of further development. Another problem with the second option is that refinements and improvements in the technology normally made on the basis of early, limited use would either not have been available at all or would have required replacing a full complement of the technology. The third option was the one chosen in the case of renal dialysis, as well as with most other developing resources (e.g., the artificial heart). Once the technology was fully developed, Congress obviated further allocation decisions (at least for the present) by establishing a federal program to finance dialysis for all patients in need of it.

In general, three distinct but interrelated issues arise at this social level:

1. access to health care services
2. the structure of health care organizations, including the dramatic increase in involvement of for-profit agencies in the health care "industry"
3. the issue of costs in health care.

2.1 Access to Health Care Services

When someone suffers from a disease condition against which medical science is powerless, the situation is tragic and disturbing. However, even more disturbing, albeit in a different way, is someone suffering from a disease condition for which the resources exist to relieve the suffering, and yet the person lacks access to these resources that could help him.

An especially dramatic example of this is the incident portrayed by Edward Albee in the one-act play *The Death of Bessie Smith*, the account of a renowned blues singer who collapsed on the street just outside a Memphis hospital and was denied life-saving treatment because she was black and the hospital was "for whites only." The injustice of such a blatant and deliberate denial of access is obvious.

This incident would not likely occur today anywhere in the United States. Courts have firmly upheld the requirement that any hospital maintaining an emergency department must render aid to anyone presenting with a condition that requires urgent attention, regardless of race or ability to pay.

Interesting to note is that no corresponding duty applies to those who supply other basic life needs. If someone starves to death on the steps of a bakery or dies of exposure next to a hotel, the baker or hotel operator does not face legal liability. An important part of the reason for this difference in accountability stems from the difference in the acknowledged role of the providers. Baking and hotel management are not professions with a self-declared dedication to service. In contrast, an inherent goal in the enterprise of medicine is the attempt to meet *all* medical needs. Thus there is still reason for concern and careful examination of the circumstances when *any* remediable medical need goes unmet for lack of access to the appropriate services. Even if this is not the result of deliberate acts of injustice, it still constitutes a tragedy within society. How can such situations be avoided? Who is responsible for correcting it? In particular, in the attempt to close any gaps of access to services, what is the responsibility of the individual physician, health care institutions, and the government?

The President's Commission for the Study of Ethical Problems in Medicine and Biomedical and Behavioral Research sets forth the following as an "ethical standard" against which the justice of existing structures and programs should be measured: "Access for all to an adequate level of care without the imposition of excessive burdens" (President's Commission 1983a, 1).[4]

2.1.1. The Current Situation In the United States at present, the extent to which gaps in access to medical care exist is far from obvious. For example, the President's Commission (1983a, 67) reports that

> the number of physician visits per year, whether in response to perceived illness or for health maintenance reasons, is a key indicator of access to care. During the past few decades the increased use of services by traditionally underserved groups, especially the poor and racial and ethnic minorities, has been dramatic. Aggregate data, unadjusted for differences in need, show a substantial narrowing of the disparities in physician visits among population groups over the past 15 years. The poor now pay on average as many visits to physicians per year as the nonpoor. Blacks, on average visit the physician at rates comparable to whites.
>
> When the data are adjusted to consider differences in health status, however, these patterns change. Once visits are adjusted by perceived health status, the poor make fewer visits to a physician each year than the nonpoor, and blacks visit a doctor less frequently than whites of comparable health status.

One member of the Commission filed a dissenting statement to this report that questioned the significance of these data:

> This "adjustment" is capable of various interpretations, one of which might be that it is meaningless and another that there are fewer hypochondriacs among the poor and blacks. It certainly cannot mean that the poor and the blacks are denied equitable opportunities to visit a doctor. (President's Commission 1983a, 201)

There were other indications of unmet medical needs reported by the Commission. The physician visits made by patients with insurance coverage average 154% the number made by those without it (or, to put the point in reverse, the visits made by those *without* coverge average only 65% of all *with* coverage); and the hospital days for those with insurance averages 191% the number for those without insurance coverage (and thus the days for those *without* coverage average only 52% of those *with* coverage) (President's Commission 1983a, 101–102).

---

4. A summary of the recommendations from this report is included in Appendix 11.3.

The site of physician interactions also shows variance. A person with an income of less than $5,000 per year is twice as likely as one whose annual income is over $15,000 to have last seen a doctor in a hospital emergency room or out-patient department instead of a private office. Blacks are 2-½ times as likely as whites to have last encountered a physician in a hospital clinic setting. (p. 75)

Significant differences are also found in the severity of illness at the point of initial treatment:

> Data from the National Cancer Institute reveal that white patients have a higher percentage of their cancers diagnosed at an early stage than black patients do. Furthermore, "paying" patients have their cancers diagnosed in an earlier stage more often and have better survival rates than indigent "nonpaying" patients. Women who are considered to be at a higher risk of cervical cancer (particularly poor, black women aged 45–64 living in nonmetropolitan areas) are less likely than other women to have had a Papanicolaou (Pap) test to screen for that disease.
>
> A study of 5000 patients hospitalized for a variety of conditions found marked differences in the severity of illness at admission among those publicly and privately insured. In another study, patients insured under private plans were more likely to be hospitalized in earlier stages of their condition than those publicly insured. Public beneficiaries diagnosed as having appendicitis, for example, were twice as likely as those covered by commercial insurance to have their disease be at an advanced stage when they were admitted to a hospital. A similar study compared the severity at hospital admission of 21 medical or surgical conditions that require hospitalization at the earliest possible stage; it found that publicly insured patients were more likely than privately insured patients to be admitted with conditions in advanced stages. (President's Commission 1983a, 74—footnotes omitted)

In discussing the relationship between payment sources and health care, it is useful to know the size of the various payment groups (Table 5-1).

Table 5-1 Health Care Coverage by Type, 1980

	Number, in millions	% of Total
Private	161.2	69.8
Medicare	21.7	9.4
Medicaid	15.2	6.6
Medicare and Medicaid	6.1	2.6
VA, CHAMPUS	5.3	2.3
Uninsured	21.5	9.3
Total	231.0	100.0

President's Commission (1983a, 91).

While the interpretation of these data is subject to considerable dispute, it does underscore the importance of access to health care services. Of special concern are the 21.5 million Americans who lack any form of assistance in paying the rising costs of health care. These are the people most likely to have pressing medical needs go unmet due to lack of access to the health care system.

2.1.2 What Is the Goal? In addressing the access issue, however, questions arise. First, what exactly is the goal sought? Paul Starr (President's Commission 1983b) distinguishes between

1. availability of services
2. nonexclusionary policies and conduct
3. access to services
4. use of services
5. results of services.

He illustrates the differences between the first and third items in this passage:

> The right to postal service is a right of availability, not of access: The government guarantees to transmit mail in and out of communities, but not that you will have enough money to send letters. Insofar as there is a right of access to the U.S. mail, it is a right of communities rather than individuals. (The government does, however, guarantee to deliver your mail if somebody else has paid the postage.) On the other hand, local government typically provides fire protection regardless of your ability to pay, in part because of the risk to others. Some aspects of medical care, such as the control of contagious diseases, have long been considered like fire protection; providing access to those who cannot afford services has been understood as a matter of community welfare. Other aspects of medical care have been treated more like the postal service: Government has been willing to acknowledge a right of availability, but not necessarily of access. (This seems to have been the premise of the Hill-Burton hospital construction program.) (President's Commission 1983b, 7)

It is an enormous puzzle to decide *which* of these five goals should be addressed in trying to promote more adequate health services.

A. Availability The easiest of the items to address, this is quite remote from the concerns with which we began. Governmental programs such as the Hill-Burton act can be used to subsidize construction of hospitals and other health care facilities. Capitation subsidies to medical schools can increase the supply of practitioners. However, if those in need are barred from using resources and/or lack the *means of access* to them, no benefit is derived from their mere presence.

B. Nonexclusion Exclusionary policies are illustrated by the Bessie Smith case described earlier. Blatant forms of exclusion can be addressed by law and social policy, but more subtle forms of discrimination may remain, and these are much more difficult to root out.

Furthermore, there are other forms of selection that are less obviously unjust. Must VA hospitals admit any citizen, or is it appropriate for them to limit their services to veterans? Could a sectarian hospital be established specifically to serve the medical needs of a particular group (e.g., Jehovah's Witnesses) and then justly serve members of the founding group exclusively? Can a hospital justly treat only certain diseases or offer exclusive types of care?

C. Access   There are three primary barriers to access to services:

1. money to pay the costs of treatment
2. time to submit to treatment
3. transportation to the site of treatment.

These barriers are more difficult to overcome than barriers to availability or exclusionary policies, as shown by the struggles over the last several decades to devise a social policy for financing health services for those in need. Furthermore, eliminating these barriers may not achieve the ultimate goal, as shown by the next point.

D. Use   Correlation studies show that even if availability and means of access are fully equalized, the rate of use varies from one population to another. Many initially assume this to be unjust until the rate of use is equalized. Indeed, if you look at Section 2.1.1, you will note that most of the indicators of unmet needs cited by the President's Commission deal with *use*. To some extent this reaction to discrepancies of use makes sense: the differences in rate of use might, in part, reflect subtle exclusionary conduct within the institutions. However, the differences reflect, in part, health beliefs and attitudes of the subculture in question. Perhaps these beliefs and attitudes have been influenced by past practices of discrimination and lack of access to health services. However, insistence on eradicating these defining beliefs as the price for achieving some ideal goal of justice violates the integrity of the cultural subgroup.

E. Results   Since it is the importance of *health* needs that prompts concern with justice, it seems natural to set a standard in terms of states of health as the goal to be sought. The problem is that even if all barriers to availability and access to health care resources are removed—and indeed, even if use were equalized—perfect health for the population as a whole would not necessarily result. Health care does not directly *produce* health in the same way that bestowing money produces wealth. Individual, cultural, and perhaps genetic differences lead to different outcomes from the same level of services.

Should society insist on equality of access even though it does not effect equal result? If so, what are we trying to equalize?

2.1.3 Level of Services   Furthermore, it is impossible to provide availability, access, and/or use to meet *all* needs. The cost of attempting to achieve this level of services would be prohibitive. Daniel Wikler calls this the "bottomless pit" problem and points out its three aspects:

> First, some patients use (or could use with benefits) health care of practically unlimited cost. Even these expenditures would not, in some cases, be enough to restore such patients to the average health status of the rest of the community. Second, even if these needy individuals are left untreated (to some extent), medical resources likely will continue to be concentrated on a relatively small number of patients. Finally, the health benefits achieved by these expenditures are not always great. There is nothing in the nature of disease or medical care that guarantees a proportionality of expense and benefit. Chronic diseases are so called, after all, because they go on and on regardless of medical intervention. (President's Commission 1983b, 120)

Notice the goal presupposed by Wikler: "to restore such patients to the average health status of the rest of the community." This goal, set in terms of results, raises two problems.

1. Why should we rest content with achieving the "average health status of the rest of the community?" Why not, instead, try to bring everyone up to the *highest possible* level of health, or at the very least, why not aim at one or two standard deviations *above* the mean rather than merely aiming at the mean? These are questions of justice and need to be addressed in a public debate focusing on principles of justice. (Parallel questions arise for goals set in terms of availability, access, or use.)
2. Talk of specifying a certain level of overall health status suggests that there are clear-cut ways to *measure* this. Complexities and uncertainties in measurement pose theoretical difficulties for stating goals, over and above the ethical difficulties mentioned in item 1.
   a. Measures traditionally used to determine *result* include personal perceptions of illness, number of sick days in a given period (i.e., days of work or school missed due to illness or days spent in bed), and gross health measures such as infant mortality, etc. All these pose great theoretical difficulties.
   b. If *availability* is the goal, the level sought would be specified in terms of ratios of hospital beds, professionals, etc., to population. These benchmarks are often derived from current average rates of use, but these may be distorted by existing vagaries of access, and thus their soundness as indicators of ideal goals is questionable.
   c. Specifications of levels of services in terms of *access* could focus on 1) barriers to be addressed, or 2) the range of services to be made available, or 3) the procedure to be employed in deciding in each

particular case what services to make available. The choice among these, as well as issues about specifying the content of each, poses theoretical problems.

d. *Use* measures raise theoretical difficulties when attempts are made to correlate them with need.

Pellegrino and Thomasma (1981, 242) offer the following priorities under a general goal of access:

[1] Primary health care, and specifically its first-contact component, seems the minimal health care claim a citizen may make on a society of our kind. It takes precedence over other forms of care because of its universality and its intensely human dimensions, and because it is the critical point of first entry into the entire system of health care. It is fundamentally a form of personal security, and one of the benefits which ought to follow on the formation of society. Following this would be [2] access to treatments which can effect a radical cure or prevent occurrence of a disease entirely. Next would come [3] the care and containment of established serious diseases for which no radical cure is available; then [4] the more expensive, highly complex procedures of dubious or unproven benefit; and last, [5] treatment for disorders with minimal disability, which, though distressing, are not incapacitating and need only symptomatic treatment or self-care.
A nation must determine how far down this list it will go, given its resources and the expectations its form of society engenders. Whether health is preferred to other human services will depend largely on how far down the list of health priorities one wants to go. Since sanitation, housing, nutrition, and environmental safety contribute to health, they might well take precedence over health care items lowest on the list. In fact, they might take precedence over primary care as well.

As stated earlier, the President's Commission proposes a standard of "an adequate level of care." After examining several ways in which this notion might be defined (President's Commission 1983a, 35–42), the Commission leaves the definition to be worked out through the political process:

The Commission cites these alternatives as examples of possible initial approaches to approximating an adequate level of health care that should be available to all Americans. There are both theoretical and practical differences between these approaches, yet each has something to offer, separately and together. For the purpose of health policy formulation, general theories as well as ordinary views of equity do not determine a unique solution to defining adequate care but rather set some broad limits within which that definition should fall. It is reasonable for a society to turn to fair, democratic political procedures to make a choice among just alternatives. Given the great imprecision in the notion of adequate health care, however, it is especially important that the procedures used to define that level be—and be perceived to be—fair. (President's Commission 1983a, 42)

2.1.4 How to . . . ?   The most difficult question is how to achieve the goal once it has been defined. An extensive variety of approaches is available. Each must be examined, not only to measure its probable effectiveness and efficiency in achieving the goal, but for its impact on other values. One's sense of the magnitude of the problem (based upon interpretation of the data in Section 2.1.1) dictates the sense of urgency with which one approaches this issue and there are a number of approaches possible.

A. Laissez Faire   This would allow existing forces to continue to act without any added interference by government or other influences,[5] in hopes that the conscience, compassion, and standards of professionals and the responsibility of institutions will lead to changes that correct existing deficiencies in availability, access, and/or use of health services.

B. Moral Suasion   A more active approach would be to strengthen these inherent tendencies through moral suasion. One means to accomplish this is to call the attention of professionals to these issues and corresponding professional responsibilities (as is being done in these pages). Another is to enunciate professional responsibilities in the form of codes of professional ethics (as the ACP Ethics Manual does, as you will see shortly). Public opinion may have impact here through general public discussion of these issues.

C. Private Subsidies   There are mechanisms in the private sector that could provide for expanded access, etc. *Private charities* could provide for the needs of those whose access, etc., to health care is deficient. Charitable organizations currently play a vital (if small) role here, but a greater initiative would require a radical expansion of their present efforts.

Cost shifting by professionals and health care institutions is a mechanism for subsidizing care for patients who cannot pay. This amounts to a (privately levied) "sick tax." (Public and private hospitals have used this mechanism for years as a way of providing care for indigent patients.)

D. Government Subsidies   Local, state, and federal governments could work within the existing system to "fill in the gaps" of access, etc. This has been the dominant thrust of most past governmental action in this country, from the Hill-Burton program to increase availability of hospitals to Medicare and Medicaid programs which pay (at least in part) for access to services for certain groups. One key problem with this approach is that it rarely occurs without regulation of the system receiving the subidies.

---

5. Another approach, not discussed at length here, is to attempt to *remove* existing external influences on the present system. Among the many practical and theoretical problems that attend this option is the thorny task of sorting out which elements *count* as "external interferences" and which have been internalized into the system. For example, are licensure and associated restrictions against practice by unqualified healers an external interference?

E. Government Manipulation   Government could deliberately contribute forces of its own to work within the system to move it in the desired direction. This can take a number of forms: The *"carrot-and-stick"* *approach* follows naturally from government subsidization of elements of the system. The next step is to tie these funds to certain regulations, as has been done from the beginning with the Medicare and Medicaid programs. This linkage is seen even more explicitly in the program of prospective funding in terms of diagnosis-related groups (DRGs). Admittedly, one can avoid the impact of these regulations by not taking advantage of the subsidies to which they are attached. (However, it may not be possible thereby to return entirely to the *status quo ante*, because other means of providing for this population, such as charity support or volunteer assistance, may have dried up with the onset of government subsidy programs.)

Direct regulation would not be escapable in the same way. By the same token, government may not have strong basis for influence if its edicts are not tied to reimbursement or some other state function. The forms of direct regulation include

1. bureaucratic regulation
2. court rulings
3. statutory law.

F. Nationalization of the Health Care System   In this, the most radical approach, the government would assume full responsibility for health care delivery. Health care institutions would be run by the government and health care professionals would become employees of the state. Patients would become, in effect, wards of the state.

The President's Commission (1983a, 4) asserts the following on the role of government in this effort:

> **When equity occurs through the operation of private forces, there is no need for government involvement, but the ultimate responsibility for ensuring that society's obligation is met, through a combination of public and private sector arrangements, rests with the Federal government**. Private health care providers and insurers, charitable bodies, and local and state governments all have roles to play in the health care system in the United States. Yet the Federal government has the ultimate responsibility for seeing that health care is available to all when the market, private charity, and government efforts at the state and local level are insufficient in achieving equity.

This approach favors government subsidies to fill the gaps after the private sector has done all it can to provide full access to health care services.

The individual practitioner also has some responsibilities here. The ACP Ethics Manual addresses these in the following comments:

> Like any other good citizen, the physician should strive for the well-being of the community and of society. He should work toward ensuring the availability of adequate medical care for all individuals and should support community health endeavors.

In addition, the physician has [the] following special obligations:

1. To be aware of the availability and accessibility of health services to the people of the area in which he practices and to participate in reasonable efforts to correct defects in such availability and accessibility. [ACP 1984a *(Manual)*, 18–19; 1984b *(Annals)*, 135–136]

The physician may be technically free to select his patients to the exclusion of those who cannot pay, but as a professional he has a moral obligation to contribute some of his services to the neglected and underprivileged and to give good medical care to all his patients irrespective of their ability to pay.

When care is free, every effort must be made to preserve the dignity and self-respect of the patient. The indigent patient should receive equal care and be treated with the same respect and thoughtful concern as the patient who can pay for services. [ACP 1984a *(Manual)*, 8–9; 1984b *(Annals)*, 132]

We agree with these statements and add that physicians have a responsibility to take a leadership role in the public debate proposed by the President's Commission. A professional understanding of needs and priorities is an essential ingredient in policy formulation. If this viewpoint is not forcefully represented, less acceptable values may prevail (see Blendon and Altman 1984).

Decisions about location and form of practice ought to be influenced by considerations of medical need and not wholly by personal preferences. But frequently the problem is a combination of "How can you keep them down on the farm . . .?" and "Make hay while the sun shines." Physicians must balance considerations of medical need with their own and their family's needs, e.g., to

1. earn enough to pay back medical school debts (This is likely to be especially urgent in an atmosphere of impending dramatic changes in cost and financing of medical education. Since it may become impossible to meet these obligations in the future, it seems urgent to medical school graduates to recoup educational expenses as rapidly as possible.)
2. provide access to cultural opportunities for themselves and their families
3. provide for the style of life to which they have become accustomed.

Medical school and residency faculties can significantly influence the choice of practice location by helping students achieve a workable match between these needs and their desire to serve. On the other hand, faculty can train students *away* from a choice of practice in an area of unmet needs by creating an aura around academic medicine as the only respectable form of practice. One mechanism by which this is done is the disparagement of the "LMD" (local MD). Given the sneer with which these initials are usually spoken, it is hardly surprising that students and residents do not aspire to the title.

2.2 The Monetarization of Medicine

Any effort to close existing gaps in access to or use of health care services will undoubtedly take money, which brings us to the role of money in medicine.

Although expressed in cynical terms, the following statement by sociologist Erving Goffman captures the traditional view of money in the profession of medicine:

> There is a double sense in which a [professional] fee is not a price. Traditionally a fee is anything other than what the service is worth. When services are performed whose worth to the client at the time is very great, the server is ideally supposed to restrict himself to a fee determined by tradition—presumably what the server needs to keep himself in decent circumstances while he devotes his life to his calling. On the other hand, when very minor services are performed, the server feels obliged either to forego charging altogether or to charge a relatively large flat fee, thus preventing his time from being trifled with or his contribution (and ultimately himself) from being measured by a scale that can approach zero. When he performs major services for very poor clients, the server may feel that charging no fee is more dignified (and safer) than a reduced fee. The server thus avoids dancing to the client's tune, or even bargaining, and is able to show that he is motivated by a disinterested involvement in his work. And since his work is the tinkering kind, which has to do with nicely closed and nicely real physical systems, it is precisely the kind of work in which disinterested involvement is possible: a repair or construction job that is good is also one that the server can identify with; this adds a basis of autonomous interest to the job itself. Presumably the server's remaining motivation is to help mankind as such. (Goffman 1961, 326–327—footnotes omitted)

Compare the foregoing to the following statement, which contains many of the same elements expressed in different terms:

> Most doctors are basically honest and conscientious individuals who began their professional careers motivated more by scientific interest and idealistic goals than by profit motives. Most doctors come to realize early in their careers that they will not become rich practicing medicine. They may hope to achieve a better-than-average income, but it is the intangible rewards of practice, closely associated in doctors' minds with humanitarian achievement and the striving toward a goal of ideal service to their patients, that brought most physicians into medicine in the first place, and, ultimately, that keeps them there. (Nourse and Marks 1963, 59)

Factors on both sides of the physician-patient relationship contribute to this attitude of downplaying its financial components. For physicians, professional standards reinforce their predisposition to concern themselves less with the money to be gained from their practice than with 1) the intrinsic fascination of the technical task itself (what Nourse and Marks call "scientific interest" and Goffman calls "disinterested involvement in his work" or "tinkering"), and 2) a concern to help people who are in need (what Goffman calls a motivation "to help mankind as such'' and Nourse and Marks describe as ''a goal of ideal service to their patients'').

On the patient's part, there are two key considerations that subordinate attention to finances: 1) There is a generally shared recognition that the ''commodity'' being dealt with is *beyond price*; i.e., it would be improper to assign a monetary value to one's life or health. 2) Furthermore, the relationship itself is more a personal relationship than a commercial transaction; i.e., it is so intimate and deals with matters so momentous that it goes beyond matters appropriate for contractual negotiations and bargaining and requires instead *trust*. Goffman acknowledges these elements:

> The server's attachment to his conception of himself as a disinterested expert, and his readiness to relate to persons on the basis of it, is a kind of secular vow of chastity and is at the root of the wonderful use that clients make of him. In him they find someone who does not have the usual personal, ideological, or contractual reasons for helping them; yet he is someone who will take an intense temporary interest in them, from their own point of view, and in terms of their own best interests. As one student of human affairs suggests:
>
>> As defined in this culture, the expert is one who derives his income and status, one or both, from the use of unusually exact or adequate information about his particular field, in the service of others. This ''use in the service of'' is fixed in our industrial-commercial social order. The expert does not trade in the implements or impedimenta of his field; he is not a ''merchant,'' a ''collector,'' a ''connoisseur,'' or a ''fancier,'' for these use their skill primarily in their own interest. [Harry Stack Sullivan, ''The Psychiatric Interview,'' *Psychiatry*, XIV (1951), p. 365.]
>
> It therefore pays the client to trust in those for whom he does not have the usual guarantees of trust. (Goffman 1961, 327–328)

Notice that these points have all been made with reference to *motivations*. This indicates that at issue here are *character judgments* rather than either *judgments of moral obligation* or *evaluative judgments*.[6] Yet the other two forms of judgment are lurking in the background. The corresponding judgment of moral obligation is tacitly assumed: it goes without saying that it would be morally wrong for a physician to act in a way that serves no purpose beyond increasing his or her personal income, e.g., to recommend and carry out a medical procedure that does not serve the best interests of the patient. Evaluative judgments are incorporated into the central character judgment: what is questionable about a ''profit motive'' orientation is the value one assigns to money relative to interest in medical science and the welfare of one's patients.

---

6. To refresh your memory about the distinctions between these three kinds of judgments, see Chapter 2, Section 2.1.

The point is that an excessive concern for money is unseemly in a professional, just as it would be, for example, in parents whose dominant thought throughout the years of child raising was how the child would provide for them in their declining years. Another example of this might be "stage parents," who put their children through audition after audition in hopes of income and/or vicarious glory for themselves. These are the wrong reasons to have children: one ought to care about them *for themselves*, not merely for the *benefits* they might bring. This is true even if the motive never affects action: in the case of parents, even if it does not influence the career guidance they give to their child; in the case of physicians, even if it never prompts them to do a single lucrative but unnecessary procedure.

But, of course, there is the added danger that it *will* affect action, especially in borderline cases. When faced with the decision, for example, whether to order an additional diagnostic test to confirm a diagnosis, a physician with profits uppermost in mind may be influenced to do the procedure since her income will thereby be enhanced, whereas a physician whose dominant interest is the welfare of the patient might refrain from inflicting this added risk. And precisely because medical decisions are so much a matter of judgment, it is exceedingly difficult for observers to know to what extent this factor has influenced choice.

Two important implications follow:

1. An ongoing discipline of examination of one's motives is an important element in the moral life. Along with reviewing the rights and wrongs of past actions, one should honestly face the pattern of motives that prompt action and examine them in terms of ethical and professional character ideals.

2. One must avoid, not merely the *fact* of impropriety, but also its *appearance*, since observers may assume the worst if any basis for a conflict of interest exists. The only check against being misled by a conflict of interest is the interior influence of professional standards and personal ethical discipline, which by its interiority is invisible to the observer. "Man judges by outward appearances. . . . ." (I Samuel 16:7).

This latter element addresses what is most disturbing about the incursion of for-profit corporations into the health care field. The check of professional standards is lacking, and thus the danger is increased that individual ethical standards will be subordinated to the profit motive.

2.2.1 What's a Nice Profession Like You . . . ?   Arnold Relman forcefully sets out the dangers here (and also offers a partial solution) in an influential essay entitled, "The New Medical-Industrial Complex":

> What I will call the "new medical-industrial complex" is a large and growing network of private corporations engaged in the business of supplying health-care services to the patient for a profit—services heretofore provided by nonprofit institutions or individual practitioners.

Can we really leave health care to the marketplace? Even if we believe in the free market as an efficient and equitable mechanism for the distribution of most goods and services, there are many reasons to be worried about the industrialization of health care.

1. In the first place, health care is different from most of the commodities bought and sold in the marketplace. Most people consider it, to some degree at least, a basic right of all citizens. It is a public rather than a private good, and in recognition of this fact, a large fraction of the cost of medical research and medical care in this country is being subsidized by public funds. . . .

2. A second feature of the medical-care market is that most consumers (i.e., patients) are not "consumers" in the Adam Smith sense at all. As Kingman Brewster recently observed, health insurance converts patients from consumers to claimants, who want medical care virtually without concern for price. . . .

3. There are other unique features of the medical marketplace, not the least of which is the heavy, often total, dependence of the consumer (patient) on the advice and judgment of the physician. . . .

All these special characteristics of the medical market conspire to produce an anomalous situation when private business enters the scene. A private corporation in the health-care business uses technology often developed at public expense, and it sells services that most Americans regard as their basic right—services that are heavily subsidized by public funds, largely allocated through the decisions of physicians rather than consumers, and almost entirely paid for through third-party insurance. The possibilities for abuse and for distortion of social purposes in such a market are obvious.

It seems to me that the key to the problem of overuse is in the hands of the medical profession. With the consent of their patients, physicians act in their behalf, deciding which services are needed and which are not, in effect serving as trustees. The best kind of regulation of the health-care marketplace should therefore come from the informed judgments of physicians working in the interests of their patients. In other words, physicians should supply the discipline that is provided in commercial markets by the informed choices of prudent consumers, who shop for the goods and services that they want, at the prices that they are willing to pay.

But if physicians are to represent their patients' interests in the new medical marketplace, they should have no economic conflict of interest and therefore no pecuniary association with the medical-industrial complex. (Relman 1980, 963, 966–967)

There is no doubt that the involvement of for-profit corporations in the health field is a mushrooming phenomenon. As one author estimates (using a somewhat wider definition of "medical-industrial complex" than Relman employs):

> As of early 1983 listed corporations already owned approximately 11 percent of the nation's 5,900 community hospitals. They also had possession of 66 percent of nursing homes and chronic care facilities.
> . . . of the $317 billion spent on health care in 1982, fully $118 billion turned up as corporate revenues for the companies of the Medical-Industrial Complex. (Wohl 1984, 19)

2.2.2 Implications for the Future   Starr (1982, 428–439), Ginzberg (1984), and others point out that the influence of the corporate invasion of the health services "industry" has extended far beyond the for-profit institutions, and certainly beyond the selected institutions that Relman singles out in his essay. A "marketing mentality" and new concepts of institutional structures have emerged in *all* health care institutions.

Paul Starr (1982, 428) insists that "medical care in America now appears to be in the early stages of a major transformation in its institutional structure, comparable to the rise of professional sovereignty at the opening of the twentieth century." He explains that

> the change goes beyond the increased penetration of profit-making firms directly into medical services. By the growth of corporate medicine, I refer also to changes in the organization and behavior of nonprofit hospitals and a general movement throughout the health care industry toward higher levels of integrated control. Five separate dimensions need to be distinguished:
>
> 1. *Change in type of ownership and control:* the shift from nonprofit and governmental organizations to for-profit companies in health care
> 2. *Horizontal integration:* the decline of freestanding institutions and rise of multi-institutional systems, and the consequent shift in the locus of control from community boards to regional and national health care corporations
> 3. *Diversification and corporate restructuring:* the shift from single-unit organizations operating in one market to "polycorporate" and conglomerate enterprises, often organized under holding companies, sometimes with both nonprofit and for-profit subsidiaries involved in a variety of different health care markets
> 4. *Vertical integration:* the shift from single-level-of-care organizations, such as acute-care hospitals, to organizations that embrace the various phases and levels of care, such as HMOs
> 5. *Industry concentration:* the increasing concentration of ownership and control of health services in regional markets and the nation as a whole. (Starr 1982, 429)

2.2.3 Exercise: Professional Responsibilities INSTRUCTIONS: Look over the statements below. *Step 1*. Discard those with which you disagree entirely. *Step 2*. Go back over those remaining, two by two, and decide 1) whether the two statements are consistent and, if so 2) whether each statement *adds* something important to the other. If the answer to either of these questions is "No," discard one of the statements. Continue in this way until you have assembled a set of statements describing a *complete, consistent,* and *acceptable* policy to deal with financial conflicts of interest in medical practice. (You may add statements of your own or amend some of these.) *Step 3*. Look up the source of the statements you chose (given at the end of the chapter, p. 250) and see whether you chose from a single policy source or you assembled your view from a mixture of sources.

1. If physicians are truly not to have conflicting financial interests as they deliver their services, they should not be in the position of charging fees for services.

2. The physician should avoid any business arrangement that might, because of personal gain, influence his decisions in patient care. Activities of physicians relating to the business aspects of his own or his group's practice should be guided by the principle that such activities be intended for the reasonable support of that practice and for the effective provision of quality care for patients. Similarly, activities relating to the provision and maintenance of research and educational endeavors of his group or institution should be guided by the same principle.

3. For a physician to own shares in a drug company or in a hospital in which he practices does not constitute unethical behavior of itself, but it does make him vulnerable to the accusation that his actions are influenced by such ownership. The safest course is to avoid any such potentially compromising situations.

4. The guiding principle of the medical profession is to serve humanity. Financial gain should be a secondary consideration. Therefore personal financial interest should never override patient welfare in decision making.

5. The patient has the right to obtain information as to any relationship of his hospital to other health care and educational institutions insofar as his care is concerned. The patient has the right to obtain information as to the existence of any professional relationship among individuals, by name, who are treating him.

6. In any conflict which might develop between the physician's financial interest and his responsibilities to a patient, the patient's welfare must be the guiding consideration.

7. So long as the care of patients is not compromised, there is no objection on ethical grounds to a physician being engaged in any proper business unrelated to his medical practice.

8. If physicians are to represent their patients' interests in the new medical marketplace, they should have no economic conflict of interest and therefore no pecuniary association with the medical-industrial complex.

9. Critics . . . will probably point out that even without any investment in health-care businesses, physicians in private fee-for-service practice already have a conflict of interest in the sense that they benefit from providing services that they themselves prescribe. That may be true, but the conflict is visible to all and therefore open to control. Patients understand fee-for-service and most are willing to assume that their doctor's professional training protects them from exploitation. Furthermore, those who distrust their physicians or dislike the fee-for-service system have other alternatives: another physician, a prepayment plan, or a salaried group.

10. Groups of consumers shopping for health care packages should be informed in advance about restrictions on seeking care from providers outside health care panels.

2.2.4 Physician Payment Systems   Another element of the financial aspect of health care is the system by which physicians are paid. Review the following description of possible methods of payment; you then will be asked to reflect upon this issue.

The possible ways of paying doctors for medical care are fee-for-service, salary, capitation, and case payment. None are linked inextricably to any way of organizing a country's medical services. National health insurance systems and national health services can be found using each of the payment methods, but national health services tend to use the more predictable device of salary and to avoid fee-for-service. . . .

Fee-for-service is payment for each medical procedure. Under "service benefits" or "direct payment" methods, the third party—i.e., the sick fund or the health service—pays the doctor directly, and the patient usually pays him nothing. Under "cash benefits" or "reimbursement" methods, the patient pays the doctor and subsequently regains all or most of the fee from the third party.

Capitation is a fixed annual payment for each person on a list regularly assigned to a doctor. The physician gives all necessary care to the members on the list who come to him. Even if a person never visits him, the doctor automatically collects the capitation fee; even if a person has many medical problems, the doctor usually can collect no more than the capitation fee. Patients usually pay nothing to the doctor.

Salary is a fixed amount of money scaled according to the rank of the job and paid according to the amount of time the doctor gives. Patients usually pay the doctor nothing. Some arrangements allow the doctor to collect fees from the third party, in addition to the salary given for basic care.

Case payments are fixed sums given the doctor for giving a patient all necessary care. They differ from capitation fees, which are paid for persons on a list regardless of illness. Case payments differ from fee-for-service in that payments are not itemized by procedure and totaled. The few case payment systems use the service benefits principle: the third party pays the doctor, and the patient pays nothing. (Glaser 1970, 25)

2.2.5 Exercise: Payment Systems

A. *Your Reaction*

1. How do *you* want to be paid?
2. Is case payment acceptable to you? Why or why not?
3. Who should control how you are paid?
   a. the hospital
   b. the government
   c. the insurance company
   d. your spouse
   e. other (specify): _____
4. Is the fee-for-service structure of payment so important to you that you are willing to avoid participation in any form of prepayment plan?

B. *General Analysis* It cannot be denied that the problems pointed out by critics of the existing fee-for-service, cost-reimbursement system of payment are genuine cause for concern. They include

1. high cost
2. overreliance on technology and technique
3. gaps in access, etc., to services not covered by some form of assured care (especially with third-party reimbursement that obscures out-of-pocket expenses)
4. failure to meet the perceived needs of patients, i.e., electrochemical reductionism vs. care and sensitivity.

What must be questioned, however, is whether these problems are the ineluctable result of irresistible forces inherent in the payment system. Instead they may result 1) from *exploitation* of the system by practitioners who do not abide by professional standards of behavior (the "black hats") and/or 2) from forces in the society independent of the medical payment system. These possibilities are usually not considered when alternative payment systems are examined. It is assumed that these new systems will be operated wholly by "white hats" and in a vacuum of external forces. But, of course, that is unlikely to happen.

As a corrective, look at the alternatives in a realistic light: assume a mixture of white and black hats, much like you would find in today's medical community (in any relative proportion that you choose to postulate). Then, on the basis of this assumption, answer the following questions for each of the payment systems described in Section 2.2.4.

1. If one intended to "game" the system, what would be the strategy to follow? How do the possible forms of exploitation vary from system to system?

2. Project the likely *consequences* of the typical forms of abuse of the system. Are there significant differences in these from one system to another?

3. Look back at the four problems listed earlier (and other parallel problems that come to mind). For each system, consider whether each problem is likely to be:
   a. removed entirely and impossible to recur
   b. relieved somewhat but not removed entirely
   c. unchanged
   d. exacerbated somewhat
   e. exacerbated greatly.

4. Describe the impact within the system of the social forces behind these problems (e.g., the general lack of deep concern for the underprivileged, fascination with technology and technique, unrealistic patient expectations of what medicine can accomplish).
   a. How does this differ from one system to another?
   b. Are there *safeguards* in the system to minimize the negative impact of these forces? If so, what are they?

5. What would it be like to be a "white hat" under each system? What changes (if any) in professional standards would each require? What changes (if any) would each make in the nature of the physician-patient relationship? (For example, what practical truth is there to the adage: "He who pays the piper calls the tune"? What differences might institutional forms of payment make to one's loyalty to patients?)

6. What incentives would you need to *continue* to be a white hat?

2.3 Cost Control

The monetarization of medicine, in turn, may exacerbate the problem of rising costs, which brings us to the issue of cost control.

2.3.1 The Problem

The good news is that modern medicine can work miracles. The bad news is that it is very expensive and that many health expenditures do not seem to yield benefits worth their cost. Medical expenditures in the United States (in 1982 dollars) rose from $503 per capita in 1950 to $776 in 1965 (the last pre-medicare, pre-medicaid year) and to $1,365 in 1981, 10.5 percent of gross national product.

. . . Hospital care expenditures alone showed even more dramatic increases, rising from $153 per capita in 1950, to $257 in 1965, and to $563 in 1981. (Aaron and Schwartz 1984, 3, 139)

Of course, it is difficult to tell how much is *too much* to spend for health care. A comparison of worldwide figures may shed some light:

. . . The available data indicate striking differences in the levels of current total public expenditures on health for capital and operating purposes, with average figures of $2.60 per capita per year in the poorest countries (1.1 per cent of the gross national product), $19 in middle-income developing countries (1.2 per cent of the gross national product), and $469 in industrialized countries (4.4 per cent of the gross national product). The combined public and private health expenditures in the United States and several northern European countries are close to $1,000 per capita per year—more than 100 times the level in the poorest group of countries. At the other extreme, a few of the poorest countries—Bangladesh, Ethiopia, Indonesia, and Zaire—have annual public expenditures on health of only $1 per capita. (Evans et al. 1981, 1122)

There are other figures of interest: total health expenditures in western European countries were much higher than ours—in West Germany, 12.8% of the gross national product (GNP) in 1978; in Sweden in the same year, 11.3% of the GNP. In contrast, Great Britain's expenditures totaled only 5.4% of the GNP in 1978 and were actually reduced slightly to 5.3% of the GNP by 1980—at which time the U.S. expenditures were 9.4% of a much higher GNP.

These differences among developed countries do not appear to have a direct effect on overall health status. Indeed,

crude indicators of health status put Britain abreast or slightly ahead of the United States. Life expectancy at birth for men was 70.2 years in Britain in 1979 and 69.9 years in the United States; British baby girls born in 1979 could expect to live 76.2 years, and their American counterparts about 1 year more. During the first year of life babies born in 1979 died at the rate of 12.9 per thousand in Britain and 13.1 per thousand in the United States. (Aaron and Schwartz 1984, 12)

It is also difficult to ascertain the relative contribution of various elements of the health care system to the cost differentials and increases. Physicians' income is often cited as a factor, yet this accounts for less that 20% of the total health care cost. Hospital costs have increased far faster than other components and now comprise more than 46% of the total national health care expenditures, but this in itself is made up of many elements. "Big-ticket" technologies are a dramatic focus of attention, but their role is disputed. Moloney and Rogers (1979, 1414) argue:

> If the annual operating costs of the nation's four most widely heralded large technologies (CT scanning, electronic fetal monitoring, coronary by-pass, and renal dialysis) were reduced by half—a dramatic rationing—the net savings to the nation would equal less than 1 per cent of last year's bill for health care.

These authors claim that a much more significant contributor to health care costs are "low-cost services such as laboratory tests and x-rays rather than a shift to the use of big, expensive technologies for diagnosis or treatment."

2.3.2 Comparison with British Health Care System An illuminating study of issues in cost containment is the comparison of the U.S. and British health care systems by Aaron and Schwartz (1984). They compared rates of use and costs for 11 medical services:

1. bone marrow transplantation
2. cancer chemotherapy
3. CT scanners
4. coronary artery surgery
5. diagnostic x-rays
6. hemodialysis
7. hemophilia treatment
8. hip replacement
9. radiotherapy
10. total parenteral nutrition
11. intensive care beds.

They summarize their conclusions as follows:

> The British, on a per capita basis, buy less than Americans of many of the technological procedures discussed in this part of the book. They provide the same volume of care only for radiotherapy, bone marrow transplantation, and the treatment of hemophilia. At the other end of the spectrum lies coronary artery surgery; the British do only 10 percent as many procedures per capita as Americans. In a few instances, such as cancer chemotherapy, differences in clinical judgment may possibly explain all the differences between the number of patients cared for in Britain and in the United States. But in the case of such procedures as coronary artery surgery and CT scans, resource limits have led the British to sacrifice some medically beneficial information or treatment. The political process implicitly concluded that the benefits were worth less than the value of alternative objects of public expenditure.

The British would have had to spend an additional $1.030 billion around 1980 to have provided full care [i.e., the same level as the U.S.], and a total of $2.395 billion if intensive care is included. These amounts may seem modest by American standards or compared with the range of improvements that could be achieved. But it represents roughly an 8 percent increase over British hospital expenditures in 1980, 18 percent if intensive care is included. In a system that has managed annual growth in real outlays of only 1.5 percent a year, however, such increases would require a major change in the priority attached to health care. It is precisely such a change that neither Labour nor Conservative governments since 1975 have been prepared to make.

The most striking aspect of these comparisons is that the pattern of rationing evident in Britain is so uneven: Britain provides some services in negligible quantities and some at nearly the same levels as found in the much less constrained U.S. system. (Aaron and Schwartz 1984, 74–76)

This rationing is accomplished in Britain by a combination of several mechanisms. First, the central government sets an overall health services budget annually—usually increased little in real dollars over the previous year. This is allocated among individual hospitals and other health care institutions through a series of bureaucracies at the national and regional levels.

Second, within the hospital, allocations are usually made by the senior consultants, a group of physicians who work exclusively in one institution and are salaried by it. Capital expenditures, allocations of beds by clinical services, and similar decisions are explicitly regulated by these consultants. "Nominally, there are no limits on the physician's ability to command pharmaceutical supplies. But in fact, financial stress results in sharp real restraints on the physician's nominal clinical freedom" (Aaron and Schwartz 1984, 55). For example,

in one large teaching hospital, we learned, the clinical interests of a consultant led to a steady growth in his expenditures on TPN [total parenteral nutrition]. As others began to prescribe it, rising costs pushed the hospital pharmacy over its budget. To make room for the TPN, the chief pharmacist cut back on maintenance, staff, and other services. Eventually the medical staff imposed a limit on TPN service. . . . In the end, the staff decided to allow a maximum of six adult patients at a time to receive TPN. (Aaron and Schwartz 1984, 55)

Finally, the primary care physician serves as gatekeeper in the rationing process. Older patients in renal failure are not referred for kidney dialysis. Instead, they are told that "nothing more can be done." If any are bold enough to seek out a dialysis center on their own (and remarkably few do so), they are likely to be accepted for treatment, in spite of a general agreement not to provide dialysis for patients over age 55 or so. (Aaron and Schwartz believe this form of rationing would not likely succeed in the United States. Patients would not accept the gatekeeper's denial of access to advanced care without protest.)

2.3.3 Professional Responsibilities   Physicians have not failed to show concern for the issue of cost increases. As one indication of professional interest, the index for the latter half of 1984 (volume 311) of the *New England Journal of Medicine* contained 28 articles under the heading "Cost."

The central question here is what the role of the physician should be in the attempt to control health care costs. Should these decisions be made by others in the society, or should the responsibility for making them be the physician's?

A. Dr. Jekyll and Citizen Hyde   The ACP Ethics Manual proposes a dual role for physicians: as citizens, a zeal for holding down health care costs, but as physicians, an equally forceful zeal for providing every beneficial resource for patients.

Patient Advocacy and Conflicting Interests

Under the covenant of personal medical care the physician is ordinarily the advocate and the champion of his patient, upholding the patient's interests above all others. All too frequently, however, the physician is forced to serve conflicting interests. For example, . . . he may at one moment serve society in the painful but necessary task of allocating limited resources, and in the next moment, quite properly, reverse his role and function as the patient's advocate under these circumstances. The patient's welfare must always be the physician's prime concern, but no one can avoid these moral dilemmas. In such cases the physician must act with sensitivity and without duplicity making it clear to the patient and understanding it himself when other interests are being served and to what extent secrecy and trust have been infringed. [ACP 1984a (*Manual*), 13; 1984b (*Annals*), 134]

Obligations of the Physician to Society

Like any other good citizen, the physician should strive for the well-being of the community and of society. He should work toward ensuring the availability of adequate medical care for all individuals and should support community health endeavors. In particular, he should seek to use all health-related resources in a technically appropriate and effective manner and to husband limited resources. . . .

In addition, the physician has [the] following special obligations:

4. To be aware of the limitations of health services resources, such as material and personnel, and to participate with others in exercising restraint in the expenditure of these resources.
5. To be aware of the costs of care and to provide care in the most efficient manner. [ACP 1984a (*Manual*), 18–19; 1984b (*Annals*), 135–136]

Resource Allocation

The physician has a particular responsibility to his patient in a world of increasingly limited financial resources. The guiding principle must be that the physician should concentrate his energy and attention on providing the patient with the best possible medical care within the context of practicing humanistic, scientific, efficient medicine. In the event that external pressures resulting from limited institutional resources prevent the physician from providing optimal care, he must decide whether it is appropriate to advise the patient of the nature of the situation. In the final analysis, no external factors should interfere with the dedication of the physician to provide optimal care for his patient. [ACP 1984a (*Manual*), 31; 1984b (*Annals*), 266]

The puzzling question is whether the roles of citizen and physician can be kept separate in the way this position requires. Can Citizen Hyde become Dr. Jekyll without the inappropriate attitudes of the former role infecting the latter? For example, can a physician who spends the morning forcefully endorsing cost-containment goals abandon this attitude in the afternoon upon encountering a patient who is obviously abusing himself and the health care system? Can the principle of loyalty to one's patients be fully honored unless one *does* shed these attitudes entirely?

B. Patron Saint Some commentators feel that these two roles cannot be combined appropriately. Thus they put the entire emphasis on the side of Dr. Jekyll and patient advocacy, leaving it to others to serve as Mr. Hyde:

> Physicians can help control costs by choosing the most economical ways to deliver optimal care to their patients. They can use the least expensive setting, ambulatory or inpatient, in which first-class care can be given. They can eliminate redundant or useless diagnostic procedures ordered because of habit, deficient knowledge, personal financial gain, or the practice of "defensive medicine" to avoid malpractice judgements.
>
> However, it is society, not the individual practitioner, that must make the decision to limit the availability of effective but expensive types of medical care. . . . If society decides to ration health care, political leaders must accept responsibility. David Owen, who is both a political leader in Britain and a physician, believes that "it is right for doctors to demand that politicians openly acknowledge the limitations within which medical practice has to operate." I agree and would add that doctors are entitled to lobby vigorously in the political arena for the resources needed for high-quality health care. (Levinsky 1984, 1575)

C. Dancing (as gracefully as possible) to Another's Tune The following commentator agrees with the substance of much of the previous position, although his attitude is quite different. He suggests that a process of external limitations on resources could work fairly smoothly.

> A major concern is whether attempts to control the use of health-care resources will affect the health of the population. Opinions differ concerning this question, and no one knows the answer with certainty. Some health experts contend that it is possible to cut expenditures substantially without seriously affecting health. They claim that some care—say, 10 per cent—is actually harmful to patients, that they

would be better off without it. It is not difficult to believe that another 10 per cent has a relatively low yield even though there may be a slight benefit. Thus, *if* cuts were concentrated on the 20 per cent that had a negative or low yield, the overall effect on health would be small. But that is a big "if." Two major problems stand in the way of such an outcome. First, much of medical practice lacks a firm, quantified, scientific base; therefore no one can be certain just which care should be cut. Second, even as clinical experience and systematic research reveal which hospital admissions, operations, x-ray procedures, prescriptions, and the like can be forgone without harm (or even possible benefit) to patients, there is no guarantee that medical practice will be modified accordingly. Media hype, irrational patient preferences, distortional insurance coverage, and perverse incentives for health care professionals and institutions may result in a pattern of care that is far different from the ideal.

What needs to be done? First, the nation's practitioners, hospitals, and academic medical centers must launch a major effort to identify the benefits that patients receive from the various components of the $400 billion that is spent annually for health care. Second, experts on health-care policy need to continue to press for reforms in organization and finance that will lead patients to want, and health professionals to deliver, more cost-effective care.

. . . For physicians to have to face these trade-offs explicitly every day is to assign to them an unreasonable and undesirable burden. The commitment of the individual physician to the individual patient is one of the most valuable features of American medical care. It would therefore be a great mistake to turn each physician into an explicit maximizer of the social-benefit/social-cost ratio in his or her daily practice.

. . . Health-plan managers, hospital administrators, insurance-company ex-ecutives, and govenmental officials will . . . make difficult decisions about the allocation of scarce resources. This shift in the locus of decision making will inevitably reduce the power of practicing physicians.[7] To the extent that these decisions set the constraints within which individual practitioners function, however, there will be less need for them to ration care to their patients explicitly. (Fuchs 1984, 1573)

D. Professional Discretion   Other commentators maintain that the most satis-factory locus of decision in limiting resources is in the framework of clinical decision making:

These new medical techniques require a shift in standard medical practice. Instead of stopping treatments when all benefits cease to exist, physicians must stop treatments when marginal benefits are equal to marginal costs. But where lies the point at which marginal costs equal marginal benefits? And who is to make this ethical decision—the patient, the doctor, some third-party payer? And how

---

7. It is hoped that this new decision locus will not be less pertinent to patients' needs.—*Authors*

do we as a society decide that we cannot afford a medical treatment that may marginally benefit someone?

. . . One answer is that third-party payers can write rules and regulations concerning what they will and will not pay for and can prohibit their clients from buying services that are not allowed under the private or public insurance systems. This is essentially how the British have kept health-care spending at half the American level.

Such a procedure works, but it works clumsily, since no set of rules can be adjusted to the nuances of individual medical problems. It will be far better if American doctors begin to build up a social ethic and behavioral practices that help them decide when medicine is bad medicine—not simply because it has absolutely no payoff or because it hurts the patient—but also because the costs are not justified by the marginal benefits. To do this we are going to have to develop and disseminate better information on the cost effectiveness of alternative medical techniques for treating different ailments. Some small fraction of what we now spend on health care could be better spent to determine the limits of health-care expenditures under different circumstances.

The medical profession now has professional norms concerning what constitutes bad medical practice. Those norms have to be expanded to include cases in which high costs are not justified by minor expected benefits. If such norms are developed and then legally defended against malpractice suits, it just may be possible to build up a system of doctor-imposed cost controls that will be much more flexible than any system of cost controls imposed by third-party payers could be. But if the medical profession fails to do this, sooner or later the United States will move to a system of third-party controls. Something will have to be done. (Thurow 1984, 1569, 1571)

Intriguing to consider is whether a limitation imposed by third parties would be more palatable to the public than one imposed by physicians. The responsible agent may have to bear a significant brunt of criticism, for in a field as inexact as medicine, attempts to limit treatments are bound to have negative outcomes in some cases.

Hiding from the public the rationing effects of these decisions would clearly be dishonest. Calabresi and Bobbit (1978) indicate that it is not uncommon to shield the implications of what they call "tragic choices" from conscious awareness, because people find it intolerable to admit that they are willing to put a price on human life. This is another conflict of fundamental values, similar to the question of whether to inform a patient of a diagnosis of terminal illness. Here the question is whether to impose an unpleasant awareness upon the society as a whole. It must be decided whether peace of mind is worth the price of self-deception and/or dishonesty toward others. It will be difficult to reach a social consensus on the issues of justice involved in these choices, but it would be self-defeating to *assume*, before making any attempt at an explicit social consensus, that one is impossible.

2.3.4 Exercise: Cost-Control Measures   Continue the exploration of realistic assumptions begun in Section 2.2.5. Consider various cost-containment approaches, answering the following questions about each:

1. What are the possibilities for exploiting the system?
2. What are the likely consequences of exploitation?
3. What safeguards against abuse are inherent in the system?
4. What tendencies are inherent in the system that would sacrifice other values (e.g., justice, compassion, professionalism) in pursuit of cost control?
5. What cost-control strategy do you find most satisfactory overall? Why?
6. *Test Case: The Self-Insured Patient.* Nowadays most patients either have third-party sources of payment (at least for hospital expenses), or it is obvious that they will become a "write-off." Occasionally, however, a patient makes a serious commitment to pay the costs of his care from his own pocket.
   a. Do you find yourself more conscious of cost in choosing diagnostic tests, etc., for this sort of patient than with insured patients?
   b. If so, reflect on the differences. There are three possibilities:
      1) The level of care this patient receives is substandard, and that which others receive is quality care.
      2) The differences between these patients make no difference to the quality of their care.
      3) The level of care this patient receives is optimal, and other patients are really overtreated.
   c. Which is most often the case, in your judgment?
   d. Could the treatment received by the self-insured patient serve as a model for cost-appropriate medicine? If not, perhaps it could serve as a negative example, i.e., as a *limit* that cost-control measures should not be allowed to reach.

2.3.5 DRGs, PPOs, and Other Alphabetical Mysteries[8]   Social forces have already set in motion programs to attempt to control costs. These have given rise to a confusing variety of acronyms, as well as to more serious frustrations in clinical decision making. And yet the public appears not to recognize the negative consequences of rationing health care. A typical reaction is an article that appeared in Scripps-Howard Newspapers on the first anniversary of the implementation of DRGs, concluding:

---

8. PPO: Preferred-provider organization.

The year-old federal program that tells hospitals how much they can charge Medicare patients for specific treatments is credited with curbing hospital costs after a 17-year-long climb. . . . With surprising unanimity, federal and hospital officials agree the new payments formula is dramatically changing the way hospitals care for their patients. (Kirkman 1984)

Claims made in the article are cited below (with the article's explanations) and are followed by questions not examined in the article (or in much of the other public reaction to health care cost containment):

1. ITEM: "Hospital prices this year have risen only 4.8 percent, compared with 12 percent last year and 19 percent annual increases in the late 1970s."

2. ITEM: "The average hospital stay has declined from 9.5 days a year ago to 7.5 days."

   Explanation: "Hospitals no longer are admitting patients early and keeping them a couple of extra days to fatten the hospitals' Medicare payments."

   Question: a) To what extent was a desire "to fatten the hospitals' Medicare payments" an influence in admission and discharge decisions in the past? b) What should a physician do with regard to patients for whom complications make it *medically advisable* to keep them in the hospital longer than the standard formula allows?

   Explanation: "If a hospital unnecessarily delays a patient's care for one day, it now costs the hospital $500 to $600 the hospital no longer can recover."

   Question: What should a physician do if he or she judges that the patient's medical condition dictates postponing the next diagnostic test until tomorrow, although this will delay the patient's care one day and thereby cost the hospital $500 to $600 that the hospital no longer can recover?

   Explanation: "The old hospital game of admitting patients on Friday to fill up the hospital with paying customers is a thing of the past."

   Question: a) To what extent was the desire "to fill up the hospital with paying customers" an influence in admission and discharge decisions in the past?" b) What should a physician do if he judges that this patient is too sick to be cared for adequately at home over the weekend, but the surgical team cannot be assembled until Monday [especially given recent staff cutbacks (see item 3)]?

   Explanation: "We're bringing patients into the hospital now on the day they're due for surgery, not the night before."

Question: This necessitates leaving preparations for surgery to the patient. a) Are patients willing and able to accept this responsibility (e.g., to avoid taking anything by mouth after midnight, to give oneself an enema, to initiate presurgical antibiotics and other medicines)? b) If a patient forgets or misunderstands these instructions and harm results, should the hospital be immune from liability for damages?

Explanation: "Our doctors are getting patients in and out of the hospital more quickly."

Question: This requires cutting corners on the "margin of safety": discharging patients at a stage when the odds of their escaping complications are (e.g.) 80% instead of the past practice of waiting until a stage at which the odds reached (e.g.) 95%. Is the cost savings worth this added risk?

3. ITEM: "Hospitals have laid off tens of thousands of employees, the first time staffs have been cut since World War II. . . . Most hospitals are reducing their staffs by attrition, but there have been some big layoffs at some hospitals, mostly nurse's aides, lab technicians, dietary workers, and maintenance workers."

Question: Can the quality of care be maintained at a satisfactory level with the reduced staff? Is the cost savings worth this added risk and inconvenience?

4. ITEM: "[H]ospital medical committees are providing cost data to their physicians so doctors can see whether they're making or losing money for the hospital. Physicians who are chronic money losers are given 'little talks' by the committees and advised to mend their expensive ways."

Question: How should a physician respond to such a "little talk"? If the physician is convinced that she has developed a pattern of practice that is in the best interests of her patients, to what degree should the physician be willing to modify (compromise?) this to "make money for the hospital"?

5. ITEM: In some hospitals, "doctor's requisition forms for X-rays and tests now show doctors how much each procedure costs."

Question: To what extent *should* the cost of a test be a factor in the physician's choice?

6. ITEM: Some hospitals "no longer admit patients with minor illnesses and injuries who would have been hospitalized in the past. Instead, the hospital treats these patients in the emergency room or out-patient clinics."

Question: a) Is this shift medically advisable? b) Are people willing to accept the added risk of complications that results from this policy? Should physicians and hospitals be immune from liability for harm that results from this policy? c) Are people willing to assume the added burden of care for family members that results from this policy? (For example, "He must have absolute bed rest for 48 hours. He cannot even get up to go to the bathroom. Elevate his leg at a 45° angle. Check his blood pressure every hour, day and night. If you note any change in mental status, call an ambulance immediately!") d) Whose responsibility is it to decide whether the patient can safely be cared for outside the institution—the hospital, the family, the patient, the physician?

It is not clear how PPOs ensure that the physician bent on financially exploiting the system will not continue to do so. This sort of arrangement depends on cost shifting plus an expanded market as strategies for success, from the provider's point of view. There are no additional assurances or guidelines to ensure upholding quality of care. It may be tempting to bring about cost savings by lowering quality of care. The ideal, of course, is to do away with unnecessary interventions and to keep beneficial ones. But to say this amounts to no more than advising the inquiring investor to "buy low and sell high." There is the danger in all these systems that the individual will be sacrificed for the sake of controlling cost. The show of concern for the welfare of the individual patient may be no more than a facade. One test of these systems will be their response to expensive rescue strategies. A certain number of these may be undertaken for symbolic purposes, or they may be avoided as "not worth the cost."

3 Reviewing Your Expectations

These questions are thorny and complex. Issues of justice, professional standards, and social expectations are woven together. Medicine's importance is demonstrated by the zeal with which people attempt to ensure ready access to health-care services for themselves and those they care about.

Ultimately, your position on these issues will depend on your fundamental principles, values, and expectations. Go back to Chapter 1 and review the sets of expectations you enunciated, starting with the exercise in Section 1.1.

Consider the following questions.

1. Have your expectations altered as a result of working through this material? Note any changes.

2. Do you see possibilities you did not recognize before for frustration of expectations in medical practice? If so, think of ways to avoid these difficulties.

3. Do your expectations enable you to set priorities among the elements considered in this chapter?

   a. If so, what position do they lead you to?
   b. Are you satisfied with this position, or will you alter your expectations?

4. In light of your expectations from your professional life and changing definitions of what is medically important in our society, do you see a need to participate in political activity? If so, what sort of group would you find most appropriate and comfortable to work within?

   a. American Medical Association
   b. medical specialty organization
   c. voluntary organization of health care providers
   d. church group
   e. political party

Discuss the pros and cons of each of these groups as instruments to achieve your goals. Do you plan to discuss these issues on an ongoing basis as part of a group that has *patients* among its members, or will you keep these discussions "within the circle" of the profession?

By thinking these questions through, you can develop a coherent, comprehensive, and personally acceptable basis for confronting these issues, and for the decisions you are likely to face in your medical practice.

Sources of Items in Exercise, Section 2.2.3

1. Elaine L. Allen, M.D., letter, *New England Journal of Medicine*, 304:232, 1981.
2. ACP 1984a (*Manual*), 21; 1984b (*Annals*), 137: "Commercialization of Medicine and Other Conflicts of Interest."
3. ACP 1984a (*Manual*), 14; 1984b (*Annals*), 134: "Personal Conflicts of Interest."
4. A paraphrase of a sentence in *Current Opinions–1984*, Section 4.04: "Health Facility Ownership by Physician" (pp. 14–15); the section is quoted in full in Chapter 3, Section 3.3.3. [NOTE: This statement is criticized by Relman (1980, 967–968).]
5. American Hospital Association (1972): "Patient's Bill of Rights." A similar provision is contained in the statement "Health Facility Ownership by Physician" in *Current Opinions–1984*, which is quoted in Chapter 3, Section 3.3.3.

6. Cf. *Current Opinions–1984*, Section 4.04: "Health Facility Ownership by Physician" (quoted in Chapter 3, Section 3.3.3.) Cf. "In the case of personal conflicts the moral edict is clear. The physician must avoid any personal commercial conflict of interest that might compromise his loyalty and treatment of the patient. Collusion with nursing homes, pharmacists, or colleagues for personal financial gain is morally reprehensible" [ACP 1984a (*Manual*), 14; 1984b (*Annals*), 134: "Personal Conflicts of Interest"].

7. ACP 1984a (*Manual*), 21; 1984b (*Annals*), 137: "Commercialization of Medicine and Other Conflicts of Interest."

8. Arnold S. Relman, "The New Medical-Industrial Complex" (1980, 967).

9. Arnold S. Relman, "The New Medical-Industrial Complex" (1980, 968).

10. Authors' construction—but it sounds much like desirable insurance company policy.

References

Aaron J, Schwartz WB: *The Painful Prescription: Rationing Hospital Care.* (Brookings Institution, Washington DC, 1984).

Alexander S: They decide who lives, who dies: Medical miracle puts a moral burden on a small committee. *Life* 9:102ff, November 1962. Reprinted in: Hunt R, Arras J (eds) *Ethical Issues in Modern Medicine* Mayfield Publishing, Palo Alto CA, 409–424, 1977.

ACP: *See* American College of Physicians.

American College of Physicians: *Ethics Manual.* American College of Physicians, Philadelphia, 1984a.

————: American College of Physicians Ethics Manual. *Ann. Intern. Med.* 101:129–137, 263–274, 1984b.

Blendon RJ, Altman DE: Public attitudes about health-care costs: A lesson in national schizophrenia. *N. Engl J. Med.* 311:613–616, 1984.

Calabresi G, Bobbit P: *Tragic Choices: The Conflicts Society Confronts in the Allocation of Tragically Scarce Resources.* WW Norton, New York, 1978.

Childress F: Who shall live when not all can live?" *Soundings* 53:339–355, 1970.

Evans JR, Hall KL, Warford J: Shattuck Lecture—Health care in the developing world: Problems of scarcity and choice. *N. Engl. J. Med.* 305:1117–1127, 1981.

Fried C: *Medical Experimentation: Personal Integrity and Social Policy.* American Elsevier, New York, Chapter 5, 1974.

Fuchs R: The "rationing" of medical care. *N. Engl. J. Med.* 311:1572–1573, 1984.

Ginzberg E: The monetarization of medical care. *N. Engl. J. Med.* 310:1162–1165, 1984.

Glaser A: *Paying the Doctor: Systems of Remuneration and Their Effects.* Johns Hopkins University Press, Baltimore, 1970.

Goffman E: *Asylums: Essays on the Social Situation of Mental Patients and Other Inmates.* Doubleday, Garden City NY, 321–386, 1961.

Judicial Council of the American Medical Association: *Current Opinions of the Judicial Council of the American Medical Association–1984.* American Medical Association, Chicago, 1984.

Kirkman D: Medicare costs: New payments formula curbs hospital prices. *The Knoxville News-Sentinel,* October 1, A2, 1984.

Levinsky G: The doctor's master. *N. Engl. J. Med.* 311:1573–1575, 1984.

Moloney W, Rogers DE: Medical technology—A different view of the contentious debate over costs. *N. Engl. J. Med.* 301:1413–1419, 1979.

Nourse AE, Marks G: *The Management of a Medical Practice.* JB Lippincott, Philadelphia, 1963.

Pellegrino ED, Thomasma DC: *A Philosophical Basis of Medical Practice*. Oxford University Press, New York, 1981.

President's Commission for the Study of Ethical Problems in Medicine and Biomedical and Behavioral Research. *Securing Access to Health Care. Vol. 1: Report*. US Government Printing Office, Washington DC, 1983a.

————: *Securing Access to Health Care. Vol. 2: Appendices: Sociocultural and Philosophical Studies*. US Government Printing Office, Washington DC, 1983b.

————: *Securing Access to Health Care. Vol. 3: Appendices: Empirical Legal, and Conceptual Studies*. US Government Printing Office, Washington DC, 1983c.

Ramsey P: *The Patient as Person*. Yale University Press, New Haven CT, Chapter 7, 1970.

Relman AS: The new medical-industrial complex. *N. Engl. J. Med*. 303:963–970, 1980.

Starr P: *The Social Transformation of American Medicine*. Basic Books, New York, 1982.

Stedman's Medical Dictionary, ed 24. Williams & Wilkins, Baltimore, 1982.

Thurow, LC: Learning to say "no." *N. Engl. J. Med*. 311:1569–1572, 1984.

Wohl S: *The Medical Industrial Complex*. Harmony Books, New York, 1984.

Further Reading

Abrams N, Buckner MD (eds): *Medical Ethics: A Clinical Textbook and Reference for the Health Care Professions*. The MIT Press, Cambridge MA, Sections I.J (79–90) and III.E (559–585), 1983.

Annas GJ, Glantz LH, Katz BF: *The Rights of Doctors, Nurses, and Allied Health Professionals: A Health Law Primer*. Ballinger, Cambridge MA, 1981.
See especially Chapter XIV: "Advertising and Compensation."

Basson MD: Choosing among candidates for scarce medical resources. *J. Med. Philos*. 4:313–333, 1979.

Childress JF: Priorities in the allocation of health care resources. *Soundings* 62:256–274, 1979.

Cooper MH: *Rationing Health Care*. Halsted Press, London, 1975.

Enthoven AC: *Health Plan: The Only Practical Solution to the Soaring Cost of Medical Care*. Addison-Wesley, Reading MA, 1980.

Fried C: Rights and health care—Beyond equity and efficiency. *N. Engl. J. Med*. 293:241–245, 1975.

Fuchs VR: *Who Shall Live? Health, Economics, and Social Choice*. Basic Books, New York, 1974.

Glover J: *Causing Death and Saving Lives*. Penguin Books, New York, 1977.

Hiatt HH: Protecting the medical commons: Who is responsible? *N. Engl. J. Med*. 293:235–241, 1975.

Judicial Council of the American Medical Association: *Current Opinions of the Judicial Council of the American Medical Association–1984*. American Medical Association, Chicago, 1984.
2.03 Allocation of Health Resources
2.08 Costs
2.16 Unnecessary Services
2.17 Worthless Services
4.04 Health Facility Ownership by Physician
6.00 OPINIONS ON FEES AND CHARGES
8.00 OPINIONS ON PRACTICE MATTERS

Katz J, Capron AM: *Catastrophic Diseases: Who Decides What?* Russell Sage Foundation, New York, 1975.

Knowles JH (ed): *Doing Better and Feeling Worse: Health in the United States*. WW Norton, New York, 1977.

McNerney WJ: Control of health-care costs in the 1980's. *N. Engl. J. Med*. 303:1088–1094, 1980.

Mechanic D: Rationing health care: Public policy and the medical marketplace. *Hastings Cent. Rep.* 6:34–37, December 1976.

Outka G: Social justice and equal access to health care. *The Journal of Religious Ethics* 2:11–32, Spring 1973.

Patient selection for artificial and transplanted organs. *Harvard Law Review* 82:1322–1342, 1969.

Pellegrino ED: Medical morality and medical economics. *Hastings Cent. Rep.* 8:8–12, August 1978.

Reich WT (ed-in-chief): *Encyclopedia of Bioethics.* Macmillian and the Free Press, New York, 1978.

Advertising by Medical Professionals (Havighurst CC)

Aging and the Aged
   I. Theories of Aging and Anti-aging Techniques (Harflick L)
   II. Social Implications in Aging (Neugarten BL)
   III. Ethical Implications in Aging (Christiansen D)
   IV. Health Care and Research in the Aged (Young EWD)

Decision Making, Medical (Murphy EA)

Drug Industry and Medicine (Coulter HL)

Food Policy (Henriot PJ)

Health Care
   I. Health-Care System (Lee PR, Emmott C)
   II. Humanization and Dehumanization of Health Care (Howard J)
   III. Right to Health-Care Services (Jonsen AR)
   IV. Theories of Justice and Health Care (Branson R)

Health Insurance (Riesenfeld SA)

Health Policy
   I. Evolution of Health Policy (Strickland SP)
   II. Health Policy in International Perspective (Anderson O)

Hospitals (Williams KJ)

Justice (Feinberg J)

Kidney Dialysis and Transplantation (Fox RC, Swazey JP)

Life—I. Value of Life (Singer P)

Rationing of Medical Treatment (Childress JF)

Social Medicine (Silver GA)

Technology—III. Technology Assessment (Walters L)

Robertson JA: *The Rights of the Critically Ill.* Bantam Books, New York, 1983.
See especially Chapter XII: "Costs and Allocation of Scarce Resources."

Scarce medical resources. *Columbia Law Review.* 69:620–692, 1969.

Schwartz WB, Joskow PL: Medical efficacy versus economic efficiency: A conflict in values. *N. Engl. J. Med.* 299:1462–1464, 1978.

Stone DA: Physicians as gatekeepers: Illness certification as a rationing device. *Public Policy* 27:227–254, 1979.

Titmuss R: *The Gift Relationship.* Vintage Books, New York, 1971.

Veatch RM, Branson R: *Ethics and Health Policy.* Ballinger, Cambridge MA, 1976.

Weinstein MC, Stason WB: Foundations of cost-effectiveness analysis for health and medical practices. *N. Engl. J. Med.* 296:716–721, 1977.

More About Ethical Theories

In this appendix the introduction to fundamental concepts and principles of ethical theory begun in Chapter 2 is continued. The focus will be on general ethical theories. As you saw in Chapter 2, the resources of ethical theory are necessary to supplement guidelines developed by the professional community. There is a long tradition of theorizing on matters of values and ethics in Western culture, although in most cases this has only recently been applied to health-care issues. The discussion will deal with the theories in the abstract and explore their application to health care and to the issues discussed throughout the text.

One goal of this text is to help you become more aware of your own personal values and fundamental ethical principles, and one of the best ways to accomplish this is for you to pay attention to the way your own thinking "resonates" or "clashes" with various positions described in this appendix. These positions represent a spectrum of different ethical theories. Don't think, however, that you have to adopt one of these classical theories "whole hog." It may be possible to combine elements of different theories into a consistent, working ethical system. However, not *all* combinations of these theories are consistent, so you will need to proceed carefully with attempts to create a hybrid system of thought.

You will find it useful to review the discussion in Chapter 2, Section 2.1 for some terminology that is important here, i.e., the distinction between evaluative obligation, and character judgments.

1 Utilitarianism and Other Goal-Based Theories

1.1 Teleologism, the Goal-Based Approach

In this view the basis of duties and rights (i.e., obligation judgments) lies in the *consequences* of our actions. The main task of the moral life is to produce as much good as we can through our actions while at the same time avoiding and eliminating harm or bad to the extent possible. More formally, the basic guiding principle of teleologism can be stated thus:

> Of all the alternatives open to a given agent at a given time, the one she or he *ought* to perform is the one that produces the greatest balance of good over evil for the

255

members of the moral reference group. If two or more alternatives are equally optimific (i.e., create an equivalent balance of good over evil or bad but greater than any other alternative), then the agent *ought* to perform one or the other of these and it would be equally *right* to perform either of them.

In contrast, *deontological* approaches maintain that the basis of duties and/or rights is to be found in something *other than* evaluating the consequences of our actions. Extreme forms of deontologism (e.g., Kant's view) hold that consequences do not have *any influence at all* in determining duties and/or rights. (Some forms of deontologism will be examined in detail in Section 2. For now, it is sufficient to grasp this fundamental difference between these two approaches in order to have an alternative to teleologism to consider as you read this section.)

There are at least three important questions that this guiding principle of teleologism leaves unanswered: 1) Who is to be included in the moral reference group? 2) What is to count as good and bad? 3) What *sort* of alternative is to be considered? Is the standard to be applied to specific actions, one at a time, or can it be used to formulate rules or policies for actions of certain *kinds?*

The answers to these three questions distinguish different forms of teleological or goal-based theories. In the following sections you will look at some different answers that have been given to each of these questions.

1.2 The Moral Reference Group

Who counts, morally? Whose welfare do we, as moral agents, have a responsibility to promote? The answer to these questions determines the "moral reference group."

A full spectrum of answers to these questions has been given in the history of Western philosophy and theology. At one extreme is *egoism*. In this view the only person toward whom each agent has any moral responsibility is *him-* or *herself*. Each person ought to do all he can to promote his own welfare (and to avoid harm to himself), but he has no obligations toward *anyone* else at all. The proponent of egoism does not necessarily mean any harm to others and may have no objection if others prosper. She merely sees no obligation to assist others. This is an extreme ethic of individualism. Each person is to look out for herself.

At the opposite extreme is the view we might call *vitalism,* which considers *all* living creatures to be members of the moral reference group. This would entail that we have a responsibility as moral agents to promote the good and minimize harm for all living things; thus plants and the lower animals are regarded as fully equal in importance to ourselves and our fellow humans. One who held this view would face a moral dilemma at the thought of having to kill a flower in order to make a medicine to save a human life. Or he might find it troubling to think that his lymphocytes are killing bacteria. [This is one way in which "sanctity of life" principles might be interpreted, as they figure prominently in the issues of suicide and abortion (see Chapter 4).]

Intermediate positions, between the extremes of egoism and vitalism, will limit membership of one's moral reference group to some identifiable set of individuals. For example, *racism* is the view that only persons with a certain racial heritage count as members of the moral reference group. *Sexism* says the same about members of one gender. *Nationalism* counts only fellow-citizens of one's nation as members of the moral reference group.

One way to explain what is wrong with racism and sexism is to consider what would be required to *justify* these positions. To begin, one would have to give reasons why the particular individuals included in the group *do* matter enough that responsibilities arise to promote their welfare. (Without this argument, the egoist position wins the debate by default.) But then, one would also have to give reasons why our responsibilities *end* with the group singled out. What is the difference between these individuals and others, and why should this trait be considered as grounds for ignoring the welfare of those not included in the "in-group"? Clearly, it will not be easy to locate any trait with all three of these requisite features: 1) being common to all members of the moral reference group, 2) not shared with any individual outside the group, and 3) having the proper moral significance to justify the proposed differences in the way we act toward the parties.

There is one particular intermediate position that should be noted at this point, since it plays an influential role in the ethical thinking of many health-care professionals. This is the view that professioinals owe a special responsibility toward *their patients* that they do not owe to other individuals who may be in equal or greater need of their services. The law often recognizes something similar to this difference in responsibility. Thus, for example, (in most states) a physician or nurse who drives by an auto accident is under no legal requirement to stop and render assistance. Similarly, a new patient who shows up at a physician's office may be turned away without treatment. (Recall the provision from Section VI of the 1980 AMA Principles of Medical Ethics: "A physician, except in emergencies, shall be free to choose whom to serve.") However, once the physician has accepted someone as a patient, to deny that person treatment when it is needed may invite legal charges of "abandonment." Professional ethics and personal conscience extend still further this sense of duty within an established professional-patient relationship. A professional is expected to go "all-out" for his or her patients. The justification for singling out this group as special is found in the nature of the professional-patient relationship that has been established. Some implications of this view of a limited moral reference group are examined in connection with the discussion of the physician-patient relationship in Chapter 1, as well as in connection with the "moral center" of medicine in Chapter 3.

The doctrine of the moral reference group most widely held in Western thought falls somewhere between the wide-ranging principle of vitalism and the special-interest views of sexism, etc. There is some controversy about precisely how to formulate it, so three variants are offered here; think about how the differences between them might affect issues such as abortion and the definition of death:

1. *Humanism:* The moral reference group includes all *human beings,* and only *human beings.*
2. *Personalism:* This view, which is closely related to humanism, states that the moral reference group includes all *persons,* and only *persons.*
3. *Universalism:* The moral reference group includes all *sentient* (i.e., conscious) *creatures,* and only *sentient creatures.*

In the past these three principles often have been carelessly lumped together as if there were no significant differences between them. Part of the reason for this was the belief that the reference groups all designated the same set of individuals, i.e., human beings = persons = sentient creatures. However, recent discussions have shed doubt on this presumption of equivalence. Animal-rights advocates point out that the lower animals are *sentient,* even though they are neither *human beings* nor *persons.* Science fiction literature introduces the possibility that there might be extraterrestrial creatures we would classify as *persons* although they are not *human beings.* Furthermore, it is a serious issue for debate whether permanently comatose patients should be considered to be *persons* or *sentient,* although they undoubtedly remain *human beings.*

For present purposes, look at the elements these three views have in common and see how they would combine with various answers to the other two primary questions about teleologism. Differences between them can then be considered in connection with specific, concrete issues.

1.3 Theories of Value

The second question left open by the guiding principle of teleologism deals with evaluative issues: what counts as good (and thus to be promoted), and what counts as bad (and thus to be avoided or minimized)? Without an answer to this question, the teleological approach cannot give us guidance in particular choices we must make. We would not know *what aspect* of the consequences counts for and against the alternative.

Suppose, for example, one were invited to take part in a certain activity and were told only that it would have the effect of causing certain body tissues to increase in size and quantity. No reasonable judgment can be made about whether the activity is worth the effort until we know *what* tissue is being referred to and whether an enlargement would be valuable or not. Is it muscle tissue, so that the result would be a healthier, more robust appearance? If so, then it might be worth pursuing. Is it brain tissue, so that the result would be increased intellect? Then, again, it might be worthwhile. On the other hand, is it fatty deposits, so that the result would be obesity? Or is it tumor tissue, so that the result would be suffering and death? Obviously, the value of the consequences makes all the difference.

Let us look at some different answers that have been given to this question of what things have value.

1.3.1 Subjective Preference   Many people would contend that it is at once both futile and presumptuous to attempt to develop a general *theory* of value. Such an attempt is thought to be futile because value judgments are regarded as totally subjective and individualistic. "Everybody is unique, and each of us has our own set of values and preferences." Thus any effort to state a list of "true" values is presumptuous, because whoever developed the list would be imposing his or her own subjective preferences upon others.

The only sound alternative, then, would be to make subjective preference the *standard* of value and to orient teleological positions toward maximizing the satisfaction of preferences and minimizing their frustration. This is the approach that many contemporary economists, sociologists, and psychologists take in their analyses of values, especially as applied in social planning. However, this is not an inevitable conclusion, nor is it obviously the best approach to take.

The fundamental problem with the subjective-preferences approach is that it overlooks the possibility that some of our preferences may be mistaken. "*Mistaken?*" you may say. "That sort of statement just proves what was said earlier about an objectivist approach being presumptuous! How could anything be more presumptuous and judgmental than to call someone's preferences 'mistaken'?" Nevertheless, presumptuous or not, we must acknowledge that subjective preferences can sometimes be mistaken.

Let us explain. In Chapter 2, Section 2.1, two sorts of evaluative judgments are exemplified. They are commonly referred to as *instrumental,* for those that are good as a means to some chosen end, and *intrinsic,* for those that are good in and of themselves. It is possible for one to be mistaken about *both* kinds of values.

Think back to the case cited in the Review Exercise at the end of Chapter 2 (Section 3.2). The *end* that the child's parents have chosen and are pursuing in this situation is to restore their daughter to health. The *means* they have chosen to reach this goal include 1) bringing their daughter to a health-care professional for treatment, and 2) demanding "rather abruptly" that the practitioner prescribe antibiotics for their child.

A. Instrumental values.   In making this specific demand, the parents have not selected "the best means to their chosen end." An antibiotic will not be effective in restoring their daughter to health. At best, it will make no difference at all in her recovery ("She will be well in seven days with the drug, without it recovery will take a week"), and it might even impede progress toward the goal through its side effects or if the child has a drug reaction. So, the parents have made a *mistaken* judgment of instrumental value. Here, as in many such situations, others may be in a better position than the parents to judge instrumental values. Furthermore, it does not seem presumptuous to point out that they may be mistaken in this way. A part of what is involved in making judgments of instrumental value is making factual *predictions* about what various alternatives are likely to achieve. And it is a fact of life that we are not all completely knowledgeable about all aspects of the world. This is why we rely on experts such as the health-care practitioner—to supplement our own knowledge.

"Okay," you may say, "Perhaps we can say that instrumental values are sometimes mistaken. But the same does not hold true for intrinsic values. Those are *entirely* a matter of the individual's own subjective preference. Nobody else can presume to tell me what is important to me!"

B. Intrinsic values. If it seems impossible to question the end chosen by the parents in the case study, perhaps this is only because it is, in fact, appropriate. But suppose they had chosen another end instead. Would we always be inclined to accept it as appropriate, no matter what it was? To take an admittedly extreme example,[1] suppose the parents brought the child to the pediatrician with the request that the physician "do something" to arrest the growth process in their daughter, giving the explanation: "We love her so much the way she is right now that we do not want to see her change!" Surely this is an inappropriate and unreasonable goal, not only because it is *impossible* to achieve (although this may be reason enough to condemn it), but because it is unreasonable even to *attempt* or to *want* to achieve it. Or suppose, as an alternative, that they announced, "If you do have to give our daughter any medicine, it must be either pink or green. That is the color scheme in our bathroom, and we insist that the contents of the medicine cabinet match the rest of the decor. If you prescribe anything else, we will not have it in the house." To elevate the goal of a coordinated decor to a status equal with the health needs of their daughter is clearly inappropriate and unreasonable.

We trust that these examples have convinced you in principle that there can be mistaken judgments of intrinsic value. Now we are in a position to consider whether a *theory* of value might be stated, to guide us in choosing correct values and avoiding mistaken ones.

---

1. We choose extreme and hypothetical examples here to make our point as strong as possible. The claim we are arguing against says that *no* intrinsic value claim can be said to be mistaken. That claim will be refuted if *any* are shown to be mistaken.

1.3.2 Hedonism   The theory of value most discussed in the history of Western philosophy is *hedonism*, which holds that the one and only thing intrinsically good is *pleasure*, and the one and only thing intrinsically bad is *pain*.[2] Initially this approach may appear just as subjective as leaving judgments to individual preference, but it can be shown as somewhat of an improvement. A hedonist view provides a basis for criticizing some specific goals as mistaken: hedonist goals involve *predictions* about what would bring the person pleasure (or avoid pain), and any prediction can be criticized as being incorrect. Thus, we could criticize the parents' demand for antibiotics in the original version of our case study on the grounds that, all things considered, they are unlikely to be made happy by this choice. If the child were to suffer side effects from the drug, the parents would clearly be unhappy, and evidence of the drug's ineffectiveness for the child's condition also would do nothing to enhance the parents' happiness, in even the best situation imaginable. Similarly, we could criticize the goal of arresting the growth of their child on the grounds that this would not really make them happy, on balance, even if it could be achieved. They would be quite likely to regret their choice at some point in the future, when they would realize how they were depriving themselves (not to mention their daugher) by foreclosing future stages of maturation and development. In the final example, the effects on the child's health of foregoing needed medication, just because it does not match the decor, would be unlikely to maximize the parents' happiness: could they really enjoy their coordinated color scheme if their child's suffering from this illness lingered on and on?

The hedonist theory has other strengths to recommend it. The disvalue of pain is especially well recognized in the health-care setting, where enormous efforts are directed at palliation. And the value of pleasurable states seems to require no defense: to experience them is *ipso facto* to recognize their value as goals worth pursuing.

Philosophers who favor hedonism have had great hopes for its usefulness as a practical basis for individual and social planning. For example, Jeremy Bentham (an eighteenth century English philosopher) proposed a schema he was convinced would allow precise, quantified measurements of pleasure and pain. His proposal included the following parameters:

---

2. Although there are subtle differences between the terms "pleasure" and "happiness," we will ignore them here and use the two words interchangeably.

A. Four Measures of the Intrinsic Value of an Individual Experience

1. Intensity   Some measure of the immediately felt degree of pleasure or pain. For example, the excruciating pain from a kidney stone is considerably more intense than the discomfort of a mild rash. Or the pleasure one receives from watching an uproarious slapstick comedy is more intense than the pleasure of hearing a mildly amusing joke.

2. Duration   Measuring how long the feelings of pleasure or pain last. For example, in considering the unpleasant side effects of a certain medication, one must compare how long they will last to how long the pain of illness will last if the medication is not taken.

3. Certainty   A measure of how likely one is to receive the type of feelings from a certain activity. For example, for a surgical treatment it is fairly certain that one will experience discomfort as the incision heals, whereas the effectiveness of the surgery in relieving one's original source of discomfort may be more or less uncertain.

4. Propinquity   A measure of how much effort one must make to achieve the feeling-state. For example, the satisfactions (and related physical-training effects) from swimming are more remote for most people than those of walking or jogging, since they must travel some distance to a pool in order to swim, whereas they could run in their own neighborhood.

B. Two Measures of the Instrumental Value of an Individual Experience

5. Fecundity   The probability of the experience being followed by additional sensations of the same kind. For example, if one enjoys learning to play tennis, this will be a fecund or fruitful pleasure because it also equips one to gain the enjoyments of playing the game later. If some self-destructive behavior is painful, this will be a fecund pain, since it will cause additional pain later from its destructive effects.

6. Purity   The probability of it *not* being followed by sensations of the *opposite* kind. For example, the "morning after" hangover makes last night's state of inebriation an impure pleasure. The discomfort associated with surgery, on the other hand, is impure pain, since it may bring relief from the original complaint as a consequence.

C. One Measure of the Social Dimension of Experience

7. Extent   The number of people affected by the pleasure. For example, a public health measure that relieves some painful state for many people will be greater in extent than an individual procedure that affects the state of health and happiness of only one person.

Bentham proposed as an agenda for the social sciences that they develop objective measures for these parameters as a way of calculating the solution to social problems. Some social scientists have undertaken this task, and some progress along these lines has been made (most notably in economics), but we are still far from achieving the comprehensive "hedonic calculus" that Bentham envisioned.

Furthermore, it is not clear that such an achievement will ever be possible. Establishing objective standards for measuring these parameters is notoriously difficult. The measure that is especially difficult is intensity. It is extremely difficult for one to compare two different pains or pleasures of *one's own* with respect to intensity, i.e., is the pain of today more or less intense than the one I experienced yesterday?; the difficulty is even greater for interpersonal comparisons, i.e., is *my* pain of today more or less intense than *your* pain of yesterday? Anyone who has worked with patients in pain knows the difficulty of judging its intensity. The health sciences have developed some descriptive terms that may help in classifying degrees of pain, but these are still far from precise. For example, one classic textbook of diagnosis says the following:

> *Quality.* Three qualities of pain are recognized: (1) *bright, pricking,* often described as sharp, cutting, knifelike, lightning-like, (2) *burning,* also reported as hot or stinging, and (3) *deep, aching* variously called boring, pounding, sore, heavy, constricting, gnawing.

> *Severity.* Precise measurements of the intensity of pain are impractical for a clinical examination, but meaningful approximations can be obtained from the patient's descriptions and the examiner's observations. The patient is asked to liken the severity of the pain to some common experience such as a toothache, menstrual cramps, labor pains, or a sore throat. Intense pain is usually accompanied by physiologic signs perceptible to the examiner and often noted by the patient, such as facial expressions, bodily postures (protecting a limb by holding it, flexion of the thighs upon the belly for severe abdominal pain), reduced bodily activity, sweating, pallor, dilatation of the pupils, elevation of the blood pressure and acceleration of the heart rate, retching and vomiting. (DeGowin and DeGowin 1976, 31–32)

This is vague, and nothing this detailed has been done with regard to pleasures.

In addition to these difficulties with measurement, there is another serious difficulty with hedonism as a *working* theory of value that makes it largely unacceptable for applying ethics to health care. The problem is that there are values that do not *appear* to be rooted in pleasure and pain; thus, even if a theoretical account of these values could be constructed in hedonist terms, the result would be too abstract and too far removed from the basis of our ordinary valuation of these things to be of any *practical* usefulness.

For example, we value knowledge at least to some extent; research scientists have dedicated their lives to pursuing this value. It is true that knowledge can often be useful in promoting pleasure and preventing pain. To this extent, its value might be accounted for in hedonist terms. But is this the whole story? What about "basic" research of a sort not likely to lead directly to the cure of disease or to other socially beneficial applications? Here knowledge seems to be sought "for its own sake," "as an end in itself," and not as a means to pleasure or prevention of pain. The standard hedonist reply is to point to forms of pleasure and pain that may be involved even in this sort of knowledge: 1) there is always the *possibility* that some beneficial application will stem from the knowledge in question; and, anyway, 2) the researcher gets satisfaction from the accomplishment of bringing this knowledge to light and/or from contemplating this new insight. But this type of account is the sort of abstract and remote result mentioned earlier. If the link between pleasure/pain and values is as esoteric as this, it is not clear how the criterion of hedonism can be of any use in making health-care decisions.

This hypothesis about the uselessness of a hedonist theory of value can be tested further by attempting to apply it to some of the specific issues discussed throughout this text. Meanwhile, let us continue our search for a satisfactory theory of value for use in health-care decisions.

1.3.3 Quality of Life   A more promising theory of value for health-care ethics stems from the notion of ''quality of life'' (QOL). This is often little more than a slogan, but it contains elements that can be developed—with thoughtful analysis—into a value basis for decision making.

In our ordinary thinking, we tend to approach the concept of QOL from the negative side. In the health-care context we speak of ''diminished QOL'' that results from disabling injuries or through the pain and suffering of lingering illness. In other contexts we speak of the ''lowered QOL'' in terms of air pollution in our cities and crime in the streets.

However, judgments about positive values can readily be derived from this catalogue of disvalues. If the *loss* of a certain ability *diminishes* one's QOL, then it must be because the *possession* of that ability previously made a *positive contribution* to one's QOL. For example, if paralysis diminishes one's QOL, then mobility must be regarded as a positive contribution to the QOL of those of us fortunate enough to have escaped a paralyzing injury.

By continuing in this way—that is, by listing the disvalues that diminish QOL and then stating their positive correlatives—a catalogue of values that make positive contributions to QOL can be generated. The list might be continued by thinking about the constituents of our own life and listing those elements that make it ''worth living.'' We could add to the list still further by listing our aspirations— things we would like to *add* to our life that we think would make it even more worthwhile. If the resulting list were too full of specifics, we might try to generalize it by looking for abstract common features within the specific things we value as contributions to QOL.

If each of us undertook such a project independently, the resulting lists would contain largely (but not entirely) the same items. For example, look at the following list generated by a pair of social scientists who conducted a several-stage process, much along the lines described above, to develop a list of features with direct bearing (some positively, others negatively) upon QOL. They had respondents list relevant items and (after the lists had been consolidated) rank them in terms of relative importance. Their conclusions are summarized below [adapted with permission from Dalkey (1972, 71)]:

Relative Importance	
15.0	Love, caring, affection, communication, interpersonal understanding; friendship, companionship; honesty, sincerity, truthfulness; tolerance, acceptance of others; faith, religious awareness.
11.5	Self-respect, self-acceptance, self-satisfaction; self-confidence, egoism; security; stability, familiarity, sense of permanence; self-knowledge, self-awareness, growth.
10.0	Peace of mind, emotional stability, lack of conflict; fear, anxiety; suffering, pain; humiliation, belittlement; escape, fantasy.
9.5	Sex, sexual satisfaction, sexual pleasure.
8.0	Challenge, stimulation; competition, competitiveness; ambition; opportunity, social mobility, luck; education, intellectual stimulation.
8.0	Social acceptance, popularity; needed, feeling of being wanted; loneliness, impersonality; flattering, positive feedback, reinforcement.
7.0	Achievement, accomplishment, job satisfaction; success; failure, defeat, losing; money, acquisitiveness, material greed; status, reputation, recognition, prestige.
6.0	Individuality; conformity; spontaneity, impulsive, uninhibited; freedom.
6.0	Involvement, participation; concern, altruism, consideration.
6.0	Comfort, economic well-being, relaxation, leisure; good health.
5.0	Novelty, change, newness, variety, surprise; boredom; humorous, amusing, witty.
3.5	Dominance, superiority; dependence, impotence, helplessness; aggression, violence, hostility; power, control, independence.
2.0	Privacy.

Surely all of us can "resonate" with this listing. Even though we might dispute some of the groupings and rankings, we can appreciate the significance of the values being expressed.

Consider some other listings. The well-known "self-actualization" theory of Abraham Maslow (1968) can be viewed as an attempt to characterize the QOL concept. Maslow postulates five levels of needs and claims that one takes an interest in satisfying those at the next higher level when—and only when—those on a lower level are set. The five levels are

1. survival
2. security
3. belongingness
4. esteem
5. self-actualization.

The social philosopher John Rawls constructs much of his theory of justice on the basis of a list of "primary goods," which he describes and lists in the following passage:

> Suppose that the basic structure of society distributes certain primary goods, that is, things that every rational man is presumed to want. These goods normally have a use whatever a person's rational plan of life. For simplicity, assume that the chief primary goods at the disposition of society are rights and liberties, powers and opportunities, income and wealth. (Later on, in Part Three the primary good of self-respect has a central place.) These are the social primary goods. Other primary goods such as health and vigor, intelligence and imagination, are natural goods; although their possession is influenced by the basic structure [of society], they are not so directly under its control. (Rawls 1971, 62)[3]

It would take us too far afield to attempt to critique these lists, reconcile the differences between them, and consolidate them into a single coherent theory of QOL. Thus, we must be satisfied with drawing upon one or more of these lists in analyzing the QOL elements in concrete cases.

When you stop to consider its implications, the concept of "quality of life" has some very interesting features. First, although it clearly relates to the notions of happiness or pleasure and subjective preference, it is not coincidental with any of these notions. We would expect that improving one's QOL would increase one's happiness and the degree to which one's subjective preferences are met, but this is by no means automatic. To achieve these goals, the agent must make use of the opportunities and abilities that constitute his or her QOL. For example, one may have the native ability to learn a foreign language, and training programs provided by the community may be accessible and affordable; but unless one takes advantage of these opportunities, one will never receive the pleasure of learning a language, or satisfy the desire to learn it. In other words, QOL appears to indicate certain *fundamental* conditions necessary as prerequisites for happiness or preference-satisfaction, rather than these states themselves.

Second, QOL standards offer a perspective for evaluating individual subjective preferences or choices in pursuit of happiness or pleasure. Many of an individual's choices and preferences have as their object constituents of the individual's QOL. (For example, almost everybody desires to be healthy and thus makes choices that would enhance health.) Other choices and preferences are individual idiosyncrasies or tastes that are neutral with respect to the individual's QOL. (For example, whether a person prefers a decor that is pink and green or one that is blue and beige does not make any difference to his QOL.) Still other choices, however, (such as the parents' desire to arrest the growth and development of their child, or their preference for decor above the health needs of their child) will be evaluated as misguided or mistaken precisely because they are *antithetical* to the individual's QOL.

---

3. Later in his book, Rawls develops what he calls a "full theory of the good," which amounts to a theory of subjective preferences corrected by rational deliberation.

Third, QOL considerations are not "subjective," although they are "subject-oriented." As Nicholas Rescher points out:

> Information of the sort available not necessarily to the person himself but to an expert outsider provides the crucial basis for judgment. However, this information is in large measure not something general and universalizable; it will hinge critically upon the specific data regarding the characteristic makeup of the particular individual at issue. (Rescher 1972, 20–21)[4]

1.4 Act vs. Rule Approach

The third general question to be answered by a teleological or goal-based theory is whether the standard is applied to individual concrete actions or more generally for formulating *policies* for action in all situations of a certain type.

Think back to the case from Chapter 2, Section 3. Having assessed all the particulars of this specific case and diagnosed a viral infection, the physician weighed the pros and cons of prescribing an antibiotic and decided against it. Must she then perform this same detailed evaluation each time a similar case arises? Or would it be better to have a general policy: "Do not prescribe antibiotics when clinical signs indicate a viral condition" or "Prescribe antibiotics whenever . . ." (and attempt to spell out the conditions under which an antibiotic would be appropriate)?

Some traditional ethical theorists argue for each of these approaches. The arguments on both sides are largely put in terms of goal-based considerations themselves. The primary arguments in favor of a rule or policy approach are those that appeal to efficiency and consistency.

1. To calculate *all* possible effects on *all* members of the moral reference group for *each* such decision would take *enormous* amounts of time. It would be a great time-saver to work through this sort of calculation once for each class of situation and henceforth act on the policy arrived at as a result of this calculation.
2. Even more serious than the time consumed by a thoroughgoing act approach is the danger that some relevant factor will be overlooked on some occasions, which might make a significant difference to the decision.
3. Consistency is not only a canon of reason, but also a moral virtue.[5] If the doctor were to refuse the parents' request for antibiotics today, and yet give another set of parents a prescription tomorrow in virtually identical circumstances, she could properly be charged with inconsistency or "unfairness." (Think of a child's reaction to such a perceived inconsistency in the actions of a parent, and you will see the moral relevance of this notion: "But you said yes to Johnny when he asked the *very same thing* yesterday! You like

---

4. Implications of this point in connection with QQL judgments are discussed in Chapter 4.
5. The popular aphorism notwithstanding, it is not always a "hobgoblin of little minds."

him best!'' In general, children are very sensitive to moral principles—especially those that serve their own interests.)

On the other side, the primary argument in favor of an act approach is that it is more sensitive to the specific factors in the situation and thus more likely to be morally correct than an approach in terms of general policies. Consider the process of clinical diagnosis in the case. The analog to a rule or policy approach in moral decision making might be for the physician to have a clinical policy: "All sore throats are assumed to be viral infections." But this would never be acceptable as an approach to clinical decision making. The physician is expected to examine all the particular elements of this specific case and take them into account in arriving at a specific diagnosis of *this* child's sore throat. Why should the process of moral decision making be any less thorough than this? It is certainly no less important to arrive at the correct moral decision than it is to arrive at the correct clinical decision.

1.5 Applying Goal-Based Theories

To summarize this discussion of goal-based theories, let us consider how one would go about making a decision in their terms. The steps leading to a decision will be presented in schematic form, then you will be asked to apply them in some detail in the Review Exercise that follows. The decision steps are somewhat different for an act approach and for a rule approach, so they are sketched separately.

1.5.1 Act Approach

1. *Step 1: Consider the concrete situation in which you are about to act.* Since this is an *act* approach, you cannot make any sort of general determination about what kind of action is always (or generally) appropriate. You can only determine what you ought to do in the specific situation. In other (different) situations, it might turn out that you should do something quite different.

2. *Step 2: Enumerate all the alternatives for action open to you in the situation at hand.* Here the great danger is that you will prejudge the whole investigation by omitting possibilities you find unappealing. For example, in arguments about sexual questions, people may refuse to consider the possibility of abstinence from sexual intercourse. "That would be impossible," they say. What they *mean* is that it would be unpleasant. But we need to determine just *how* unpleasant it would be. It might turn out that all other alternatives are even less desirable in the long run. And if this is the result, then it follows that sexual abstinence is what ought to be practiced.

3. *Step 3: Predict all the consequences each of these alternatives are likely to have as they affect any member of the moral reference group.* The danger here is that crucial factors will be left out. You must consider *all* the effects of the alternatives, even those in the distant future and those that are very much indirect. You should also estimate the *probability* of occurrence for each consequence. The more remote the probability, the less weight the consequence should carry in your decision.

This is obviously an *enormous* undertaking—far more than could be accomplished in deciding what to do in a specific situation. However, it is the ideal of rational decision making under this model, so we must attempt to come as close to it as possible.

4. *Step 4: Evaluate these consequences.* Apply the theory of nonmoral value you find most plausible. Determine how much intrinsic value and how much intrinsic disvalue each of the actions themselves contain. Then determine the value and disvalue of each of the consequences. (This will be the instrumental value of the action.) Finally, sum these evaluations to determine the final or total value of the action.

5. *Step 5: Compare the alternatives.* The alternative with the greatest final value, i.e., producing the greatest balance of good over bad, is the one you should undertake.

1.5.2 Rule Approach

1. *Step 1: Enumerate all the possible policies or rules for action in the situation at hand.* Here you must think *beyond* the specific situation and begin to determine how you would act in *all situations similar to this one in relevant respects.*

2. *Step 2: Predict all the consequences each of these policies are likely to have (if implemented) on any member of the moral reference group.* Here again, the task is enormous. One advantage of a rule approach, however, is that one can come closer to carrying out this step. On issues of social policy, mechanisms such as "environmental impact statements," "risk assessments," or "technology assessments" are attempts to do what is required here.

3. *Step 3: Evaluate these consequences.*

4. *Step 4: Compare the alternatives and choose the rule or policy that maximizes the balance of good over bad.*

1.6 Review Exercise: Goal-Based Theories

Now *you* are asked to approach a decision in terms of a goal-based theory. In particular, the exercise will follow an act approach. For purposes of this exercise, the process will be simplified considerably, since a full-scale analysis would take much too long. However, be sure to include enough detail in your work to test whether you understand the complexities of this approach to ethical decisions. Consider the following case.

1.6.1 Case: "Don't Tell the Doctor!"

A young unmarried woman (age 17) was admitted to the hospital with excessive uterine bleeding, which she explained was connected with her monthly period. She stated that this had occurred several times over the course of the past year and was of great concern to her.

A student nurse, of the approximate age of the patient, was caring for her the day after admission. After the student had established rapport with her, the patient confided to the student that she had been certain she was pregnant and had taken some medication that she had been told would bring about an abortion. She insisted that she did not want anyone—not even the doctor—to know about this.

She asked the student to promise not to tell anyone, particularly not the doctor. (Adapted from Tate 1977, case 15)

What should the nursing student do?

1.6.2 Questions As you answer the following questions, keep in mind all you have read in this appendix, especially the steps of an act-approach analysis as sketched in Section 1.5.1.

1. What *can* the student nurse do? What alternatives are open to her? List as many alternatives for action in this situation as you can. (Remember: Do not limit yourself to the obvious, or to those actions you already feel would be morally acceptable. The point here is to acquire material for ethical analysis in the stages to follow.)

2. For purposes of this exercise, choose a moral reference group and defend your choice.

3. For purposes of this exercise, choose one of the theories of nonmoral value discussed in this appendix and defend your choice. Choose any *two* of the alternatives for action you enumerated in question 1 (including the one you are initially inclined to favor) and list as many of their morally relevant consequences as you can.

4. Label each of the consequences you listed in terms of your estimate of their probability:

++ = highly likely to occur
+ = likely to occur
+/− = as likely not to occur as to occur
− = unlikely
− − = highly unlikely

5. Evaluate the consequences in terms of your theory of nonmoral value. Use the following labels:

Pro+ = extremely good
Pro = moderately good
Neut = neutral
Con = moderately bad
Con+ = extremely bad

Be sure to indicate the basis of these evaluations in your discussion.

6. Compare the alternatives. Explain which you think should be chosen by comparing the weights of the evaluations you listed above.

7. Reflect on this process. Do you find yourself comfortable with this way of arriving at a decision? Why or why not? What morally relevant elements (if any) seem to be *left out* in this process?

2 Deontological Theories

2.1 Duty-Based Theories

This approach proposes a very different way of making moral decisions than the process you have just worked through. Instead of weighing and balancing the values in the situation, a duty-based theory examines the situation for moral factors of a different order. This can be shown most clearly through an example.

2.1.1 Side Constraints Suppose a person had borrowed $50 from a friend to tide her over an urgent financial crisis, on the firm promise that she would pay him back that afternoon. He explained that it was important that she pay him back today because he planned to go to the ballet that night, and he would need the money to pay for the tickets. Now she has scraped together the $50 and is on her way to pay her debt when she runs into an old friend with a hard-luck story. He has lost his job here in town several weeks ago, and all his savings have been exhausted in providing for himself and his family while he looked (unsuccessfully) for another job. As a result, he and his family (which includes a couple of appealing small children) have not eaten in more than 24 hours. He has a promise of a job in another city, but he has no money for bus fare to get there or for living expenses for himself and his family until his first paycheck.

And here she stands with $50 in her pocket that she knows her creditor friend plans to spend on ballet tickets. How can this use of the money begin to compare, on any goal-based analysis, with the good it could do in the hands of her other friend who is down on his luck? Surely the *best* use she could make of the money is to give it to this friend and leave her creditor without the resources to go to the ballet.

Of course, a goal-based theory must take into account *all* the consequences of the action, and so she must consider the anger her creditor is likely to feel when he discovers she has caused him to miss the ballet, the loss of any opportunity on her part to borrow money from him again in the future, and other such factors. But these must be balanced against the disappointment felt by the other friend's children when he tells them he was unsuccessful in finding any money to buy supper, and the sensations of hunger they experience at going without supper, etc. Thus it still appears that the balance of good over evil would be maximized by giving the money to the friend with a problem instead of to the creditor.

A duty-based theorist would claim that balancing the amount of good and evil that would follow from each use of the money is the wrong way to approach this decision. It is not *open to the agent* to determine what is the best use she could make of this money, the deontologist would insist. The fact is she made a *promise* to repay the debt, which means she ought to give the money to the creditor, even if a better use for it comes along. This, after all, is the *point* of his having extracted the promise from her: to ensure she would not merely consider his plan to use the money as one candidate among others for the best way for her to spend this money. He loaned her the money only on the basis of the assurance that she would repay him that afternoon *even if a better use for the $50 occurred to her.*

In other words, moral factors such as the duty created by the promise to repay the loan serve as "side constraints" on our goal-based calculations. They restrict our freedom to choose, not only to serve our own interests, but also to attempt to maximize the balance of good over evil for others as well.

2.1.2 Absolute Duties According to some deontological theories, these side constraints (or, at least, certain ones) cannot be overridden by *any sort of consideration whatever*. This claim has a certain initial plausibility, for example, in connection with very serious moral principles such as:

1. It is wrong to kill an innocent person.
2. It is wrong to tell a lie.
3. It is wrong to do physical harm to an innocent person.

Charles Fried expresses his view of the absolute or categorical character of these norms in the following:

> It is part of the idea that lying or murder are wrong, not just bad, that these are things you must not do—no matter what. They are not mere negatives that enter into a calculus to be outweighed by the good you might do or the greater harm you might avoid. Thus the norms which express deontological judgments—for example, Do not commit murder—may be said to be absolute. They do not say: "Avoid lying, other things being equal" but "Do not lie, period." This absoluteness is an expression of how deontological norms or judgments differ from those of consequentialism. (Fried 1978, 9–10)

2.1.3 Responsibility for Consequences   This duty-based approach may sound extremely harsh. Is a person to let himself be murdered, for example, when he could save his life by a "little, white lie"? From what has been said so far, it might seem that one must, according to this theory. However, there are several ways in which the harsh aspects of this view can be toned down a bit. One of them is especially important in some discussions of medical ethics, so it is worth describing at this point.

The basic idea behind the *principle of double effect* is that one's actions may have multiple effects (often more than the two suggested by the name of the principle) and one's moral relationship to the consequences may not be the same in all cases. This point may be put in terms of obligation judgments or character judgments. In its obligation-judgment form, the claim would be that not all ways of bringing about the same consequence are equally morally *right* or *wrong*. In character terms, the point is that one is not equally *responsible* morally for all the consequences of what one does or fails to do.

Consider the following situation: Tom chooses a piece of pie from the cafeteria line and eats it. This action may have a number of effects: 1) it increases the profits of the cafeteria owner; 2) it increases the calorie content of Tom's diet; 3) it pleases the cook, who looks out of the kitchen and sees the relish with which Tom eats the pie; 4) since this is the last piece of this kind of pie available in the cafeteria and since you are behind Tom in the line, it deprives you of your favorite dessert.

Is this action of Tom's right or wrong? Is he morally blameworthy for it, or what?

The teleologist would sum the value of these consequences and rule that it is morally right and praiseworthy if this action brought about a greater balance of good over evil than anything Tom could have done in the situation. Otherwise, it is morally wrong and blameworthy.

But the deontologist proponents of the principle of the double effect would maintain that it makes a difference what one's *relationship* is to each of the effects. It matters, in particular, which effect(s) of Tom's action *entered into his delib-*

eration when he decided to act. If he made the decision to choose the pie *in order to* increase the profits of the cafeteria owner (because he had heard that the establishment was in financial trouble) or *in order to* please the cook (because he knew she frequently looks out of the kitchen and is always especially happy to see someone enjoying her pies), then our assessment of both the action and the agent would be favorable. We would judge that he did a good thing and that he is a good person for having done that thing.

On the other side of the ledger, he can hardly be held morally responsible for depriving you of your favorite dessert since (let us suppose) he did not know either that this was your favorite or that this was the last piece available. Moral responsibility also may be negligible for some consequences he *does* know about in advance, i.e., increasing the calorie content of his diet. After all, the benefit to the cafeteria owner's financial solvency or the cook's self-respect seems to be worth the harm that might come to Tom from a few added calories.

However, suppose we discovered that Tom *did* know he would be depriving you of your favorite dessert by choosing the piece of pie; and indeed, suppose he confessed that this is precisely what motivated him to choose the pie and eat it with such relish. Then our moral evaluation of the action and the agent would be quite different. To act *in order to* deprive you of the pie is morally wrong (since it is a spiteful act), and Tom would be blameworthy for acting in this way.

We see, then, that two acts with identical consequences can differ in moral quality. The difference depends on the relationship of each of these consequences to the intentions of the agent in acting.

This distinction might be employed to temper the harshness of an absolutist theory of obligation. It is absolutely and always wrong to kill, but what this means is that one may never *directly* or *intentionally* bring about the death of another. However, there might be occasions where one might do something that results in the death of another as an unintended *side effect* of an acceptable action. And this might be morally justified. For example, a direct abortion is ruled impermissible in this tradition. However, excision of the cancerous uterus of a pregnant woman is permissible, even though the death of the fetus is foreseen as a side effect. This has obvious relevance for issues of life and death discussed in Chapter 4. In particular, it sheds light on the distinction drawn by the AMA Judicial Council between *letting* a terminally ill patient die and *intentionally* causing death. (For the full context, see the opinion entitled "Terminal Illness" quoted in Chapter 4, Section 2.1.)

The doctrine of double effect can be stated formally as follows:

1. The act to be done must be good in itself or at least indifferent, i.e., it must *not* be intrinsically wrong.
2. The good intended must not be obtained by means of the evil effect.
3. The evil effect must not be intended for itself, but only permitted.

4. There must be a proportionately grave reason for permitting the evil effect.
5. There must be no alternative course of action available to the agent that would produce the same, or an equivalent, good effect while avoiding the evil.[6]

2.1.4 *Prima Facie* Duties One serious problem with an absolutist view is that moral rules may conflict with one another. If one holds that it is absolutely and always wrong to tell a lie and also to do physical harm to an innocent person, what is one to do if a situation arises in which the only way to *prevent* physical injury to an innocent person is through telling a lie?[7]

One way of dealing with this sort of problem is to deny that moral rules are absolute. Instead, they may be taken to hold *prima facie* or "other things being equal." This means that nothing other than *another moral rule* could override them. It would not be justified to ignore a moral duty because you found it inconvenient, or because you did not want to do what it dictates. However, when two moral rules conflict (as in the preceding example, where the only way to avoid bringing physical injury to an innocent person is to tell a lie), then the weight or stringency of the conflicting rules must be determined, and the weightier or more stringent rule takes precedence.

Many of the issues in biomedical ethics involve conflicts of duties, so you will have plenty of occasion to work with this way of viewing moral rules in discussions of concrete issues. This is roughly the approach illustrated in the discussions of concrete cases throughout this book. Note especially its use in Chapter 4, Section 2.4.

2.2 Kant's Deontological Theory

Immanuel Kant is often taken to be the paradigm deontologist. He maintains that it is absolutely and always wrong to treat persons "merely as a means and not at the same time as an end in themselves" (Kant 1959). This phrase is far from clear on the surface, however. What all is ruled out? Let us explore its meaning.

To treat someone as an end is to respect the ends or goals that she has set for herself. Thus, Kant maintains that we should never impose anything on a person against her will. We may even have a positive obligation to do what we can to help her further her goals. To do otherwise implies she is not important; in the extreme case, it may amount to treating her in the way we would treat an inanimate object—as nothing more than a means to our goals.

---

6. For further discussion and critique of this doctrine, see Glenn C. Graber (1979, 65–84).

7. Actually, absolutists would either 1) deny that such a situation could arise and/or 2) try to avoid personal responsibility for the physical injury that resulted from truth-telling through an analysis using the doctrine of double effect.

The most dramatic cases of using someone as a means would be those in which the person is treated exactly as one would treat an inanimate object. Small children, for example, may not hesitate to step on their father in order to reach objects that would otherwise be too high for them. (He forgives them, because they are very young and do not know better, but he probably fervently hopes they will learn better before they reach a size that would make this practice harmful to him.) In slapstick comedies, one person will sometimes duck behind another to avoid the cream pie that is hurtling toward him. These are paradigm cases of "treating someone as a means only."

Only slightly removed is the act of getting someone to do what you want through deceit or coercion (something we probably all have done at some time or other). Here you know that the other person has no desire to do the things in question. (If the person did want to do it, neither deceit nor coercion would be needed, simply a polite request.) But you do not let the person's unwillingness stop you from getting what you want. You "use" the person by appealing to goals that she *does* have: the desire not to be harmed, in cases of coercion; a variety of goals, in cases of deceit.

It should be pointed out that you still would be using the other person *as a means* if you got her to do the thing through a polite request. However, in this case, you would not be using her *merely* as a means. By offering her the chance to decline the request, you acknowledge respect for her wishes and thus treat her *as an end* as well as a means. Kant sees nothing wrong in this sort of action.

The question to ask, then, in applying Kant's criterion to specific decisions is: In what you are considering doing here, are you acknowledging the goals and desires of the other person(s) or are you treating them merely as a means to your own goals? Answering this question may still require considerable interpretation, but it is a starting point for moral analysis of concrete situations.

As some authors point out (Benjamin and Curtis 1981, 34), Kant's theory of obligation cuts across the subcategories of deontological theories. The criterion we have just considered is probably best interpreted as a *rights-based theory*. However, Kant insisted that this formulation was exactly equivalent to the "universal law" formulation of the Categorical Imperative, which is clearly a duty-based criterion.

2.3 Ross' List of *Prima Facie* Duties

Another important theory of moral obligation that you may find useful in considering ethical dimensions of medical practice is the theory of Sir David Ross (1930). He sets out a list of *prima facie* duties in the following passage (emphasis in italic is added):

> (1) Some duties rest on previous acts of my own. These duties seem to include two kinds, (a) those resting on a promise or what may fairly be called an implicit promise, such as the implicit undertaking not to tell lies which seems to be implied

in the act of entering into conversation (at any rate by civilized men), or of writing books that purport to be history and not fiction. These may be called the *duties of fidelity*. (b) Those resting on a previous wrongful act. These may be called the *duties of reparation*. (2) Some rest on previous acts of other men, i.e., services done by them to me. These may be loosely described as the *duties of gratitude*. (3) Some rest on the fact or possibility of a distribution of pleasure or happiness (or of the means thereto) which is not in accordance with the merit of the persons concerned; in such cases there arises a duty to upset or prevent such a distribution. These are the *duties of justice*. (4) Some rest on the mere fact that there are other beings in the world whose condition we can make better in respect of virtue, or of intelligence, or of pleasure. These are the *duties of beneficence*. (5) Some rest on the fact that we can improve our own condition in respect of virtue or of intelligence. These are the *duties of self-improvement*. (6) I think that we should distinguish from (4) the duties that may be summed up under the title of "not injuring others." No doubt to injure others is incidentally to fail to do them good; but it seems to me clear that *non-maleficence* is apprehended as a duty distinct from that of beneficence, and a duty of a more stringent character. (Ross 1930, 21)

2.4 Review Exercise: Deontological Theories

1. Analyze the case from Section 1.6.1 from the point of view of *either* Kant's theory *or* Ross's list of *prima facie* duties. a) For Kant's theory, the question to ask is which alternative would involve everyone being treated as ends in themselves and not merely as means. b) For Ross's theory, 1) choose *one* of the alternatives for action, 2) explain which of Ross's *prima facie* duties relate to it, and 3) explain which set of duties has the greater stringency.
2. Which appears initially more plausible to you: a) the view of moral rules as absolute and exceptionless, or b) the *prima facie* view of moral rules? Defend your answer, including examples of how the views would differ in practice.
3. Is Ross's list of *prima facie* duties *complete?* Try to think of rules that should be added to the list to make it adequate to deal with moral issues in health care.

2.5 Conclusion

In this appendix you have surveyed a number of ethical theories. These provide the resources for grappling with concrete issues. The ideal may be a theory everyone could agree upon and that would yield a clear answer to every dilemma we encounter. However, as you have seen, this is not possible. Instead, you have examined a variety of theories, each having strengths and weaknesses, and each having some ambiguities that will cause difficulties in applying it to concrete health-care issues. Keep these difficulties in mind as you use these theories in future discussions.

References

Benjamin M, Curtis J: *Ethics in Nursing.* Oxford University Press, New York, 1981.

Dalkey NC: *Studies in the Quality of Life. Delphi and Decision-Making.* DC Heath, Lexington MA, 1972.

DeGowin EL, DeGowin RL: *Bedside Diagnostic Examination,* ed 3. Macmillan, New York, 1976.

Fried C: *Right and Wrong.* Harvard University Press, Cambridge MA, 1978.

Graber GC: Some questions about double effect. *Ethics Sci Med* 6:65–84, 1979.

Kant I: *Foundations of the Metaphysics of Morals* (originally published 1785), Beck LW (trans), Bobbs-Merrill, Indianapolis, 1959.

Maslow AH: *Toward a Psychology of Being,* ed 2. Van Nostrand, New York, 1968.

Rawls J: *A Theory of Justice.* Harvard University Press, Cambridge MA, 1971.

Rescher N: Welfare: *The Social Issues in Philosophical Perspective.* University of Pittsburgh Press, Pittsburgh, 1972.

Ross WD: *The Right and the Good.* Clarendon Press, Oxford, 1930.

Tate BL (project director): *The Nurse's Dilemma: Ethical Considerations in Nursing Practice.* International Council of Nurses, The Florence Nightingale International Foundation, Geneva, 1977.

Further Reading

Beauchamp TL, Childress JF: *Principles of Biomedical Ethics,* ed 2. Oxford University Press, New York, 1983.
Two authors who hold different fundamental theories of ethics approach issues on the basis of principles they can agree upon.

Fletcher J: *Morals and Medicine.* Beacon Press, Boston, 1954.
A teleological approach to a variety of ethical issues in medicine. Fletcher is the author who coined the term "situation ethics" in an earlier book with that title.

Frankena WK: *Ethics,* ed 2. Prentice-Hall, Englewood Cliffs NJ, 1973.
An excellent summary and analysis of the range of ethical theories.

Office of Research and Monitoring, Environmental Studies Division: *The Quality of Life Concept: A Potential New Tool for Decision-Makers.* Environmental Protection Agency, Washington DC, 1973.

Reich WT (ed-in-chief): *The Encyclopedia of Bioethics.* Macmillan and the Free Press, New York, 1978.
Bioethics (Clouser KD)
Double Effect (May WE)
Ethics
    I. The Task of Ethics (Ladd J)
    II. Rules and Principles (Solomon WD)
    III. Deontological Theories (Baier K)
    IV. Teleological Theories (Baier K)
    V. Situation Ethics (Fletcher J)
    VI. Utilitarianism (Hare RM)
    VII. Theological Ethics (Carney FS)
    VIII. Objectivism in Ethics (Gert B)
    IX. Naturalism (Wellman C)
    X. Non-Descriptivism (Hare RM)
    XI. Moral Reasoning (Foot P)
    XII. Relativism (Wellman C)
Law and Morality (Brody BA)
Life—II. Quality of Life (Reich WT)
Natural Law (D'Arcy E)
Obligation and Supererogation (Bole TJ III, Schumaker M)
Religious Directives in Medical Ethics
    I. Jewish Codes and Guidelines (Trainin IN, Rosner F)
    II. Roman Catholic Directives (Haring B)
    III. Protestant Statements (Derr TS)
Rights
    I. Systematic Analysis (Feinberg J)
    II. Rights in Bioethics (Macklin R)

Veatch RM: *A Theory of Medical Ethics.* Basic Books, New York, 1981.
A comprehensive approach to medical ethics from a deontological perspective.

Summaries of the Reports from the President's Commission for the Study of Ethical Problems in Medicine and Biomedical and Behavioral Research

1. Making Health Care Decisions: The Ethical and Legal Implications of Informed Consent in the Patient-Practitioner Relationship[1]

1. Although the informed consent doctrine has substantial foundations in law, it is essentially an ethical imperative.

2. Ethically valid consent is a process of shared decisionmaking based upon mutual respect and participation, not a ritual to be equated with reciting the contents of a form that details the risks of particular treatments.

3. Much of the scholarly literature and legal commentary about informed consent portrays it as a highly rational means of decisionmaking about health care matters, thereby suggesting that it may only be suitable for and applicable to well-educated, articulate, self-aware individuals.

   Whether this is what the legal doctrine was intended to be or what it has inadvertently become, it is a view the Commission unequivocally rejects.

   Although subcultures within American society differ in their views about autonomy and individual choice and about the etiology of illness and the roles of healers and patients, a survey conducted for the Commission found a universal desire for information, choice, and respectful communication about decisions. Informed consent must remain flexible, yet the process, as the Commission envisions it throughout this Report, is ethically required of health care practitioners in their relationships with all patients, not a luxury for a few.

4. Informed consent is rooted in the fundamental recognition—reflected in the legal presumption of competency—that adults are entitled to accept or reject health care interventions on the basis of their own personal values and in furtherance of their own personal goals.

---

1. U.S. Government Printing Office, Washington, DC, 1982; vol. 1:2–6.

Nevertheless, patient choice is not absolute.

—Patients are not entitled to insist that health care practitioners furnish them services when to do so would violate either the bounds of acceptable practice or a professional's own deeply held moral beliefs or would draw on a limited resource on which the patient has no binding claim.

—The fundamental values that informed consent is intended to promote— self-determination and patient well-being—both demand that alternative arrangements for health care decisionmaking be made for individuals who lack substantial capacity to make their own decisions. Respect for self-determination requires, however, that in the first instance individuals be deemed to have decisional capacity, which should not be treated as a hurdle to be surmounted in the vast majority of cases, and that incapacity be treated as a disqualifying factor in the small minority of cases.

—Decisionmaking capacity is specific to each particular decision. Although some people lack this capacity for all decisions, many are incapacitated in more limited ways and are capable of making some decisions but not others. The concept of capacity is best understood and applied in a functional manner. That is, the presence or absence of capacity does not depend on a person's status or on the decision reached, but on that individual's actual functioning in situations in which a decision about health care is to be made.

—Decisionmaking incapacity should be found to exist only when people lack the ability to make decisions that promote their well-being in conformity with their own previously expressed values and preferences.

—To the extent feasible, people with no decisionmaking capacity should still be consulted about their own preferences out of respect for them as individuals.

5. Health care providers should not ordinarily withhold unpleasant information simply because it is unpleasant. The ethical foundations of informed consent allow the withholding of information from patients only

   —when they request that it be withheld, or

   —when its disclosure *per se* would cause substantial detriment to their well-being.

   Furthermore, the Commission found that most members of the public do not wish to have "bad news" withheld from them

6. Achieving the Commission's vision of shared decisionmaking based on mutual respect is ultimately the responsibility of individual health care

professionals. However, health care institutions such as hospitals and professional schools have important roles to play in assisting health care professionals in this obligation.

The manner in which health care is provided in institutional settings often results in a fragmentation of responsibility that may neglect the human side of health care. To assist in guarding against this, institutional health care providers should ensure that ultimately there is one readily identifiable practitioner responsible for providing information to a particular patient. Although pieces of information may be provided by various people, there should be one individual officially charged with responsibility for ensuring that all the necessary information is communicated and that the patient's wishes are known to the treatment team.

7. Patients should have access to the information they need to help them understand their conditions and make treatment decisions. To this end the Commission recommends that health care professionals and institutions not only provide information but also assist patients who request additional information to obtain it from relevant sources, including hospital and public libraries.

8. As cases arise and new legislation is contemplated, courts and legislatures should reflect this view of ethically valid consent. Nevertheless, the Commission does not look to legal reforms as the primary means of bringing about changes in the relationship between health care professionals and patients.

9. The Commission finds that a number of relatively simple changes in practice could facilitate patient participation in health care decisionmaking. Several specific techniques—such as having patients express, orally or in writing, their understanding of the treatment consented to—deserve further study.

Furthermore, additional societal resources need to be committed to improving the human side of health care, which has apparently deteriorated at the same time there have been substantial gains in health care technology. The Department of Health and Human Services, and especially the National Institutes of Health, is an appropriate agency for the development of initiatives and the evaluation of their efficacy in this area.

10. Because health care professionals are responsible for ensuring that patients can participate effectively in decisionmaking regarding their care, educators have a responsibility to prepare physicians and nurses to carry out this obligation. The Commission therefore concludes that:

    —Curricular innovations aimed at preparing health professionals for a process of mutual decisionmaking with patients should be continued and strengthened, with careful attention being paid to the development of methods for evaluating the effectiveness of such innovations.

—Examinations and evaluations at the professional school and national levels should reflect the importance of these issues.

—Serious attention should be paid to preparing health professionals for team practice in order to enhance patient participation and well-being.

11. Family members are often of great assistance to patients in helping to understand information about their condition and in making decisions about treatment. The Commission recommends that health care institutions and professionals recognize this and judiciously attempt to involve family members in decisionmaking for patients, with due regard for the privacy of patients and for the possibilities for coercion that such a practice may entail.

12. The Commission recognizes that its vision of health care decisionmaking may involve greater commitments of time on the part of health professionals. Because of the importance of shared decisionmaking based on mutual trust, not only for the promotion of patient well-being and self-determination but also for the therapeutic gains that can be realized, the Commission recommends that all medical and surgical interventions be thought of as including appropriate discussion with patients. Reimbursement to the professional should therefore take account of time spent in discussion rather than regarding it as a separate item for which additional payment is made.

13. To protect the interests of patients who lack decisionmaking capacity and to ensure their well-being and self-determination, the Commission concludes that:

—Decisions made by others on patients' behalf should, when possible, attempt to replicate the ones patients would make if they were capable of doing so. When this is not feasible, decisions by surrogates on behalf of patients must protect the patients' best interests. Because such decisions are not instances of personal self-choice, limits may be placed on the range of acceptable decisions that surrogates make beyond those that apply when a person makes his or her own decisions.

—Health care institutions should adopt clear and explicit policies regarding how and by whom decisions are to be made for patients who cannot decide.

—Families, health care institutions, and professionals should work together to make health care decisions for patients who lack decisionmaking capacity. Recourse to the courts should be reserved for the occasions when concerned parties are unable to resolve their disagreements over matters of substantial import, or when adjudication is clearly required by state law. Courts and legislatures should be cautious about requiring judicial review of routine health care decisions for patients who lack capacity.

—Health care institutions should explore and evaluate various informal administrative arrangements, such as "ethics committees," for review and consultation in nonroutine matters involving health care decisionmaking for those who cannot decide.

—As a means of preserving some self-determination for patients who no longer possess decisionmaking capacity, state courts and legislatures should consider making provision for advance directives through which people designate others to make health care decisions on their behalf and/or give instructions about their care.

The Commission acknowledges that the conclusions contained in this Report will not be simple to achieve. Even when patients and practitioners alike are sensitive to the goal of shared decisionmaking based on mutual respect, substantial barriers will still exist. Some of these obstacles, such as long-standing professional attitudes or difficulties in conveying medical information in ordinary language, are formidable but can be overcome if there is a will to do so. Others, such as the dependent condition of very sick patients or the ever-growing complexity and subspecialization of medicine, will have to be accommodated because they probably cannot be eliminated. Nonetheless, the Commission's vision of informed consent still has value as a measuring stick against which actual performance may be judged and as a goal toward which all participants in health care decisionmaking can strive.

2. Deciding to Forego Life-Sustaining Treatment: Ethical, Medical and Legal Issues in Treatment Decisions[2]

1. The voluntary choice of a competent and informed patient should determine whether or not life-sustaining therapy will be undertaken, just as such choices provide the basis for other decisions about medical treatment. Health care institutions and professionals should try to enhance patients' abilities to make decisions on their own behalf and to promote understanding of the available treatment options.

2. Health care professionals serve patients best by maintaining a presumption in favor of sustaining life, while recognizing that competent patients are entitled to choose to forego any treatments, including those that sustain life.

---

2. U.S. Government Printing Office, Washington, DC, 1983; 3–9. See also Albert R. Jonsen, "A Concord in Medical Ethics," *Ann. Intern. Med.* 99 (August 1983), 263.

3. As in medical decisionmaking generally, some constraints on patients' decisions are justified.

    —Health care professionals or institutions may decline to provide a particular option because that choice would violate their conscience or professional judgment, though in doing so they may not abandon a patient.

    —Health care institutions may justifiably restrict the availability of certain options in order to use limited resources more effectively or to enhance equity in allocating them.

    —Society may decide to limit the availability of certain options for care in order to advance equity or the general welfare, but such policies should not be applied initially nor especially forcefully to medical options that could sustain life.

    —Information about the existence and justification of any of these constraints must be available to patients or their surrogates.

4. Governmental agencies, institutional providers of care, individual practitioners, and the general public should try to improve the medically beneficial options that are available to dying patients. Specific attention should be paid to making respectful, responsive, and competent care available for people who choose to forego life-sustaining therapy or for whom no such therapies are available.

5. Several distinctions are frequently made in deliberating about whether a choice that leads to an earlier death would be acceptable:

    —The distinction between acting and omitting to act separates patients that deserve more scrutiny from those that are likely not to need it.

    —The mere difference between acts and omissions never by itself determines what is morally acceptable. Acceptability turns on other morally significant considerations, such as the balance of harms and benefits likely, the duties of others to dying persons, the risks imposed on others in acting or refraining, and the certainty of outcome.

    —The distinction between failing to initiate and stopping therapy—that is, withholding versus withdrawing treatment—is not itself of moral importance. A justification adequate for not commencing a treatment is also sufficient for ceasing it. Erecting a higher requirement for cessation might unjustifiably discourage vigorous initial attempts at treatment that sometimes succeed.

6. Achieving medically and morally appropriate decisions does not require changes in statutes concerning homicide or wrongful death, given appropriate prosecutorial discretion and judicial interpretation.

7. Primary responsibility for ensuring that morally justified processes of decisionmaking are followed lies with physicians.
   Health care institutions also have a responsibility:
   —to ensure that there are appropriate procedures to enhance patients' competence,
   —to provide for designation of surrogates,
   —to guaranteee that patients are adequately informed,
   —to overcome the influence of dominant institutional biases,
   —to provide review of decisionmaking, and
   —to refer cases to the courts appropriately.
   The Commission is not recommending that hospitals and other institutions take over decisions about patient care; there is no substitute for the dedication, compassion, and professional judgment of physicians.

Incompetent Patients Generally:

8. Physicians who make initial assessments of patients' competence and others who review these assessments should be responsible for judging whether a particular patient's decisionmaking abilities are sufficient to meet the demands of the specific decision at hand.

9. To protect the interests of patients who have insufficient capacity to make particular decisions and to ensure their well-being and self-determination:
   —An appropriate surrogate, ordinarily a family member, should be named to make decisions for such patients. The decisions of surrogates should, when possible, attempt to replicate the ones that the patient would make if capable of doing so. When lack of evidence about the patient's wishes precludes this, decisions by surrogates should seek to protect the patient's best interests. Because such decisions are not instances of self-choice by the patient, the range of acceptable decisions by surrogates is sometimes not as broad as it would be for patients making decisions for themselves.
   —The medical staff, along with the trustees and administrators of health care institutions, should explore and evaluate various formal and informal administrative arrangements for review and consultation, such as "ethics committees," particularly for decisions that have life-or-death consequences for incompetent patients.
   —State courts and legislatures should consider making provision for advance directives through which people designate others to make health care decisions on their behalf and/or give instructions about their care.

- Such advance directives provide a means of preserving some self-determination for patients who may lose decisionmaking capacity.
- Durable powers of attorney are preferable to "living wills" since they are more generally applicable and provide a better vehicle for patients to exercise self-determination, though experience with both is limited.

—Health care professionals and institutions should adopt clear, explicit, and publicly available policies regarding how and by whom decisions are to be made for patients who lack adequate decisionmaking capacity.

—Families, health care institutions, and professionals should work together to make decisions for patients who lack decisionmaking capacity. Recourse to the courts should be reserved for the occasions when adjudication is clearly required by state law or when concerned parties have disagreements that they cannot resolve over matters of substantial import. Courts and legislatures should be cautious about requiring judicial review of routine health care decisions for patients with inadequate decisionmaking capacity.

Patients with Permanent Loss of Consciousness:

10. Current understanding of brain functions allows a reliable diagnosis of permanent loss of consciousness for some patients.

   Whether or not life-sustaining treatment is given is of much less importance to such patients than to others.

11. The decisions of patients' families should determine what sort of medical care permanently unconscious patients receive.

   Other than requiring appropriate decisionmaking procedures for these patients, the law does not and should not require any particular therapies to be applied or continued, with the exception of basic nursing care that is needed to ensure dignified and respectful treatment of the patient.

12. Access to costly care for patients who have permanently lost consciousness may justifiably be restricted on the basis of resource use in two ways:

   —by a physician or institution that otherwise would have to deny significantly beneficial care to another specific patient, or

   —by legitimate mechanisms of policy formulation and application if and only if the provision of certain kinds of care to the patients were clearly causing serious inequities in the use of community resources.

Seriously Ill Newborns:

13. Parents should be the surrogates for a seriously ill newborn unless they are disqualified by decisionmaking incapacity, an unresolvable disagreement between them, or their choice of a course of action that is clearly against the infant's best interests.

14. Therapies expected to be futile for a seriously ill newborn need not be provided; parents, health care professionals and institutions, and reimbursements sources, however, should ensure the infant's comfort.

15. Within the constraints of equity and availability, infants should receive all therapies that are clearly beneficial to them. For example, an otherwise healthy Down Syndrome child whose life is threatened by a surgically correctable complication should receive the surgery because he or she would clearly benefit from it.

    —The concept of benefit necessarily makes reference to the context of the infant's present and future treatment, taking into account such matters as the level of biomedical knowledge and technology and the availability of services necessary for the child's treatment.

    —The dependence of benefit upon context underlines society's special obligation to provide necessary services for handicapped children and their families, which rests on the special ethical duties owed to newborns with undeserved disadvantages and on the general ethical duty of the community to ensure equitable access for all persons to an adequate level of health care.

16. Decisionmakers should have access to the most accurate and up-to-date information as they consider individual cases.

    —Physicians should obtain appropriate consultations and referrals.

    —The significance of the diagnoses and the prognoses under each treatment option must be conveyed to the parents (or other surrogates).

17. The medical staff, administrators, and trustees of each institution that provides care to seriously ill newborns should take the responsibility for ensuring good decisionmaking practices. Accrediting bodies may want to require that institutions have appropriate policies in this area.

    —An institution should have clear and explicit policies that require prospective or retrospective review of decisions when life-sustaining treatment for an infant might be foregone or when parents and providers disagree about the correct decision for an infant. Certain categories of clearly futile therapies could be explicitly excluded from review.

—The best interests of an infant should be pursued when those interests are clear.

—The policies should allow for the exercise of parental discretion when a child's interests are ambiguous.

—Decisions should be referred to public agencies (including courts) for review when necessary to determine whether parents should be disqualified as decisionmakers and, if so, who should decide the course of treatment that would be in the best interests of their child.

18. The legal system has various—though limited—roles in ensuring that seriously ill infants receive the correct care.

—Civil courts are ultimately the appropriate decisionmakers concerning the disqualification of parents as surrogates and the designation of surrogates to serve in their stead.

—Special statutes requiring providers to bring such cases to the attention of civil authorities do not seem warranted, since state laws already require providers to report cases of child abuse or neglect to social service agencies; nevertheless, educating providers about their responsibilities is important.

—Although criminal penalties should be available to punish serious errors, the ability of the criminal law to ensure good decisionmaking in individual cases is limited.

—Governmental agencies that reimburse for health care may insist that institutions have policies and procedures regarding decisionmaking, but using financial sanctions against institutions to punish an "incorrect" decision in a particular case is likely to be ineffective and to lead to excessively detailed regulations that would involve government reimbursement officials in bedside decisionmaking. Furthermore, such sanctions could actually penalize other patients and providers in an unjust way.

Cardiopulmonary Resuscitation:

19. A presumption favoring resuscitation of hospitalized patients in the event of unexpected cardiac arrest is justified.

20. A competent and informed patient or an incompetent patient's surrogate is entitled to decide with the attending physician that an order against resuscitation should be written in the chart. When cardiac arrest is likely, a patient (or a surrogate) should usually be informed and offered the chance specifically to decide for or against resuscitation.

21. Physicians have a duty to assess for each hospitalized patient whether resuscitation is likely, on balance, to benefit the patient, to fail to benefit, or to have uncertain effect.

    —When a patient will not benefit from resuscitation, a decision not to resuscitate, with the consent of the patient or surrogate, is justified.

    —When a physician's assessment conflicts with a competent patient's decision, further discussion and consultation are appropriate; ultimately the physician must follow the patient's decision or transfer responsibility for that patient to another physician.

    —When a physician's assessment conflicts with that of an incompetent patient's surrogate,

    - further discussion,
    - consultation,
    - review by an institutional committee,
    - and, if necessary, judicial review

    should be sought.

22. To protect the interests of patients and their families, health care institutions should have explicit policies and procedures governing orders not to resuscitate, and accrediting bodies should require such policies.

    —Such policies should require that orders not to resuscitate be in written form and that they delineate who has the authority both to write such orders and to stop a resuscitation effort in progress.

    —Federal agencies responsible for the direct provision of patient care (such as the Veterans Administration, the Public Health Service, and the Department of Defense) should ensure that their health care facilities adopt appropriate policies.

23. The entry of an order not to resuscitate holds no necessary implications for any other therapeutic decisions, and the level or extent of health care that will be reimbursed under public or private insurance programs should never be linked to such orders.

24. The education of health care professionals should ensure that they know how to help patients and family make ethically justified decisions for or against resuscitation; those responsible for professional licensure and certification may want to assess knowledge in these areas.

3. Securing Access to Health Care: The Ethical Implications of Differences in the Availability of Health Services[3]

In this Report, the President's Commission does not propose any new policy initiatives, for its mandate lies in ethics not in health policy development. But it has tried to provide a framework within which debates about health policy might take place, and on the basis of which policymakers can ascertain whether some proposals do a better job than others of securing health care on an equitable basis.

In 1952, the President's Commission on the Health Needs of the Nation concluded that "access to the means for the attainment and preservation of health is a basic human right."[4] Instead of speaking in terms of "rights," however, the current Commission believes its conclusions are better expressed in terms of "ethical obligations."

The Commission concludes that society has an ethical obligation to ensure equitable access to health care for all. This obligation rests on the special importance of health care: its role in relieving suffering, preventing premature death, restoring functioning, increasing opportunity, providing information about an individual's condition, and giving evidence of mutual empathy and compassion. Furthermore, although life-style and the environment can affect health status, differences in the need for health care are for the most part undeserved and not within an individual's control.

In speaking of society, the Commission uses the term in its broadest sense to mean the collective American community. The community is made up of individuals who are in turn members of many other, overlapping groups, both public and private: local, state, regional, and national units; professional and workplace organizations; religious, educational, and charitable institutions; and family, kinship, and ethnic groups. All these entities play a role in discharging societal obligations.

The societal obligation is balanced by individual obligations. Individuals ought to pay a fair share of the cost of their own health care and take reasonable steps to provide for such care when they can do so without excessive burdens. Nevertheless, the origins of health needs are too complex, and their manifestation too acute and severe, to permit care to be regularly denied on the grounds that individuals are solely responsible for their own health.

Equitable access to health care requires that all citizens be able to secure an adequate level of care without excessive burdens. Discussions of a right to health care have frequently been premised on offering patients access to all

---

3. U.S. Government Printing Office, Washington, DC, 1983; vol 1:3–6.

4. *President's Commission on the Health Needs of the Nation,* U.S. Government Printing Office, Washington, DC, 1953.

beneficial care, to all care that others are receiving, or to all that they need—or want. By creating impossible demands on society's resources for health care, such formulations have risked negating the entire notion of a moral obligation to secure care for those who lack it. In their place, the Commission proposes a standard of "an adequate level of care," which should be thought of as a floor below which no one ought to fall, not a ceiling above which no one may rise.

A determination of this level will take into account the value of various types of health care in relation to each other as well as the value of health care in relation to other important goods for which societal resources are needed. Consequently, changes in the availability of resources, in the effectiveness of different forms of health care, or in society's priorities may result in a revision of what is considered "adequate."

Equitable access also means that the burdens borne by individuals in obtaining adequate care (the financial impact of the cost of care, travel to the health care provider, and so forth) ought not to be excessive or to fall disproportionately on particular individuals.

When equity occurs through the operation of private forces, there is no need for government involvement, but the ultimate responsibility for ensuring that society's obligation is met, through a combination of public and private arrangements, rests with the Federal government. Private health care providers and insurers, charitable bodies, and local and state governments all have roles to play in the health care system in the United States. Yet the Federal government has the ultimate responsibility for seeing that health care is available to all when the market, private charity, and government efforts at the state and local level are insufficient in achieving equity.

The cost of achieving equitable access to health care ought to be shared fairly. The cost of securing health care for those unable to pay ought to be spread equitably at the national level and not allowed to fall more heavily on the shoulders of particular practitioners, institutions, or residents of different localities. In generating the resources needed to achieve equity of access, those with greater financial resources should shoulder a greater proportion of the costs. Also, priority in the use of public subsidies should be given to achieving equitable access for all before government resources are devoted to securing more care for people who already receive an adequate level.[5]

Efforts to contain rising health care costs are important but should not focus on limiting the attainment of equitable access for the least well served portion of the public. The achievement of equitable access is an obligation of sufficient moral urgency to warrant devoting the necessary resources to it. However, the nature of the task means that it will not be achieved immediately.

---

5. Although the Commission does not endorse devoting public resources to individuals who already receive adequate care, exceptions arise for particular groups with special ethical claims, such as soldiers injured in combat, to whom the nation owes a special debt of gratitude.

While striving to meet this ethical obligation, society may also engage in efforts to contain health costs—efforts that themselves are likely to be difficult and time-consuming. Indeed, the Commission recognizes that efforts to rein in currently escalating health care costs have an ethical aspect because the call for adequate health care for all may not be heeded until such efforts are undertaken. If the nation concludes that too much is being spent on health care, it is appropriate to eliminate expenditures that are wasteful or that do not produce benefits comparable to those that would flow from alternate uses of these funds. But measures designed to contain health care costs that exacerbate existing inequities or impede the achievement of equity are unacceptable from a moral standpoint. Moreover, they are unlikely by themselves to be successful since they will probably lead to a shifting of costs to other entities, rather than to a reduction of total expenditures.

American College of Physicians Ethics Manual: Excerpts[1]

The Relationship of the Physician to Other Health Professionals

The interests of the patient have primacy in all aspects of the patient-physician relationship. The physician should act as an advocate and coordinator of care for his patient and should assume appropriate responsibility, especially when utilizing the help of other health professionals. The physician should deal only with competent health professionals when sharing the care of the patient. Delegation of treatment or technical procedures must be limited to persons who are known to be competent to conduct them with skill and thoughtfulness; the physician who is primarily in charge of the patient's care must retain ultimate responsibility for all aspects of the patient's management. Society has identified the physician as possessing the necessary training to undertake this responsibility and has granted a specific license to exercise this authority and responsibility. This relationship is implied between patient and physician.

. . . When responsibility for a patient's care is undertaken by a physician, the physician must exercise ultimate responsibility. Degrees of responsibility must be dictated by the competence of the licensed allied health professionals and the nature of the actual practice setting. Ethical relationships must derive from a sense of mutual respect and a clear delineation of the professional relationship between the physician and the licensed allied health professionals. Competent licensed allied health professionals often add to the quality of care and comfort of patients, thereby expanding the capability of the physician. The patient should be told about the variety and availability of such services, which can be facilitated through cooperation between physicians and licensed allied health professionals.

---

1. "American College of Physicians Ethics Manual," *Annals of Internal Medicine* 101: 136, 264–266, 1984; *Manual*, 19–20, 26–30, 1984. © 1984 American College of Physicians. Reprinted with permission.

Quality of Life

Quality of life is the subjective satisfaction expressed or experienced by an individual with his current physical, mental or social situation. Assessment by a physician of a patient's quality of life can feature prominently in making clinical decisions. It is wise for physicians to be aware of the personal and subjective values that may contribute to such evaluations. Thus, the assessment may vary according to a physician's age, present health, history of personal illness, cultural background, and long-standing knowledge of the patient as a person. Clinical decisions that hinge on assessing the quality of life should be undertaken with great care and with full cognizance of the subjectivity of the assessment, with full patient participation, or, if that is not possible, with participation of knowledgeable and concerned relatives or guardian. Under ordinary circumstances, a physician's judgment about the quality of life of a patient should not be unilateral.

Care of the Hopelessly Ill

The relationship between the patient and the physician is based on trust. The physician must be vigilant in seeking objectivity in judging all matters relating to decision making, despite all external considerations. Outside pressure may derive from economic considerations, societal demands (for example, from family members) or from other professional or paraprofessional sources. An institutional ethics committee representing professionals from several disciplines (sociology, ethics, psychology, law, religion) can help by advising the physician on difficult ethical issues.

The physician has a responsibility to ensure that his hopelessly ill patient dies with dignity and with as little suffering as possible. The preference of the patient in regard to use of life-support measures should be given the highest priority. There may be circumstances in which the physician may elect to support the body when clinical death of the brain has occurred, but there is no ethical standard that dictates he must prolong physical viability in such a patient by unusual or heroic means. The lowest threshold of life may be considered a state of irreversible loss of human cognitive or communicative functions and implies that the "person" no longer exists in any significant sense of the term and that awareness of self in relation to surroundings have vanished and never will be experienced again.

Brain Death: "An individual who has sustained either [1] irreversible cessation of circulatory and respiratory function, or [2] irreversible cessation of all functions of the entire brain, including the brain steam, is dead. A determination of death must be made in accordance with accepted medical standards". (President's Commission for the Study of Ethical Problems in Medicine and Biomedical and Behavioral Research. *Defining Death.*)

Do-Not-Resuscitate Orders or No-Code Orders: "The purpose of cardio-pulmonary resuscitation (CPR) is the prevention of sudden unexpected death. Cardiopulmonary resuscitation is not indicated in certain situations, such as cases of terminal irreversible illness where death is not unexpected." [Standards and guidelines for cardiopulmonary resuscitation (CPR) and emergency cardiac care (ECC). *JAMA* 1980; 244:453–509]

Cardiopulmonary resuscitation requires the use of appropriate techniques and devices to treat sudden and unexpected cardiac or respiratory arrest by those trained in these techniques. A decision *not* to attempt resuscitation is the ultimate responsibility of the physician-of-record. Such responsibility cannot be taken over, morally or legally, by institutional committees on ethics or any other person or group of persons who may be available for advice to the physician-of-record.

A decision not to attempt resuscitation and the process of initiating and implementing such action involves clinical and ethical knowledge and judgment; necessary legal knowledge; and, at times, consideration of religious beliefs.

Initiation of the do-not-resuscitate order requires the physician-of-record to review in detail the patient's status: Is the patient terminally ill from an acute or chronic disease?

Having reviewed the data on the clinical status of the patient, the physician must make a judgment as to whether any known treatment can restore the patient to a state of reasonable comfort and function. When treatment is judged useless, writing or giving a verbal order not to resuscitate such a patient is ethical.

A corollary observation: If a physician decides that the disease process or other medical condition that the patient has would not positively be affected by the initiation of resuscitative efforts—in other words, if resuscitative efforts would only prolong the dying process—then a decision to write a do-not-resuscitate order is ethically proper.

A further corollary: It is not ethical to code a patient "do-not-resuscitate" just because he is aged.

If the patient is a mentally competent adult, he has the legal right to accept or refuse any form of treatment, and his wishes must be recognized and honored by his physician. He can decide whether he wishes to be resuscitated when faced with a terminal event. The problem should not be discussed with his family unless the patient authorizes such a discussion. If the patient signifies his preference for a do-not-resuscitate order, this preference becomes the paramount consideration. If the patient's preference is contrary to the desires of his spouse or others, the latter have no legal, ethical, or moral standing to enforce their desires unless a court declares the patient to be legally incompetent and appoints a guardian to make treatment decisions for the patient.

The physician should understand that making decisions about resuscitation does not legally require the counsel or consent of the patient's family, unless a family member is the parent of a minor child or has been appointed the guardian of the patient's person. Physicians should not breach the confidential nature of the physician/patient relationship by discussing the patient's care with persons who are not authorized by the patient to be made aware of the patient's diagnosis, prognosis, or treatment. Obviously, a competent patient can advise the physician as to with whom his care can be discussed. With the incompetent patient, however, the situation is quite different. In the absence of a medical emergency (in which case the patient's consent to treatment is implied), the physician would be well advised to recommend to the patient's family that they have one of the family appointed as the patient's guardian so that the physician will have a person to deal with who has the legal authority to make treatment decisions for the patient. Physicians should understand that mere blood relationship does not by itself allow a family member to know about or authorize the medical treatment of a patient. Local counsel should be sought to learn the exact parameters of state law on this topic.

For individuals who are mentally defective or deficient and have been declared legally incapacitated, do-not-resuscitate orders must never be written solely on the basis of the mental condition but for the same reasons as for patients who are mentally competent. Legally, when it has been adjudicated that a patient is mentally incapacitated, the only person who can act on his behalf is a guardian or conservator appointed by the court. A relative or friend has no legal right to act for a mentally incapacitated patient unless appointed by the court.

A final corollary: The Federal government and several states and regulatory bodies are recommending or requiring that hospitals maintain committees that create policies, advise physicians, or even make treatment decisions about terminally ill patients, *especially* newborns. It is too early to predict the long-term effect of such regulations or committees, but physicians are *strongly* advised to seek legal counsel about the correct state of the law in this very volatile area.

States vary in the time required to appoint a legal guardian or conservator. During that time the physician-of-record can legally exercise his judgment in the care of his incapacitated patient. The physician is the patient's advocate and has a duty to him, and to no other person, during the interim. Full discussion with the spouse or other close relatives about the indications for cardiopulmonary resuscitation, the do-not-resuscitate order, the legal aspects of such orders and the physician's role as the patient's advocate will nearly always result in a decision that is correct ethically.

When a do-not-resuscitate order has been written, the physician must ensure that the patient is as comfortable as possible. A decision to withhold supportive therapy, while ethically sound, may not be acceptable to some families for religious or other reasons. Their wishes must be considered but not necessarily followed. The physician must be the final arbiter in decisions related to a patient, placing the wishes of the patient above all other considerations.

Living Will: The so-called "living will" has excited considerable interest that will continue in the future. Physicians should be aware, however, that fewer than 20 states have enacted statutes making such documents legally enforceable and/or binding on the physician. Physicians who practice in states that have enacted living will statutes are urged to seek local legal counsel as to the exact rights and responsibilities encompassed by that state's statute. The statutes differ *markedly* between states, and one should not presume that prior experience with one state's statute will be instructive when practicing in another state.

In those states that have not enacted living will statutes or that have expressly provided that living wills are not legally enforceable within that state (even though the document may have been valid in the state in which it was executed), the physician is under no binding legal obligation to follow the instructions or information contained in the document unless the physician has specifically agreed with the patient or guardian to be bound by its content. All physicians would be well advised to be aware of the thoughts and desires of the patient expressed in the document, but need only consider that language to be instructive, and *not* determinative of the way in which the physician will treat the patient.

Of course, if the physician cannot agree with the restrictions placed on care of the patient by a living will or the statements of the patient or guardian, the physician can withdraw from the case provided that the requirements of local law and practice regarding notice to the patient, continuity of care, and so forth, have been satisfied.

Euthanasia: Active voluntary euthanasia is legally prohibited. However, euthanasia is a classic ethical dilemma that occurs when the ethical responsibility of the physician to preserve life, maintain the quality of life, or both, conflicts with his covenant with the patient who desires an end to pain and suffering that he considers no longer endurable or when immediate family members request termination of life for patients who are comatose or otherwise unable to exercise intellectual control.

The social, religious, and political implications of euthanasia have been discussed exhaustively. They remain controversial and will not be discussed here. While there is no resolution of the problem on ethical grounds, there are major legal prohibitions against euthanasia in the United States today.

Table of Cases

298

Index